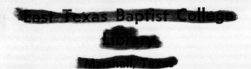

PROGRESS IN

Medical Genetics

PROGRESS IN

Medical Genetics

Volume VIII

Edited by

ARTHUR G. STEINBERG, Ph.D.

Professor of Biology, Department of Biology, and Professor of Human
Genetics, Department of Reproductive Biology, Case Western Reserve
University, Cleveland, Ohio

and

ALEXANDER G. BEARN, M.D.

Professor and Chairman of the Department of Medicine, Cornell
University Medical College, and Physician-in-Chief, The New York
Hospital, New York

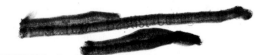

GRUNE & STRATTON

New York and London

1972

Library of Congress Catalog Card Number 60-53514
International Standard Book Number 0-8089-0723-9
Printed in the United States of America

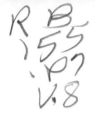

Foreword

THE BROAD DIVERSITY OF SUBJECTS which interest human genticists is well illustrated by the topics covered in Volume VIII of *Progress in Medical Genetics*. Dr. Frank Fenner (Chapter 1) introduces the volume with a most valuable and scholarly article on the genetics of animal viruses and the genetic aspects of the host response to viral infection. The relationship between chromosomal variations in somatic cells and neoplastic disease has been the subject of a long and unresolved debate which has been marked more by differing interpretation of data rather than disputation of fact. Dr. James German (Chapter 2) discusses the role of specific genes on the chromosomal stability of somatic cells and their significance in our understanding of neoplastic disease. An essay on the future of human population genetics by N. E. Morton (Chapter 3) focuses on a number of contemporary problems in human population genetics and closes with a spirited and rallying envoi.

Sir Archibald Garrod's view that genes control the synthesis of enzymes is now widely recognized as one of the keystones of genetic theory. Henry N. Kirkman discusses new concepts in our understanding of enzymatic defects in man in Chapter 4. The successful prevention of Rh hemolytic disease is one of the most spectacular advances in medical genetics of recent years. The paper by C. A. Clarke (Chapter 5) is an account of the development of the present worldwide experience in the successful prophylaxis of Rh isoimmunization. The explosive development of our knowledge of the inherited abnormalities of ganglioside metabolism is reviewed by R. O. Brady and E. H. Kolodny (Chapter 6); the importance of tissue culture and enzymatic techniques in furthering our understanding of these rare inborn errors of metabolism is fully discussed. The term hereditary dwarfism includes a large number of inherited syndromes of considerable importance to the medical geneticist; these syndromes are discussed from a clinical and genetic viewpoint by Charles I. Scott (Chapter 7).

The editors would like once again to express their sincere thanks to the authors for their willingness to undertake the responsibility of writing for *Progress in Medical Genetics* despite their already overburdened schedules.

A.G.S.
A.G.B.

Contents

CHAPTER 1

Genetic Aspects of Viral Diseases of Animals*

Frank Fenner

John Curtin School of Medical Research, Australian National
University, Canberra, Australia.

VIRUSES CONSTITUTE THE SIMPLEST LIVING SYSTEMS KNOWN, and vertebrates the most complex. Viral infections involve interactions between
these two systems, one possible consequence of which is the production of
disease. The object of this review will be to consider aspects of animal
virus genetics which are relevant to the production of viral disease, and
aspects of the host response to viral infection for which there is evidence
of genetic control. The genetics of animal viruses as such has been the
topic of recent reviews (Fenner, 1969, 1970) to which the reader is referred for a more detailed account than is possible here.

THE GENETIC MATERIAL OF ANIMAL VIRUSES

Unlike organisms, which universally rely on double-stranded DNA as
the repository of their genetic information, viruses are remarkably versatile
in their modes of inheritance. In different groups the viral genome consists
of either double-stranded or single-stranded DNA or double-stranded or
single-stranded RNA. The genome may occur in the virion either as a
single linear or cyclic molecule or as a specific aggregate of several small
nucleic acid molecules. Although our information on the nucleic acids of
many viruses is more difficult to obtain, and therefore at present less precise, than our knowledge of certain phenotypic properties such as their
morphology, it has nevertheless been apparent for several years that it
would be possible to classify viruses on the basis of the type, amount,
arrangement, and base composition of their nucleic acids in a way that
was meaningful in relation to all their other properties (Bellett, 1967a,

---

* Literature review completed August, 1970.

1967b). As our knowledge of viruses expands, it is becoming clear that the very large number of different viruses now known to infect vertebrate animals can be arranged in perhaps 20 groups on the basis of the morphology of their virions and the nature of their genomes. Such groups as have been clearly defined by these criteria are meaningful in relation to many other properties of the viruses including the pathogenesis of the diseases they cause (Fenner, 1968a). Such groupings also provide an opportunity for extracting order from a great volume of seemingly unrelated observations and allow us greatly to simplify our consideration of all aspects of virology, including those related to disease. For this reason I have tabulated the accepted or putative groups of animal viruses (Table 1).

It is clear from the data in Table 1 on the molecular weights of viral nucleic acids that the numbers of genes present in viruses of different groups vary considerably, but are always small or very small, compared with the numbers of genes in other organisms. Estimates can be made of the numbers of genes based on four assumptions: (a) that the genetic

TABLE 1.—*The Major Taxonomic Groups of Animal Viruses**

Group	Shape	Diameter, nm	Nucleic acid †	Some associated human diseases
Parvovirus	Spherical ‡	20	D:SS:2	?
Adenovirus-associated viruses	Spherical	20	D:SS:2	?
Papovavirus	Spherical	45–55	D:DS:3–5	Warts (tumors in rodents)
Adenovirus	Spherical	70–80	D:DS:20–25	Upper respiratory tract infection, conjunctivitis (tumors in rodents)
Herpesvirus	Spherical (env.) §	150–200	D:DS:70–100	Varicella-zoster, herpes simplex, cytomegalovirus infection
Poxvirus	Brick-shaped	100 × 200 × 300	D:DS:160–200	Smallpox, orf
Picornavirus	Spherical	20–30	R:SS:2–3	Poliomyelitis, aseptic meningitis, carditis, common cold
Togavirus	Spherical (env.)	50–60	R:SS:3–4	Encephalitis, yellow fever
Myxovirus	Spherical (env.)	80–120	R:SS:3(P)	Influenza
Paramyxovirus	Spherical (env.)	100–300	R:SS:7	Mumps, bronchiolitis, measles
Coronavirus	Spherical (env.)	80–120	R:?	Common cold
Rhabdovirus	Bullet-shaped (env.)	70 × 180	R:SS:5(?P)	Rabies
Leukovirus	Spherical (env.)	100–120	R:SS:10–12(?P)	Leukemia in animals
Reovirus	Spherical	70–80	R:DS:15(P)	?

*There are several other viruses distinguishable from all named groups about which knowledge is still too limited to propose a group name.

†D = DNA; R = RNA; SS = single-stranded; DS = double-stranded; 2, etc. = molecular weight in millions of daltons; (P) = genome in several pieces.

‡"Spherical," without (env.) = envelope, are icosahedral in detailed structure.

§"Spherical (env.)" indicates roughly spherical structure of enveloped virion; internal component may be icosahedral or tubular.

code is a nonoverlapping triplet code, (b) that there are no repetitive sequences, (c) that the only gene products are polypeptides, and (d) that, on average, viral polypeptide molecules contain about 200 amino acids. The first two assumptions appear to be true for all viruses, but it has been reported that, in addition to polypeptides, a few sequences of herpesvirus DNA may specify particular transfer RNAs (Subak-Sharpe et al., 1966). In ribophages (Steitz, 1969) and bacteria (Rechler and Martin, 1970), there appear to be nontranslated nucleotide sequences between the initiation and termination codons; it is not known whether the same situation holds for animal cells and animal viruses, nor what proportion of the total nucleic acid these regions comprise. Even more important is the observation that several viral polypeptides are very large and contain many more than 200 amino acids (see Skehel and Joklik, 1969). Clearly, the last two assumptions are likely to lead to overestimation of the numbers of genes.

Table 2 lists more detailed information on the nature of viral nucleic acids and on calculations of the numbers of genes present in viruses of different groups based (a) on these assumptions, and (b) on possible physical genes, viz., the numbers of different fragments found in virions

TABLE 2.—*Estimates of the Numbers of Genes in Various Animal Virsues*

			Number of genes	
Group	Prototype virus	Nucleic acid *	By convention †	By product ‡
Parvovirus	Minute virus of mice	D:SS:1.7(1)	8	
Papovavirus	Polyoma, papilloma	D:DS:3(1, cyclic)	7	1 = 25%
		D:DS:5(1, cyclic)	13	
Adenovirus	Adenovirus type 2	D:DS:23(1)	60	9 = 29%
Herpesvirus	Herpes simplex	D:DS:100(1)	250	9 = 11%
Poxvirus	Vaccinia	D:DS:160(1)	400	
Picornavirus	Poliovirus	R:SS:2.6(1)	13	4 = 36%
Togavirus	Sindbis	R:SS:4(?2 P)	20	2 = 21%
Myxovirus	Influenza A	R:SS:3(6–7 P)	15 (7)	4 = 50%
Paramyxovirus	Newcastle disease	R:SS:7(1)	35	3 = 24%
Leukovirus	Rous sarcoma	R:SS:10(?4 P)	50	
Rhabdovirus	Vesicular stomatitis	R:SS:4(?4 P)	20	3 = 44%
Reovirus	Reovirus 3	R:DS:15(10 P)	50 (10)	8 = 68%

*D = DNA; R = RNA; DS = double-stranded; SS = single stranded; 1.7, etc. = molecular weight in millions of daltons; (1) = genome consists of one molecule; (6–7 P) = genome consists of 6–7, etc., molecules.

†Based on conventions on coding potential and average size of viral polypeptide.

‡Based on probable number of polypeptides produced (figures in parentheses are equivalent to number of pieces of RNA in their genomes), or on number of polypeptides in virion and percentage of genome accounted for by their molecular weight.

with aggregated genomes (see Smith et al., 1969). Also shown, in the last column, are current estimates of the numbers of polypeptides in the virion and the percentage of the genome these represent in terms of their total molecular weight. Calculations based either on the numbers of pieces ($\equiv$ genes) in viruses with fragmented genomes or on the total molecular weights of virion polypeptides suggest that the numbers of genes postulated on the basis of the listed assumptions are, for most viruses, much too high.

One feature of the figures in the last column is the apparent variability in the amounts of the genome devoted to specifying structural components of the virion in viruses of different groups. Part of this is doubtless due to ignorance; part is probably real. The data for the small viruses like SV40 and poliovirus are reliable and indicate that 60% of the genome specifies polypeptides that are not incorporated into the virion. These probably include, in the case of SV40 the T antigen, and with poliovirus RNA polymerase(s) responsible for replication of the viral RNA. With the large deoxyriboviruses, a large part of the genome is available for specifying nonstructural proteins but only a few of these have been characterized so far, e.g., thymidine kinase and DNA polymerase in poxviruses (McAuslan, 1969) and thymidine kinase in herpesviruses (Buchan and Watson, 1969).

Transcription and Translation

It is worth devoting some attention to transcription and translation of the genetic message of animal viruses because the novel nature of many viral genomes presents interesting problems which may be unfamiliar to geneticists concerned with organisms.

Deoxyriboviruses

Viruses containing a single double-stranded DNA molecule would appear, at first sight, to present no novel problems, and indeed a range of mRNAs of different sizes appears to be transcribed and then translated into polypeptides on cytoplasmic polyribosomes (McAuslan, 1969). As will be described below, the polycistronic message encoded in the viral RNA of picornaviruses appears to be translated into a single giant precursor polypeptide molecule which is subsequently cleaved into the several viral polypeptides. A comparable sort of posttranslational cleavage may occur with some poxvirus proteins (Katz and Moss, 1970). The polypeptides of the poxvirus core appear to be formed by cleavage of a high molecular weight precursor by a process that occurs relatively slowly during the maturation of virions. The cleavage is inhibited by refampicin but, with a rifampicin-resistant mutant, cleavage and maturation occur normally.

In herpesvirus-infected cells, RNA may be transcribed from the viral DNA template in the nucleus as a very large molecule which is cleaved before its cleavage products become associated with cytoplasmic polyribosomes as viral *m*RNA (Wagner and Roizman, 1969).

The poxviruses and other deoxyriboviruses which multiply in the cytoplasm, like frog virus 3 (Granoff et al., 1966), pose a problem as to the origin of their transcriptase, for cellular DNA-dependent RNA polymerase appears to be restricted to the nucleus. With the poxviruses, transcription is carried out by a virus-coded enzyme which is a component of the virion (Kates and McAuslan, 1967). It has been assumed that the cellular DNA-dependent RNA polymerase transcribes the genome of the other deoxyriboviruses, which multiply in the nucleus. This must be true for the papovaviruses, because their purified DNA is infectious (Dulbecco and Vogt, 1963), and possibly for adenovirus-associated viruses, because their DNA is infectious if inoculated on adenovirus-infected cells (Hoggan et al., 1968). The question as to whether the transcriptase is a cellular or a viral enzyme should perhaps be reexamined with adenoviruses and herpesviruses, whose DNAs have not been shown to be infectious.

RIBOVIRUSES

Current work is revealing a variety of different mechanisms of transcription and translation amongst the riboviruses.

Viral RNA Is the Messenger RNA

With poliovirus, the model virus of the picornavirus group, the purified viral RNA is infectious, and in in vitro systems it can be shown to act as messenger RNA (Warner et al., 1963). However, unlike ribophage RNA in bacterial cells, where chain-initiating and chain-terminating nucleotide sequences occur (Zinder et al., 1966), there is no evidence for punctuation of the message in poliovirus-infected cells (Jacobson and Baltimore, 1968; Summers and Maizel, 1968), or in cells infected with several other picornaviruses (Holland and Kiehn, 1968; Kiehn and Holland, 1970). In these cases the viral RNA appears to act as a polycistronic messenger which is translated in its entirety into a single very large ($\sim$220,000 daltons) polypeptide (Jacobson et al., 1970; Kiehn and Holland, 1970). This is broken down by a series of "posttranslational cleavages" into the characteristic viral polypeptides. The 14 viral polypeptide peaks originally observed in polyacrylamide gels prepared from poliovirus-infected cells

(Summers et al., 1965) did not include this very large precursor molecule, but several of the "noncapsid viral proteins" are now recognized to have been intermediate cleavage products.

Posttranslational cleavage occurs with several different picornaviruses and in many kinds of cell lines and primary cell cultures (Kiehn and Holland, 1970). The cleavage points are specific for each virus and the same in many different host cells. The properties of the cleavage enzyme are being studied. It is not sensitive to actinomycin D and does not cleave host cell proteins. The enzyme could be virus-coded, or it could be a preformed host enzyme which is activated or released by the virus.

In contrast to this evidence for high specificity of cleavage, studies with different mutants of poliovirus suggest that there may be some ambiguity in cleavage, for the calculated total molecular weight of the derived polypeptides may exceed the coding potential of the RNA, and there are substantial differences in the polyacrylamide gel pattern found with closely related mutants (Cooper et al., 1970). With poliovirus, Jacobson et al. (1970) found so many apparent identities between tryptic digest peptides of two capsid proteins (VP2 and VP4) that they suggest the possibility of different cleavage points in different molecules of the known precursor protein, VP0.

Posttranslational cleavage may also occur with Semliki Forest virus (Burrell et al., 1970), a togavirus which, like poliovirus, yields infectious RNA after suitable treatment.

These discoveries raise a question of considerable general biological interest, namely, to what extent does punctuation operate in the translation of cellular mRNAs in animal cells?

mRNA Is Transcribed from Single-Stranded Viral RNA

Results now appearing suggest that with some viruses the messenger RNA is transcribed from single-stranded viral RNA. The genome of paramyxoviruses consists of a single, very large molecule of single-stranded RNA of about 7 million daltons molecular weight (57S) which is not infectious. Cells infected with these viruses contain an amount of negative-strand (complementary) RNA in considerable excess of their content of viral RNA. This occurs in four size classes, 18, 22, 35S, and a small amount of complementary strand 57S RNA (Bratt and Robinson, 1967; Blair and Robinson, 1968). The complementary strand RNAs are found associated with polyribosomes, which suggests that they may function as messenger RNA. There is no information about how the negative strands are transcribed from the viral RNA, or as to whether the transcriptase is a virion protein.

The other two cases in which *m*RNA may be transcribed from single-stranded viral RNA involve situations in which the viral genome is certainly (with influenza virus) or probably (with vesicular stomatitis virus) an aggregate of several pieces. Influenza virus-infected cells contain an RNA polymerase that will synthesize complementary strand RNA in vitro (Scholtissek, 1969). Influenza virus-infected cells contain complementary strand RNA, which occurs as small molecules of different sizes, about one-third of which is associated with viral RNA in double-stranded replicative-form molecules and two-thirds is single-stranded (Duesberg and Robinson, 1967). In infected cells, synthesis of free complementary strand RNA precedes that of plus strand RNA, and doublestranded RNA is never found in large amounts (Scholtissek and Rott, 1970). It is not known whether the viral RNA or the free negative strands act as *m*RNA; the apparent absence of transcriptase in the virion suggests that viral RNA itself must be the messenger. In any event the fragmented nature of the genome appears to obviate the need for posttranslational cleavage.

Vesicular stomatitis virus (VSV), a rhabdovirus, may also contain several loosely linked RNA fragments in its genome. Infected cells contain complementary strand RNAs which function as *m*RNA (Huang et al., 1970). These molecules are transcribed by a viral RNA polymerase which is a component of the virion (Baltimore et al., 1970).

Viral RNA Is Transcribed into DNA

The leukoviruses have long presented a puzzling problem in relation to transcription and translation. Their replication is dependent upon initial DNA synthesis (Bader, 1966) and continued DNA function (Temin, 1964), and neither complementary RNA nor double-stranded RNA can be recovered from the cytoplasm of cells in which leukoviruses were replicating when techniques are used which regularly yield such products from cells infected with paramyxoviruses and myxoviruses (Robinson, 1967). Earlier nucleic acid hybridization experiments which suggested that leukovirus-infected and perhaps "normal" chicken cells contained DNA homologous to the viral RNA have been confirmed by Baluda and Nayak (1970), who found that cells transformed by avian myeloblastosis virus contained about four "DNA equivalents" of viral RNA per cell. The somewhat smaller amount of complementary DNA present in some "normal" chicken cells is probably due to latent leukovirus infection, which may be due to defective viruses (Huebner and Todaro, 1969; Hanafusa et al., 1970).

These anomalous results, which are peculiar to viruses of the leukovirus group, have been clarified by the discovery that the virions of these agents contain an enzyme which transcribes RNA into DNA, i.e., an RNA-dependent DNA polymerase (Temin and Mizutani, 1970; Baltimore 1970). It is presumed that this DNA copy then acts, within the cell, as the "viral" genome in relation to the production both of viral mRNAs and new viral RNA.

If this hypothesis is correct, the viral RNA should itself be able to function as a messenger, although it may well not be able to replicate itself and hence may not produce infective particles. High molecular weight RNA from leukosis virus has been shown to be template-active in a subcellular system (Říman et al., 1967), and in chicken cells this RNA induces specific antigen formation although infectious virus is not produced (Hlozžánék et al., 1970).

mRNA Is Transcribed from Double-Stranded Viral RNA

The reoviruses contain about 15 million daltons of double-stranded RNA which occurs as 10 pieces, in three size classes (Shatkin et al., 1968), as separate fragments in the virion (Millward and Graham, 1970). The reovirion contains an RNA-dependent RNA polymerase (Shatkin and Sipe, 1968). In the presence of the appropriate precursor molecules, and with virions partially degraded by removal of their outer coat, this enzyme transcribes single-stranded RNAs of size classes corresponding to the double-stranded fragments (Skehel and Joklik, 1969). This in vitro transcription occurs rapidly and in an unregulated fashion, the frequency of transcription of genome RNA fragments being inversely proportional to their molecular weight. By contrast, in the infected cell certain segments of the genome are transcribed at different rates and the frequency of translation of the resulting mRNAs is also regulated (Zweerink and Joklik, 1970). The sizes of the seven virion proteins that have been recognized correspond with the sizes of the various pieces of genome RNA (Smith et al., 1969), suggesting that in this case also no posttranslational cleavage occurs.

General Comment

Unlike bacterial cells, where punctuation mechanisms similar to those recognized for transcription from DNA (nonsense codons) also act as terminating triplets in the translation of the polycistronic viral RNAs (Zinder et al., 1966), vertebrate cells do not appear to have developed a translational punctuation mechanism. In this situation different riboviruses appear to have solved the problem of translating the message encoded in viral RNA in a variety of ways: (a) by posttranslational cleavage of a giant precursor polypeptide synthesized directly on viral RNA acting as messenger, (b) by transcription of monocristronic *m*RNAs from a number of fragments of viral RNA, each of which corresponds to one gene, or (c) by transcription first into a DNA provirus from which appropriate *m*RNAs are subsequently transcribed.

MUTATION

The nucleic acids of viruses, like those of organisms, undergo spontaneous mutations, and the mutation rate can be greatly increased by the use of chemical or physical mutagens. The hallmark of a spontaneous mutational change in a virus is its random occurrence during viral replication, demonstrable by the random distribution of mutant clones among the yields of individual cells. In three cases examined with animal viruses, plaque mutation in poliovirus (Dulbecco and Vogt, 1958), encephalomyocarditis virus (Breeze and Subak-Sharpe, 1967), and the *morph*^{r} → *morph*^{t} mutation of Rous sarcoma virus (Temin, 1961), the mutants were clonally distributed. The spontaneous mutation rates, which have been determined in a few instances only, varied between 10^{-5} and 10^{-7} per particle per duplication (Dulbecco and Vogt, 1958; Carp, 1963; Breeze and Subak-Sharpe, 1967). However, it is difficult to interpret these rates in terms of changes in the nucleotide sequence of a particular gene, because the phenotypic change observed might have been due to changes in any one of several genes. An extreme case is the white pock mutation of rabbitpox virus, a phenotype that occurs with a frequency of 1%, but is due to mutations in many genes (Gemmell and Fenner, 1960).

In every infection of a vertebrate animal, the single virion or the very small dose of viral particles that initiates the infection multiplies several million times, often in a variety of cells in which different selective pressures may operate. Many spontaneous mutations must therefore occur. Whether or not they are of any significance depends in the main upon three factors: (a) whether they are advantageous under conditions of natural selection either in the particular infected animal or for transmission to other animals, (b) whether they occur early or late in the infective process (for this will affect clone size), and (c) whether the mutant particles are transmitted to other animals. The force of natural selection operating mainly at the level of transmissibility, and not "inherent mutability," is the most important factor in determining whether or not particular sorts of mutation (e.g., to high or low virulence or to changed surface antigens) are rare or relatively common. This point will be illustrated when we consider the evolutionary histories of myxomatosis and influenza in a later section.

Until about 1964 animal virologists concentrated their attention on mutations affecting plaque or pock morphology. Since then, benefiting from the experience of bacteriophage workers, they have made extensive use of conditional lethal mutants, i.e., viral mutants which are able to grow normally or nearly normally under one set of experimental conditions but whose multiplication is blocked under other conditions. Host-dependent mutants, which fail to grow in particular host cells but do grow in others, have been investigated in a few cases. Unlike the *amber* and *ocher* mutants of bacteriophage they do not depend upon the existence of *sus* (supressor) mutations in the permissive host cell, and they have not yet been extensively utilized. Temperature-sensitive mutants, which are mis-sense mutations that produce such an alteration in the nucleotide (and therefore the amino acid) sequence that the resulting polypeptide functions normally at low but very poorly at higher temperatures, have been extensively used for the analysis of viral gene functions, and their use is increasing (see reviews: Fenner, 1969, 1970).

GENETIC RECOMBINATION

Observations with a variety of intact animals and lines of animal cells have shown that latent viral infections are very common (Fenner, 1968b). The leukoviruses in chickens (Hanafusa et al., 1970) and mice (Huebner and Todaro, 1969) constitute an extreme example. It follows that, both in laboratory experiments and under natural conditions, superinfection of cells (and therefore mixed infection) must occur frequently. Multiple infection is still more frequent, for it is clear that, when viruses spread either on the surfaces of sheets of cells or between cells in solid organs, it is usual rather than exceptional for several newly released virions to penetrate adjacent single cells. The occurrence of mixed or multiple infections raises the possibility of interactions between viruses, either between their nucleic acid molecules or between viral gene products (proteins).

Interactions between viral nucleic acid molecules constitue genetic recombination. In cases where one or both of the parental viruses is inactivated, this is called genetic reactivation. Examples of genetic recombination and genetic reactivation are set out in Table 3.

Among deoxyriboviruses, genetic recombination has been demonstrated with poxviruses and herpesviruses and between adenovirus and SV40. Among the ribovirus groups, it has been found with influenza viruses, reoviruses, vesicular stomatitis virus, poliovirus, and foot-and-mouth disease virus. Using what appear to be adequately sensitive systems, it has been looked for but not found with group A togaviruses (Sindbis and Semliki Forest virus) and with a paramyxovirus (Newcastle disease virus).

TABLE 3.—*Nucleic Acid Interaction: Genetic Recombination and Reactivation**

Phenomenon	Parent 1	Parent 2	Progeny	Comment
Genetic recombination:				
1. Between conditional lethal mutants of the same virus	A*B*C	ABC	ABC	Wild type
2. Between different strains of the same virus	ABC	AST	ABT	With influenza and vaccinia viruses
3. Between unrelated viruses (adenovirus and SV40, a special case)	ABC	XYZ	ABCYZ	Note *addition* of nucleic acid
4. Between papovavirus and host cell	ABC	123(cell)	12AB3	Integration of viral genes produces malignant cell
Cross reactivation:				
Between UV-inactivated virus and active virus of a different strain (same virus)	A̶B̶C̶	AST	ASC	Rescue of genes from inactivated parent
Multiplicity reactivation:				
Between virions of same virus inactivated in different genes	A̶B̶C	AB̶C	ABC	Viable virus produced from inactivated parents

*A, etc. = active viral genes; 1, etc. = active cellular genes; *B*, etc. = mutant gene; A̶, etc. = inactivated gene.

RECOMBINATION BETWEEN DEOXYRIBOVIRUSES

Poxviruses

Early work with two different wild-type strains of poxviruses of the vaccinia subgroup—dermal vaccinia and rabbitpox virus—showed that recombination occurred readily between them, both in conditions of mass culture (Fenner and Comben, 1958) and in the yield from single mixedly infected cells (Fenner, 1959). Subsequently experiments carried out with the very common white pock mutants of rabbitpox virus showed that many pairs of these recombined, often with high frequency (Gemmell and Fenner, 1960). Later it was discovered that some of these white pock mutants were host-dependent, in that they failed to multiply in a line of pig kidney (PK) cells (McClain, 1965). Although physiological tests showed that these PK-negative mutants were functionally heterogeneous, in that in restrictive host cells different mutants were blocked at different stages of the replication cycle (Fenner and Sambrook, 1966), they did not recombine with each other. However, PK-negative mutants do recombine with PK-positive white pock mutants (McClain and Greenland, 1965) and with *ts* (temperature-sensitive) mutants with a red pock phenotype (Padgett and Tomkins, 1968). White pock mutants of rabbitpox virus can thus be arranged into five clusters which can be ordered relative to each other by recombination frequencies, as shown in Fig. 1 (Fenner and Sambrook, 1966).

Temperature-sensitive mutants are readily obtained from stocks of rabbitpox virus grown in the presence of the mutagen 5-bromodeoxyuridine. Indeed, most viable progeny in such preparations appeared to be to some extent temperature-sensitive (Sambrook et al., 1966), although few of the mutants were sufficiently stable and nonleaky for further use. However, Padgett and Tomkins (1968) obtained 18 *ts* mutants of rabbitpox virus that were suitable for genetic experiments. Recombination occurred with all pairs tested, sometimes with low frequency (0.02%-0.2%) but often at frequencies of 10%-20%. The three mutants which had the lowest recombination frequencies also failed to show significant complementation and thus appear to form a tight linkage group. In spite of the reproducible differences in the recombination rates further mapping was not possible. Double mutants have been obtained from mixed infections involving *ts* and PK-negative mutants. These could be useful for making three-factor crosses and thus ordering the *ts* mutants, but no such experiments have been carried out.

Recombination between different members of the vaccinia subgroup of the poxviruses occurs readily (Woodroofe and Fenner, 1960; Bedson and Dumbell, 1964). Recombination between vaccinia and cowpox viruses has been used to demonstrate the separate genetic control of the histological

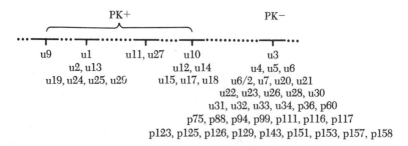

FIG. 1.—The division of the white pock (*u*) mutants of rabbitpox virus into five clusters and the order of these relative to each other. All Pk⁻ mutants fail to multiply in pig kidney (PK) cells which are permissive for the other *u* mutants and for wild-type rabbitpox virus. Among the PK⁻ mutants, *u* indicates that the mutant was first isolated as a white pock mutant on the chorioallantoic membrane, *p* indicates isolation as a PK⁻ mutant which was subsequently demonstrated to have *u* phenotype. Different PK⁻ mutants are blocked at different steps in multiplication, but they do not recombine with each other. (Reprinted by permission from Fenner and Sambrook, 1966.)

type of poxvirus cytoplasmic inclusion body, and whether virions are present or absent from these inclusion bodies (Ichihashi and Matsumoto, 1968).

Herpesvirus Group

As long ago as 1955 Wildy demonstrated recombination between different strains of herpes simplex, using mouse virulence and pock type on the chorioallantoic membrane as marker characters. It would be well worth while reexamining herpesviruses genetically, using *ts* mutants, for they are a large and important group in relation to human and animal disease and a good deal is now known about their replication (Roizman, 1969).

Adenovirus and Simian Virus 40 (SV40)

No convincing evidence has yet been presented that adenoviruses undergo recombination, probably because of the inadequacy of plaque assay methods and the failure to use suitable mutants. However, a fascinating story has emerged concerning interactions, including genetic recombination, between human adenoviruses and the papovavirus SV40. Human adenoviruses fail to produce progeny in simian cells, although the viral DNA is synthesized (Rapp et al., 1966). Yet much of the early work with human adenoviruses was carried out in monkey kidney cells, which at the time the adenoviruses were discovered were perhaps the most commonly used cell in the virus laboratory. It now transpires that human adenoviruses could multiply in these cells only because they were concurrently infected with the papovavirus SV40. Arising from this laboratory accident a variety of remarkable interactions between SV40 and adenoviruses has been observed (see reviews: Rapp and Melnick, 1966; Rapp, 1969). A variety of types of mixed virions can occur, with variable amounts of both adenovirus and SV40 DNA being enclosed within adenovirus capsids, linked by covalent bonds (Baum et al., 1966). Such particles are able to rescue superinfecting human adenoviruses of another serotype in mixed infections of simian cells, and rescue is accompanied by phenotypic mixing and transcapsidation. Detailed investigation of the SV40-adenovirus genetic hybrids has proved difficult because they occur as minority component in a mixture from which it has been impossible to separate them by cloning (because they are defective) or by biophysical means. The biophysical problem of separating the genetic hybrids from adenovirions has been partially overcome, with some hybrids, by using fixed-angle equilibrium density gradient centrifugation in cesium chloride (Baum et al.,

1970). Hybrid particles that were separable had a lower buoyant density than adenovirions, possibly because they had lost more adenovirus DNA than the amount of SV40 DNA that they had acquired.

THE MECHANISM OF RECOMBINATION WITH DEOXYRIBOVIRUSES

The foregoing summary indicates that animal virologists are still at the descriptive stage with respect to genetic interactions between deoxyriboviruses. Since all the examples studied so far involve viruses whose genome consists of a single molecule of double-stranded DNA there is no need to invoke novel mechanisms of recombination. Recombination rates are compatible with those found for bacterial viruses with large genomes, and it can be predicted that the same mechanisms that occur with bacteria and bacterial viruses will also apply to animal deoxyriboviruses.

RECOMBINATION BETWEEN VIRAL AND CELLULAR DNAS

Ever since it was discovered that cells transformed by polyoma virus failed to release infectious virus (Vogt and Dulbecco, 1962), analogies have been drawn between bacterial lysogeny and an equivalent state in virus-transformed animal cells. Integration of viral with cellular DNA has now been demonstrated with SV40 and polyoma viruses. Several types of evidence, notably the invariable presence in virus-transformed cells of T (Habel, 1965) and transplantation (Sjögren, 1965) antigens, showed that viral nucleic acid was present and expressed in all virus-transformed cells. Nucleic acid hybridization experiments have shown that cells transformed by polyoma virus, SV40, and oncogenic adenoviruses contain mRNAs homologous with the appropriate viral DNAs (Benjamin, 1966; Fujinaga and Green, 1966). Westphal and Dulbecco (1968) showed that the viral DNA in SV40 and polyoma virus-transformed cells was present in the cell nucleus, and that the number of "viral DNA equivalents" per cell varied between 5 and 60 in different transformed cell lines. A doubly transformed cell line contained 40 SV40 and 10 polyoma DNA equivalents per cell, and a line transformed by defective SV40 contained fewer DNA equivalents than lines which yielded infectious SV40 on fusion. Sambrook et al. (1968) then used biophysical methods to examine the location of SV40 DNA in the nuclei of the transformed 3T3 cells. They showed that such nuclei did not contain free viral DNA of a size similar to that present in virions and that the DNA which hybridized with virus-complementary RNA was present as a high molecular weight DNA associated with the chromosomes. Their conclusion was that the viral DNA molecules were integrated with cell DNA by alkali-stable covalent linkages, either as one large piece at a single site or at multiple sites with several individual insertions.

Indirect evidence that the viral DNA is associated with certain chromosomes has been provided by experiments with hybrid human-mouse cell lines, the human cell component of which had been transformed by SV40 (Weiss et al., 1968). Spontaneous loss of human chromosomes occurred during subsequent multiplication of the hybrid cells. This was accompanied by loss of T antigen production, but only when the great majority of the human chromosomes had disappeared, suggesting that viral DNA had been integrated either in all or in a small number of the human chromosomes in the transformed cells. Experiments leading to a similar conclusion have been carried out with polyoma virus and biochemical mutants of BHK21 cells (Marin and Littlefield, 1968).

If the genetic message of leukovirus RNA is transcribed into DNA in infected cells, as now seems likely (see p. 7), the question arises of possible integration of this DNA "provirus" (Temin, 1964b) into the cellular genome. Application of the approach used with SV40 to the leukoviruses should be possible (Baluda and Nayak, 1970) and may solve this problem.

RECOMBINATION BETWEEN RIBOVIRUSES

Influenza Virus

Recombination with animal viruses was first demonstrated with influenza virus (Burnet and Lind, 1949, 1951) and a large amount of work was carried out in the 1950s with different wild-type strains as parents (see review: Kilbourne, 1963). Since then, two types of recombination experiment with influenza viruses have yielded valuable physiological and genetic information. One group of experimenters has studied antigenic recombinants between different strains of influenza A, and the other *ts* mutants of one strain of this virus.

Prior to 1961, recombination experiments were carried out in the allantoic sac of the chick embryo. The results obtained were criticized because of cloning problems, but recombination between different strains of influenza A virus using plaque assay methods has demonstrated the validity of the early work. Using a mammalian cell line, Sugiura and Kilbourne (1966) found high frequency recombination (6% to 34% in different experiments) between two unrelated type A viruses which belonged to subtypes A0 and A1, and similar results have since been described with human and avian (Easterday et al., 1969) or equine (Kilbourne, 1968) strains of influenza A. Recombination between influenza A and influenza B has been sought, but has not been demonstrated. Likewise, in tests for genetic relatedness by molecular hybridization of viral and complementary strand RNA, there was a substantial degree of cross-hybridization between strains of influenza A of varying provenance (in time and animal source), but slight or no crossing between the influenza A strains and influenza B (Scholtissek and Rott, 1969). The commonest recombinants of type A strains have the ribonucleoprotein and hemagglutinin antigens of one parent and the neuraminidase of the other (Laver and Kilbourne, 1966). These recombinants have been exploited for studying the size and shape of the envelope proteins (Laver and Valentine, 1969), for assessing the significance of the viral neuraminidase at the cellular level (Compans et al., 1969), and in relation to protection (Schulman et al., 1968). Recombination experiments between several influenza A2 strains, including A2 Hong Kong/68, and strain A0/NWS, showed that all the cross-reactivity of the envelope antigens of the Hong Kong virus with other A2 strains resided in the neuraminidase and not the hemagglutinin (Schulman and Kilbourne, 1969). Recombination between different animal influenza A viruses (e.g., from swine and birds) has been demonstrated in intact animals as well as in embryonated eggs and cell culture (Webster, 1970).

The other approach to influenza virus genetics has been to use *ts* mutants of a strain (WSN) that plaques well on check embryo fibroblasts. Two reports have appeared (Simpson and Hirst, 1968; Mackenzie, 1970). Recombination was readily demonstrated and often occurred with high frequency, but the two groups of workers interpreted their results differently. MacKenzie reported that, with very careful attention to the experimental conditions, the recombination rates with particular pairs of *ts* mutants were reproducible (frequencies varying between 0.4% and over 6%) and additive. The higher frequencies are some sevenfold higher than would be expected for a genome of about 3 million daltons by analogy with recombination frequencies for a single round mating of T4. Simpson and Hirst found even higher recombination rates, between 6% and 20%. They interpret this in terms of assortative mating and exchange of pieces of RNA, a view 'that receives strong support from biophysical studies of the influenza virus genome, whereas MacKenzie believed that a linear "map" of the influenza virus genome could be constructed. These views are not necessarily irreconcilable if the RNA pieces are in fact aligned in some specific order in the virion.

Poliovirus

Recombination with poliovirus was first demonstrated by Hirst (1962) and Ledinko (1963). Subsequent studies on recombination are due almost entirely to Cooper and his colleagues, who used *ts* mutants of poliovirus type 1 (Cooper, 1968, 1969). Cooper found that recombination rates were of the magnitude expected by analogy with T4, i.e., always <0.9%. They were reproducible when the tests were carefully carried out (selected stocks, rigid temperature control, etc.), and map distances were additive, yielding a linear map. The ordering of mutants determined by additivity of the two-factor crosses was confirmed by three-factor crosses involving a *ts* *g*^{r} (guanidine resistant) double mutant (Fig. 2). Subsequent work (Cooper, 1970) has confirmed this picture, and has extended the map

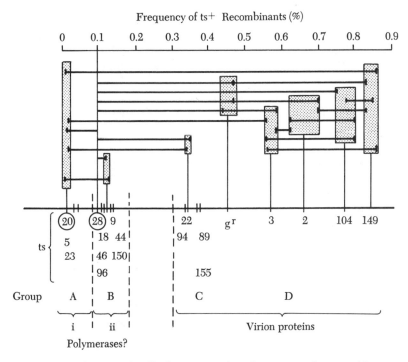

FIG. 2.—Genetic map of poliovirus type 1, based upon experiments with temperature-sensitive (*ts*) and guanidine-resistant (*g*^{r}) mutants. (Reprinted by permission from Cooper, 1968.) Upper figures represent the scale (percent recombinants); lower figures are the identification numbers of the mutants examined. Recombination frequencies are determined by two-factor crosses; the stippled boxes represent the discrepancies in the additivity of recombination frequencies. The location (to the left or to the right of all mutants with respect to *ts*28) has been found by three-factor crosses involving *ts*28 adapted to guanidine resistance (*ts*28*g*^{r}); *g*^{r} indicates the locus for its guanidine resistance. The mutants have been allocated to physiological groups. Mutants of group A (characterized by *ts*20) appear to be defective in a function needed to make or maintain double-stranded RNA; mutants of group B (characterized by *ts*28) are defective in a function needed to produce progeny RNA free of the double-stranded complex. Most of the mutants allocated to groups C and D appear to be defective in the production of a virion protein.

0.25 units to the left, with two mutants physiologically identical with $ts20$, and a dextran sulfate-resistant marker has been located close to g^r. Several new ts mutants have mapped within the existing limits and have conformed physiologically also. This fact, and consideration of the coding potential of the genome and the molecular weight of the coat proteins (equivalent to 40% of coding potential), suggests that the map may cover 70-80% of the genome.

Foot-and-mouth disease virus, another picornavirus, undergoes recombination to much the same extent as does poliovirus (Pringle, 1968).

Reovirus

Since multiplicity and cross-reactivation had been demonstrated with wild-type reoviruses of the same and different serotypes (McClain and Spendlove, 1966) it was not surprising to find that recombination could be readily demonstrated between ts mutants of reovirus type 3 (Fields and Joklik, 1969). The frequency of isolation of the mutants (2-10%, with different mutagens) and their stability suggests that most were multiple mutants. Nevertheless, when recombination tests were carried out by mixedly infecting cells at the permissive temperature and assaying the yield at permissive and restrictive temperatures, recombination between different pairs was either zero or in excess of 3% (and sometimes up to 50%). Thirty-five ts mutants were arranged in five recombination groups. Studies of RNA synthesis by the mutants agreed with grouping based on the genetic analysis.

Vesicular Stomatitis Virus

Although its properties are particularly suitable for genetic studies (good plaquing, high yield, rapid growth), the first experiments on recombination with vesicular stomatitis virus, a rhabdovirus, were not reported until this year (Pringle, 1970). One hundred and seventy-five temperature-sensitive mutants could be allocated to four complementation groups. Genetic recombination could not be detected (0.01% to < 0.001%) in crosses between different mutants within each of the two largest complementation groups, but occurred with frequencies of 0.31% and 3.4% in crosses between these groups. The time course of production of recombinants and their apparent independence of multiplicity suggested reassortment of subunits rather than crossing over.

Other Riboviruses

The only other riboviruses that have been examined for recombination are two group A togaviruses, Sindbis and Semliki Forest virus (Burge and Pfefferkorn, 1966; Tan et al., 1969), and the paramyxovirus Newcastle disease virus (Granoff, 1962; Dahlberg and Simons, 1969). No success has yet been reported in several attempts, using *ts* mutants and a sensitive system.

MECHANISM OF RECOMBINATION BY RIBOVIRUSES

In many aspects of molecular and cellular virology animal virologists have discovered that the viruses they deal with behave in a manner analogous to the bacterial viruses. However, a few notable and interesting exceptions are emerging. Genetic recombination, for example, has not been observed with ribophages, whereas with animal riboviruses two types of result have been observed. With two picornaviruses (poliovirus and foot-and-mouth disease virus) whose genome is a single linear molecule of single-stranded RNA, recombination occurs with a low frequency, compatible with recombination by crossing over, presumably between the double-stranded replicative intermediate molecules described by Bishop et al. (1969).

Recombination between mutants or strains of viruses of the myxovirus and reovirus groups, on the other hand, occurs with a very high frequency, and although there has not yet been sufficient effort to demonstrate them, double-mutant recombinants have yet to be demonstrated. It will be recalled that in these viruses the genome is an aggregate of several pieces of RNA. It seems highly likely that recombination usually occurs by exchange of pieces of RNA, possibly even by addition of a specific piece of RNA [just as "incomplete" influenza virus is associated with the absence of a specific piece of RNA (Pons and Hirst, 1969)]. It is possible, of course, that "crossing over" could occur within one piece of RNA to give low frequency recombination between different mutants of one gene.

GENETIC REACTIVATION

Table 3 also illustrates ways in which genetic reactivation can occur. An intensive study of multiplicity reactivation with rabbitpox virus (see review: Sharp, 1968) emphasizes the great important of particle aggregation in this phenomenon. This is explicable when we recall that poxviruses (and many other viruses) multiply in localized "factory" areas within the cytoplasm of large animal cells. When one or both parental viruses is unable on its own to produce an expanding factory by multiplying, genetic interactions could only occur if interacting nucleic acid molecules are brought mechanically to the same part of the cell, as they may be by clumping of the virions. Kirvaitis and Simon (1965) used the device of deliberate aggregation and dispersion of ultraviolet-irradiated particles to demonstrate multiplicity reactivation with Newcastle disease virus, but in this case the interpretation is complicated by possible effects of polyploid particles. Multiplicity and cross-reactivation are readily demonstrable with influenza viruses (Barry, 1961; Schäfer and Rott, 1961), but incomplete influenza virus (von Magnus virus) does not exhibit multiplicity reactivation (Rott and Scholtissek, 1963) because all the particles in such preparations lack one particular piece of viral RNA (Pons and Hirst, 1969).

Reoviruses inactivated by ultraviolet irradiation readily undergo multiplicity reactivation even when the virions are not clumped but are deliberately dispersed before inoculation (McClain and Spendlove, 1966). Cross-multiplicity reactivation occurred readily between all three reovirus serotypes.

The results with genetic reactivation are compatible with those observed with recombination, namely, repair by crossing over in the case of poxviruses and assortative mating to produce viable progeny in influenza virus and reoviruses. With Newcastle disease virus, in which recombination has not been demonstrated, multiplicity reactivation (which was only demonstrable after clumping of the virions) may not involve recombination as usually understood but may be an effect of the frequent occurrence of polyploid particles in this paramyxovirus.

GENE PRODUCT INTERACTIONS

Besides interactions involving viral nucleic acids, interactions between viral gene products (proteins) can occur in mixedly infected cells. Most commonly these depress the yield of one or both viruses, because of interference; sometimes the yield of one component of the mixture is enhanced above its otherwise normal level (see Fenner, 1968c). Interference often involves host-cell effects (interferon production or receptor saturation); it does not bear directly on problems of viral genetics and will not be considered here.

COMPLEMENTATION

For the geneticist, although not necessarily for the virologist, complementation is a more important phenomenon than either interference or enhancement. The term can be used in a general sense to describe all cases in which interaction between viral gene products or gene functions in multiply or mixedly infected cells results in an increased yield of infective virus of one (or both) parental types.

Complementation Between Closely Related Viruses

The gene as a unit of function can be defined by tests for complementation that determine whether two mutants, which exhibit similar phenotypes, are defective in the same function. In experimental virology, complementation between related viral mutants is useful, as a preliminary step to genetic mapping, to sort mutants into groups before doing recombination experiments. Unlike genetic recombination, complementation does not involve exchange of viral nucleic acid but reflects the fact that one virus provides a gene product in which the other is defective, so enabling both to multiply in the mixedly infected cell. Table 4 illustrates some examples. Complementation is often asymmetrical, i.e., one parental type dominates the yield.

Complementation has been observed in all situations in which recombination has been demonstrated (see above). In addition, it has proved a valuable way of classifying mutants into functional groups with Sindbis virus (Burge and Pfefferkorn, 1966) and with polyoma virus (Eckhart, 1969; Di Mayorca et al., 1969).

Poxviruses. Rabbitpox *ts* mutants showed a substantial degree of mutual complementation when inoculated together at the restrictive temperature

TABLE 4.—*Gene Product (Protein) Interaction: Complementation and Phenotypic Mixing**

Phenomenon	Parent 1	Parent 2	Progeny	Comment
Complementation:				
1. Between conditional lethal mutants in different genes	ABC ↓↓↓ abc	ABC ↓↓↓ abc	ABC and ABC	Reciprocal, both mutants rescued
2. Between defective virus and unrelated helper virus	ABC ↓ ↓ a c	BYZ ↓↓↓ b y z	ABC and BYZ	Defective virus is rescued by gene product b of helper BYZ
Phenotypic mixing:				
1. Enveloped viruses	ABC ↓ a	XYZ ↓ x	ABC/ax , XYZ/ax	Mixed peplomers in envelopes, genomes unaltered
2. Nonenveloped viruses (transcapsidation)	ABC ↓ a	XYZ ↓ x	ABC/x , XYZ/a	Heterologous capsids, not always reciprocal

*A, etc. = active viral genes; B = mutant gene; B = defective gene B; a, b, etc. = product of gene, A, B, etc.

$$\frac{ABC}{ax} = \frac{\text{Genome}}{\text{Proteins in envelope (or capsid)}}$$

(Padgett and Tomkins, 1968). There are so many genes in poxviruses that it is not surprising that only one complementation group (of three mutants) was detected amongst the 18 *ts* mutants examined.

Poxviruses also exhibit a novel form of complementation associated with their uncoating. It was found many years ago that animals inoculated with heat-killed virulent myxoma virus and an active avirulent fibroma virus (two antigenically related poxviruses) contracted myxomatosis (Berry and Dedrick, 1936). Initially this was thought to be due to "transformation" of the type Griffith and Avery had discovered with pneumococci, but experiments with a variety of poxviruses, many of which were genetically marked, showed that the heat-inactivated virus was reactivated by a nongenetic mechanism (Fenner et al., 1959). Joklik (1964) postulated that reactivation was host-cell mediated, but more recent work (McAuslan, 1969) suggests that it is due to viral complementation, the heat-damaged component probably being the viral DNA-dependent RNA polymerase which is associated with poxvirus particles (Kates and McAuslan, 1967). This sort of complementation occurs between all poxviruses that have been examined (Fenner and Woodroofe, 1960). Recently a phenomenon analogous to poxvirus reactivation has been observed with adenoviruses (Béládi et al., 1970); the mechanism has not yet been elucidated.

Papovavirus group. Recombination has yet to be demonstrated between papovaviruses, although it probably does occur between them and the cellular genome during transformation. Complementation has been used for grouping *ts* mutants of polyoma virus into functional groups (Eckhart, 1969; Di Mayorca et al., 1969), and thus for studying the mechanism of viral oncogenesis.

Picornavirus group. With *ts* mutants of poliovirus, Cooper (1965) found that complementation was demonstrable, but it was restricted to a few combinations of mutants, it was highly asymmetric, and the yield was low. It has not provided useful for either genetic or physiological studies.

Mixed infection of cells with a nonrestricted picornavirus and an unrelated guanidine-restricted picornavirus results in rescue (by complementation) of the RNA of the restricted virus (Cords and Holland, 1964a). It may be enclosed within homologous, phenotypically mixed, or completely heterologous capsids (Holland and Cords, 1964).

Togavirus group. The two group A togaviruses that have been studied genetically show remarkable differences in the efficiency of complementation. With Sindbis virus complementation was efficient (Burge and Pfefferkorn, 1966) and proved a useful method of grouping mutants in a way that corresponded with functional defects (see review: Pfefferkorn and Burge, 1968). With Semliki Forest Virus, on the other hand, complementation was hardly detectable even between the very dissimilar RNA⁺ and RNA⁻ mutants; it was useless for grouping mutants (Tan et al., 1969).

Myxovirus group. When cells were mixedly infected with two *ts* mutants of influenza virus and incubated at the restrictive temperature, the yield contained recombinant (*ts* ⁺) virus together with a much higher content of virus with *ts* phenotype than in control cells, i.e., both complementation and recombination occurred under the restrictive conditions (Simpson and Hirst, 1968; Mackenzie, 1968).

Paramyxovirus group. Dahlberg and Simon (1968) obtained 48 nitrous acid-induced *ts* mutants of NDV. By taking precautions to minimize the effects of eluted virus they were able to detect yields as low as 10^{-4} PFU per cell. Complementation tests revealed nine nonoverlapping complementation groups amongst 29 *ts* mutants. Sixteen mutants were in one complementation group.

Earlier, Kirvaitis and Simon (1965) had reported that recombination occurred between *ts* mutants of Newcastle disease virus. It is now apparent that there is no recombination at levels about $2-5 \times 10^{-5}$ (Dahlberg and Simon, 1969). The earlier results were due to the occurrence of complementing heteropolyploid particles, which may produce small plaques.

Leukovirus group. Until very recently difficulties of cloning have prevented genetic studies with leukoviruses, but recent experiments with a particular strain (B77) of avian sarcoma virus that clones readily and is not contaminated with avian leukosis virus yielded *ts* mutants (Toyoshima and Vogt, 1969). This opens up the possibility of a genetic analysis of the functions of these interesting viruses.

Unlike strain B77, most variants of both avian and murine leukoviruses that produce solid tumors (e.g., Rouse sarcoma virus and Moloney sarcoma virus) are defective (Hanafusa et al., 1963, 1964; Huebner et al., 1966). They can be rescued by appropriate coinfection of transformed nonyielder cells with avian leukosis or murine leukemia viruses respectively. The type of viral antigen in the envelope of the rescued virions is determined by the helper viruses. This has led to the concept of "pseudotypes" of these sarcoma viruses, in which the genome is that of the defective sarcoma virus and the envelope protein (which determines host-cell range) is that of the helper virus.

Complementation Between Unrelated Viruses

The occurrence of genetic recombination between adenoviruses and SV40 has already been described. Adenoviruses also exhibit a striking range of complementation reactions with other deoxyriboviruses. As already mentioned, human adenoviruses are defective in simian cells. Yields of infectious adenovirus can be enhanced more than 1000-fold if the simian cells are coinfected with either a simian adenovirus (Naegele and Rapp, 1967), SV40, or hybrid human adenovirus containing defective SV40 and adenoviral DNA (Rapp and Jerkofsky, 1967). In all cases the complementing virus appears to affect the cell in such a way that the human adenovirus genome can express its full potential for the production of infectious progeny particles.

In addition to this situation, where adenoviruses are the rescued agents, there exists a group of small icosahedral viruses which contain a small molecule of single-stranded DNA, the adenovirus-associated viruses (AAV), and which are completely dependent upon adenoviruses for their replication (Atchison et al., 1965). A canine adenovirus has been shown to complement AAV both in canine cells and in human cells, in which the adenovirus itself grows very poorly. Some adenovirus function later than T antigen production is required (Smith and Gehle, 1967). During an epidemiological survey in a children's home, AAV was isolated frequently during an 8-week period, usually from anal swabs and almost always in association with adenovirus isolations. Two AAV serotypes and 10 adenovirus serotypes were isolated, and there was no evidence of illness attributable to AAV infection (Blacklow et al., 1968).

Adenovirus 12 complements the parvovirus H1 in cells which normally restrict parvovirus growth (Ledinko et al., 1969).

Phenotypic Mixing

Following mixed infection by two viruses which share certain common features but do not necessarily belong to the same group, some of the progeny may acquire phenotypic characteristics from both parents, although their genotype remains unchanged (Table 4). For example when cells are infected with antigenically different strains of influenza virus (Burnet and Lind, 1953), with influenza virus and a paramyxovirus (Granoff and Hirst, 1945), or with a paramyxovirus and the rhabdovirus vesicular stomatitis virus (Choppin and Compans, 1970), the envelopes of some of the progeny particles contain viral antigens characteristic of each of the parental viruses. However, each virion usually contains the nucleic acid of only one of the parental viuses, so that on passage it will produce only virions resembling that parent, although with loosely enveloped viruses heteropolyploidy (genotypic mixing) may sometimes occur.

Phenotypic mixing also occurs with nonenveloped viruses if they mature in the same part of the cell (cytoplasm or nucleus). It is common in mixed infections with picornaviruses, either different serotypes of poliovirus (Ledinko and Hirst, 1961) or different enteroviruses, such as poliovirus and coxsackieviruses (Holland and Cords, 1964). In the latter instance the "mixing" of capsid proteins may be minimal; instead "transcapsidation" may occur, whereby the genome of one agent is enclosed within the capsid of the other. Phenotypic mixing has also been observed when simian adenoviruses complement human adenoviruses in simian cells; some of the progeny of such infections are doubly antigenic (Altstein and Dodonova, 1968). Transcapsidation rather than phenotypic mixing appears to be the rule with human adenoviruses after cocultivation with SV40 in monkey cells (Rapp and Melnick, 1966); often the genome which is encapsidated consists of covalently linked adenovirus and SV40 DNA.

POLYPLOIDY AND GENOTYPIC MIXING

Attention should be drawn to what can be called polyploidy and "genotypic mixing" (heteropolyploidy) in animal viruses, for either phenomenon may greatly complicate genetic experiments. Normal populations of parainfluenza virus type 1, for example, include many virions with multiple complete genomes, each enclosed within its capsid (Hosaka et al., 1966), and the same phenomenon has been demonstrated with other paramyxoviruses. Indeed it may be expected to occur with greater or less frequency with all loosely enveloped viruses that mature by budding from cellular membranes, especially among those containing tubular nucleocapsids. Clearly, if a cell were mixedly infected with genetically different forms of a particular virus, the envelope could enclose two different genomes; hence the concept of genotypic mixing, a term originally used by McBride (1962).

Such genotypically mixed virions resemble the diploid particles of bacteriophage f1 (Scott and Zinder, 1967) rather than the heterozygotes found with the T-even bacteriophages, in which the heterologous DNA is part of a single viral DNA molecule. Their existence may complicate genetic experiments; for instance, what was first reported as "recombination" between *ts* mutants of Newcastle disease virus (Kirvaitis and Simon, 1965) is apparently due to complementation by heteropolyploid particles (Dahlberg and Simon, 1969).

HOST RESPONSES TO VIRAL INFECTIONS

At the practical level the only significant feature of a virus is its power to produce disease. Since disease is one of the outcomes of virus-host interaction and involves the response of the host animal as an organism, an essay on genetic aspects of viral diseases must involve consideration not only of the genetics of viruses but also the genetics of the host response, a much more complex topic.

Many viruses show a high degree of species specificity. For example, chickenpox and smallpox are viruses of man; foot-and-mouth disease virus affects cattle; myxomatosis affects rabbits. Except for a few rodent-pathogenic mutants obtained by a laborious process of adaptation, polioviruses infect only primates, and in cell culture only primate cells. This specificity may be associated with failure of a virus to attach to, and therefore to enter, cells of a particular species of vertebrate. Or the virus may be adsorbed but not penetrate; or it may penetrate, only to have its replication blocked at some later step.

Vertebrates have evolved in a world infested with parasites and have therefore developed a variety of mechanisms to enable them to adjust to parasitic invasion with a minimum of bodily disturbance. If cellular infection and viral multiplication do occur, then a complex series of host responses come into play which in large part determine the outcome of the infection. The most clearly defined defence mechanism is the immune response, but a host of other physiological factors play a role—interferon, body temperature, nutrition, hormones etc.

MODES OF INHERITANCE OF RESISTANCE TO VIRAL INFECTIONS

Breeding experiments on the inheritance of resistance have been carried out with mice and chickens. Three types of result can be expected; the distribution of resistance expected in each case with the parental animals, F1 generation, and backcrosses is illustrated in Fig. 3. Single-gene inheritance with susceptibility dominant (Fig. 3B) occurs in cases where presence of the appropriate cellular receptor determines susceptibility. Single-gene inheritance with resistance dominant (Fig. 3A) is found in some cases where there is an intracellular block in viral multiplication. Polygenic inheritance (Fig. 3C) may occur in situations where reactions of the host organism as such are involved, e.g., the immune response, although the capacity to respond immunologically to particular antigens may be determined by a single gene (McDevitt and Chinitz, 1969; Ellman et al., 1970). The physiological basis of inherited susceptibility has been adequately demonstrated only in cases where susceptibility is determined by the presence of appropriate cellular receptor sites and resistance by their absence.

CELLULAR RECEPTORS AND SUSCEPTIBILITY TO INFECTION

The best examples of genetically controlled cellular receptors acting as the determinant of susceptibility of cell and organism are found with the

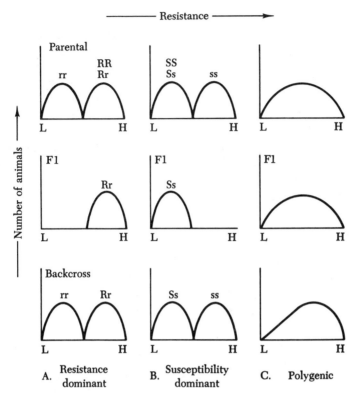

FIG. 3.—Diagram illustrating the expected modes of inheritance of resistance against an infection on three hypotheses: (A) A single pair of alleles with resistance dominant makes an important contribution. (B) A single pair of alleles with susceptibility dominant makes an important contribution. (C) Many genes affect susceptibility. *Upper curves:* Parental generations, with resistance plotted on the abscissa in arbitrary units (L = low resistance; H = high resistance). *Middle curves:* The resistance of F_1 progeny of matings of highly susceptible and highly resistant animals. *Lower curves:* The resistance of back-crosses of F_1 with suitable parental types. (Modified from Allison, 1965.)

enteroviruses. Poliovirus attaches efficiently to cultured human and monkey cells, but nonprimate cells fail to adsorb detectable amounts of virus (McLaren et al., 1959). The determining influence of such attachment on susceptibility has been demonstrated by the production of poliovirions after infection of "insusceptible" cells with poliovirus RNA (Holland et al., 1959), and by elegant experiments involving transcapsidation of poliovirus and coxsackievirus (Cords and Holland, 1964b). As described earlier, Holland and Cords (1964) had previously obtained mixed virions, in which the poliovirus genome was enclosed within the capsid of coxsackievirus B1, by double infection of HeLa cells, in the presence of the inhibitor guanidine, with guanidine-dependent coxsackievirus B1 and guanidine-sensitive poliovirus. These mixed virions infect and multiply for a single cycle in cultured mouse fibroblasts and in mice, both of which are completely insusceptible to poliovirus but are susceptible to infection with coxsackievirus. The yield consists entirely of poliovirus type 1 particles which are unable to initiate a second cycle of infection in the adjacent cells because of their lack of surface receptors for the poliovirus capsomers.

The susceptibility of chicken and mammalian cells to infection with the avian leukoviruses is determined by the affinity of viral envelope antigens for receptors in the plasma membrane (Rubin, 1965; Hanafusa and Hanafusa, 1966). However, in contrast to the situation just described for enteroviruses, the cellular receptors and viral envelope antigens do not determine viral attachment, for avian leukoviruses attach equally well to susceptible and resistant cells (Piraino, 1967; Crittenden et al., 1967; see also review by Vogt et al., 1969). However, the uneclipsed virions remain attached to the surface of resistant cells, i.e., the block occurs at the stage of penetration. This block can be circumvented by phenotypic mixing of envelope antigens (Vogt, 1967) or by cocultivation of resistant and heavily irradiated susceptible cells (Crittenden, 1968); in both cases replication occurs in the resistant cells if the leukovirus genome gains entrance.

Because of their derivation by numerous serial passages in chickens, most laboratory "strains" of avian leukoviruses are complex mixtures of several serotypes which are only now being separated and cloned, largely on the basis of cellular susceptibility. It has been possible to divide avian leukoviruses into four groups (A, B, C, and D) on the basis of their envelope proteins, either by immunological tests or by tests based on the susceptibility of cells from chickens of various genetically characterized lines (Vogt and Ishizaki, 1965; Duff and Vogt, 1969). The oncogenicity for mammals of certain stock strains of Rous sarcoma virus appears to be due to the presence of small amounts of virus of subgroup D in the stocks (Duff and Vogt, 1969).

The genetic resistance of lines of chickens to avian leukoviruses of a particular subgroup is a recessive trait controlled at a single autosomal locus (Rubin, 1965; Crittenden et al., 1967; Payne and Biggs, 1966, 1970). If the appropriate receptor is present on cells, in either heterozygotes or homozygotes, the cells and the chickens are susceptible to viruses of the subgroup involved (inheritance as in Fig. 3B).

GENETIC CONTROL OF VIRAL MULTIPLICATION

Attachment of a virus to a cell and penetration of the genome into the cell are necessary but not sufficient conditions for productive infection, and many instances have been reported of particular types of cell in which attachment, penetration, and uncoating occur normally but no infectious progeny are produced. Examples are human adenoviruses in simian cells, considered at length earlier in this review, abortive infections of pig kidney (PK) cells by PK-negative mutants of rabbitpox virus (Fenner and Sambrook, 1966), and abortive infections of cultured cells by influenza viruses (Fraser, 1967).

RESTRICTION OF HOST-DEPENDENT CONDITIONAL LETHAL MUTANTS

Among the bacteriophages, mutants (*amber* and *ocher*) have been recognized which multiply normally in certain bacterial hosts but fail to multiply in wild-type bacteria of the same species. The permissive hosts contain one or another of several suppressor genes that compensate for the effect of the phage mutations by specifying mutant transfer RNAs that translate the "nonsense" chain-terminating codons (UAG or UAA) as amino acids (Garen, 1968).

Suppressor genes of this sort have not been recognized in animal cells. If the implication of posttranslational cleavage is accepted, i.e., that punctuation codons do not operate, at least at the level of translation, then they probably do not occur in animal cells. However, a few other types of host-cell dependent mutants have been described. The best characterized are the PK-negative mutants of rabbitpox virus (McClain, 1965; Fenner and Sambrook, 1966), which multiply normally in chick cells but fail to multiply in pig cells. Different mutants are blocked at different stages of the viral multiplication cycle, some very early (before DNA replication) and others much later (at the stage of maturation). The mechanism of restriction in pig cells has not been discovered. Takemori et al. (1969) have described mutants of adenovirus 12 which failed to multiply in KB cells, and, starting from wild-type herpes simplex virus, which fails to multiply in dog kidney cells, Roizman and his colleagues (see review: Roizman, 1969) have obtained a mutant which did multiply in these cells.

These host-dependent conditional lethal mutants should be useful tools for investigating mechanisms of translation in vertebrate cells, as well as for the study of steps in viral biosynthesis.

GENETIC CONTROL OF THE SUSCEPTIBILITY OF MACROPHAGES

Macrophages play a major role in the pathogenesis of many generalized viral infections, and they may play an important role in preventing the infection of susceptible cells by viruses circulating in the blood stream. For example, Mims (1960, 1964) showed that, when influenza, myxoma, or a dermal strain of vaccinia virus was inoculated intravenously into mice, the circulating virus was rapidly cleared by the Kupffer cells of the liver. The injected viruses did not multiply in these cells, nor did they subsequently invade and multiply in the hepatic parenchymal cells. The susceptibility of the latter cells was demonstrated by the fact that all three viruses multiplied in them when the macrophage barrier was bypassed by injection of suspensions of virus directly up the bile duct.

Two examples have been reported in which macrophages from different strains of mice differ in their susceptibility to viruses, and this variation seems to be responsible for different susceptibility of the intact animals to the effects of infection with these viruses. Some strains of mice are resistant and others susceptible to infection with group B togaviruses (Sabin, 1954; Goodman and Koprowski, 1962). Resistance is dominant and under single-gene control (inheritance as in Fig. 3A). The antibody response appears to play no part in resistance, nor does the capacity of the cells of the two strains to produce interferon (Vainio et al., 1961). The only difference observed was the much greater yield of viruses from cultures of peritoneal or splenic macrophages from susceptible than from resistant mice (Vainio, 1963; Goodman and Koprowski, 1962). Variable and smaller differences were found in cultures of cells of other organs. A possible cause of the difference lies in interferon responsiveness of cells. Using congenic resistant and susceptible mice, Hanson et al. (1969) found that the resistant mice and cells derived from them were much more responsive to the inhibitory effect of interferon on group B togaviruses. The greater effectiveness of interferon was limited to these viruses.

Experiments with the same strains of mice and the murine coronavirus mouse hepatitis virus provide another example of resistance, due not to the absence of cellular receptors or differences in the immune response but to failure of the virus to multiply in hepatic or peritoneal macrophages of the resistant mice (Bang and Warwick, 1960; Kantoch et al., 1963). The block occurs after adsorption and penetration and before uncoating and eclipse (Shif and Bang, 1970a). Both virus and host cell play a role, for the genetic resistance of the resistant mice and their macrophages can be overcome by mutation in the virus (Shif and Bang, 1970b). In this case breeding experiments showed that resistance was due to a single pair of alleles with susceptibility dominant (Bang and Warwick, 1960). Resistance also depends on physiological factors and can be greatly reduced, at levels of both cell and organism, by treatment with cortisone (Gallily et al., 1964) or by neonatal thymectomy (Allison, 1965).

RESISTANCE ASSOCIATED WITH THE IMMUNE RESPONSE

Circulating antibody plays a major part in the protection of vertebrates from reinfection with viruses, especially those with a viremic phase, as has been clearly demonstrated by passive immunity experiments (Fenner, 1968d). Cell-mediated immunity is important in recovery from generalized viral infections (Blanden, 1971), and thus in the level of resistance to disease. Evidence relating the immune response with genetic differences in resistance to viral diseases is derived from studies in mice and men.

RESISTANCE OF C57B1 MICE TO POLYOMA TUMORS

Virus-induced tumors are associated with the appearance of new virus-specific transplantation antigens on the surface of transformed cells (Sjögren, 1965). There is compelling evidence that the failure of polyoma virus to produce tumors when inoculated into normal adult mice is due to early elimination of virus-transformed cells by a cellular immune response. Newborn mice, or adult mice in which the cell-mediated immune response has been abrogated by neonatal thymectomy or inoculations of antilymphocyte serum, develop tumors (see review: Law et al., 1966). When they are infected with polyoma virus, mice past the neonatal period suffer an acute generalized infection and develop high titer antiviral antibodies (Rowe, 1961). It is presumed that during such infections an unknown but small proportion of virus-cell interactions leads to cellular transformation, which is accompanied by the appearance of a new antigen on the surface of the transformed cell. In animals with defective cell-mediated immunity, e.g., newborn mice, such cells multiply without restraint to produce tumors, whereas in immunologically competent mice there is an immune response to the new cellular antigen and the transformed cells are eliminated. Such mice are then resistant to doses of polyoma tumor cells that multiply in normal mice.

In contrast to most other strains, C57B1 mice are resistant to the induction of tumors by polyoma virus even when inoculated as newborn animals. However, C57B1 organ explants are just as susceptible to polyoma virus-induced transformation in vitro (Dawe, 1965), and if C57B1 mice are inoculated with polyoma virus a few days after neonatal thymectomy they do develop tumors, although they develop normal levels of circulating antibody to polyoma virus (Law and Ting, 1965). Resistance therefore operates at the level of organism, rather than at the level of cell or organ, and appears to be due to cell-mediated immunity. C57B1 mice are known to develop immunological responsiveness to transplantation antigens at a much earlier age than most other strains of mice (Argyris, 1965). Different breeding experiments designed to determine the inheritance of the resistance of C57B1 mice to polyoma tumors have implicated one or several different genes. Jahkola's (1965) results suggest incompletely dominant resistance depending on two or three independent genes, all of which are required for the expression of resistance (inheritance as in Fig. 3C).

Schell's (1960a, 1960b) observations on the resistance of C57B1 mice to the lethal effects of mousepox virus likewise implicate the effective immune response of this strain. His preliminary breeding experiments suggested that resistance depended upon a single autosomal gene, with resistance dominant.

HUMAN IMMUNOLOGIC DEFICIENCIES

Bruton's (1952) recognition of congenital agammaglobulinemia in man opened a new chapter in our understanding of the relationship between immunity and the host response to viral and bacterial infections. Subsequent studies have revealed the complexity of "agammaglobulinemia," and several types, with characteristic immunological differences and associated differences in their response to infections, have been distinguished. In an attempt to bring order into the somewhat chaotic array of immunologic dificiency syndromes Seligmann et al. (1968) have proposed a tentative classification (Table 5) based upon syndrome analysis in terms of cellular, immunoglobulin, and functional defects, pathological characteristics, and genetic considerations. Following observations on immunoglobulin abnormalities in children with congenital rubella they draw attention to the need to consider fetal infections as a cause (rather than an effect) of some types of immunologic deficiency.

The reader is referred to the article by Seligmann et al. (1968) for detailed references. In general, it appears that syndromes in which immunoglobulin deficiencies are accompanied by normal cell-mediated immunity (e.g., infantile sex-linked agammaglobulinemia) are associated with recurrent infections with pyogenic bacteria but normal recovery from viral infections. Contrary to what would be expected on the basis of immunization experiments (Chanock, 1970), many individuals with selective IgA deficiency are healthy (Hanson, 1962), although some suffer from recurrent respiratory infections (West et al., 1962) and some from steatorrhoea (Heremans and Crabbé, 1968). In all situations in which cell-mediated immunity is defective, however, resistance to generalized viral infections is depressed (Seligmann et al., 1968). Indeed in many infants the existence of defective cell-mediated immunity has been recognized when they suffer overwhelming infection after the administration of a live virus vaccine (e.g., vaccinia; Fulginiti et al., 1966). As Table 5 shows, however, in most syndromes the immunological response is defective in several components, making analysis of the role of different arms of the immune response difficult (Fulginiti et al., 1968).

GENETIC CONTROL OF RESPONSE TO PARTICULAR ANTIGENS

The idea that certain blood groups may be related to resistance or susceptibility to infectious diseases, and indeed that their frequency in particular populations may be the result of this, has been proposed by several investigators. Among viral infections associations of susceptibility to smallpox with blood group A (Vogel et al., 1960) and of infection with influenza virus with blood group O (McDonald and Zuckerman, 1962) have been suggested, but in a critical review of published work Muschel (1966) found no well-established association.

There are, nevertheless, well-established cases of genetic control of the immune response to particular antigens or antigenic determinants in experimental animals. The genetically controlled presence of certain complement components in mice has been unequivocally demonstrated to prevent the immune response of mice to these complement components, whereas strains of mice lacking this complement component have an immune response (Cinader et al., 1964). There are several examples of linkage of the immune response to histocompatibility genes, both to simple synthetic antigens (McDevitt and Chinitz, 1969; Ellman et al., 1970) and certain mouse erythrocyte antigens (Gasser, 1969). If such an antigenic determinant were a component of an important surface antigen of a virus, the resulting immune unresponsiveness might have an important role in resistance.

MISCELLANEOUS EXAMPLES OF GENETICALLY DETERMINED RESISTANCE

Several examples of genetically determined responses to viral disease have been described which do not fit into any of the categories listed above. It will suffice to draw attention to two of these, both affecting the production of malignancies.

Meier et al. (1969) have investigated the inheritance of resistance to leukemia in mice, and find that two congenic types of HRS/J mice, which differ only with respect to one allele (*hr* or +), differ very greatly in the occurrence of leukemia. Forty-five percent of hairless (*hr/hr*) mice have leukemia by the time they are 8-10 months old, whereas the incidence of leukemia in heterozygous (*hr/+*) mice is only 1%, although both genotypes harbor murine leukovirus to high titer.

Human fibroblasts can be transformed by the papovavirus SV40. Among a number of fibroblast cell strains, those established from individuals suffering from Fanconi's anemia were found to be 10 times as susceptible to transformation by SV40 as strains established from normal individuals (Todaro, 1968).

TABLE 5.—Classification of Immunologic Deficiency Diseases of Man*

Syndrome	Immunologic Defects			Clinical features due to immunologic deficiency	Genetics
	Immunoglobulin deficiencies	Humoral antibody response	Cellular immunity responses		
Infantile sex-linked agammaglobulinemia	All classes extremely deficient	Absent or extremely deficient to all antigens	Normal	Recurrent infections with extracellular pyogenic pathogens	X-linked recessive
Selective inability to produce IgA	Both exocrine and circulatory IgA absent; others generally normal	Normal except for IgA antibodies	Normal	Bronchitis, sinusitis; enteropathy with malabsorption syndrome and steatorrhea; some such subjects remain perfectly healthy	Unknown; some may be autosomal recessive
Transient hypogammaglobulinemia of infancy	IgG primarily depressed	Generally low or absent to most antigens	Normal	Recurrent infections with extracellular pyogenic pathogens	Familial, (?) genetic
Non-sex-linked primary immunoglobulin deficiency with variable onset and expression	Immunoglobulin deficit invariably present but variable	Constant deficiency of responses to most antigens	Inconstant deficiency of responses to some antigens but not to others	Recurrent infections primarily with pyogenic pathogens; may have deficient resistance to virus and fungus infections	Possibly autosomal recessive in some
Agammaglobulinemia with thymoma	All markedly reduced	Constant deficient responses to all antigens	Constant deficiency in responses to most antigens	Recurrent infections primarily with pyogenic pathogens; may have deficient resistance to virus and fungus infections	(?) Genetic factor
Immune deficiency with thrombopenia and eczema	Immunoglobulin deficit usually present (low IgM and high IgA frequent)	Constant deficient responses to some antigens but not others	Constant deficient responses to most antigens	Frequent infections with all kinds of pathogens (pyogens, virus, fungi)	X-linked recessive
Ataxia-telangiectasia	Immunoglobulin deficit inconstant but usually present (often low IgA)	Inconstant deficiency in response to some antigens but not to others	Constant deficiency in response to some antigens but not others	Frequent sinopulmonary infections in cases with low IgA	Autosomal recessive
Primary lymphopenic immunologic deficiency	Immunoglobulin deficit invariably present but variable	Constant deficiency in responses to some antigens	Constant deficient responses to most antigens	Often die in early childhood of fungus, pneumocystis, or virus infection	X-linked recessive or autosomal recessive

Autosomal recessive alymphocytic agammaglobulinemia	All extremely deficient	Absent or extremely deficient to all antigens	Deficient responses to all antigens	Do not survive infancy	Autosomal recessive
Autosomal recessive lymphopenia with normal immunoglobulins	All normal	Antibodies present, probably deficient	Deficient responses to all antigens	Frequent virus, fungus, or pneumocystis infection	Autosomal recessive
Thymic aplasia	All normal	Many apparently deficient responses	Absent responses to all antigens	Usually die in infancy; frequent virus, fungus, or pneumocystis infection in most cases	No evidence of genetic mechanism

*Abbreviated from Seligman et al. (1968).

PRACTICAL ASPECTS OF VIRAL GENETICS

ADAPTATION OF VIRUSES TO LABORATORY HOSTS

Animal virology began as an essentially practical undertaking; it was, and still is, concerned with the prevention and control of viral diseases of man and his domestic animals. The first step to be taken before a satisfactory study can be made of the behavior of a virus, and before other than general "sanitation" can be applied as a measure for control of a viral disease, is the cultivation of the agent in question in a convenient laboratory animal or, nowadays, in cultured cells. To illustrate this, one has only to recall the rapid expansion in our knowledge of poliovirus and poliomyelitis that followed first the production of a recognizable disease in monkeys by Landsteiner and Popper 1909) awkward though these animals are for laboratory studies, and then the demonstration of its growth in cultured cells (Enders et al., 1949). By contrast, we are still abysmally ignorant about the nature of hepatitis viruses and the pathogenesis of viral hepatitis, because these viruses have so far not been cultivated.

Sometimes a virus which causes disease in man or a domestic animal grows equally well in a laboratory animal or in some type of cultured cell; e.g., cowpox virus obtained from infected cows grows as well in rabbits, on the chorioallantoic membrane of the developing egg, or in cultured cells as it does in cows. At other times the production of reproducible and recognizable changes in a laboratory animal or a cell line involves a long series of passages—a process called "adaptation." The genetics of adaptation has not been analyzed critically, but it probably depends upon a series of mutations and the selection of mutants that can grow progressively better in the new host, so that eventually a population of virus particles is obtained which is several unknown mutational steps away from the parental wild-type virus. The adapted virus may still be perfectly satisfactory for laboratory studies, but the fact that it has undergone prolonged selection and differs from the wild-type in many genes must not be overlooked.

PRODUCTION OF VIRAL VACCINES

Although the existence of specific viral enzymes, such as the transcriptases and replicases, provides an opportunity for the development of selective antiviral chemotherapy, the sheet anchor of specific prophylaxis in viral diseases will remain immunization. This can be achieved either with viruses or viral proteins used as inactivated antigens, or more frequently with live virus vaccines, which produce inapparent but immunizing infections.

The development of satisfactory live vaccines is a practical exercise in viral genetics. If a particular virus causes disease serious enough to warrant immunization, then a live vaccine must be attenuated. For the most part existing live vaccines have been obtained by empirical methods, although terminal dilution in tissue culture has been used to help ensure the genetic "purity" of the product (Sabin, 1955), and nowadays plaque purification is routinely used for this purpose. The usual procedure for obtaining an attenuated strain for human vaccination has been to passage wild-type virus serially for many passages in eggs or cultured cells, often at a lower temperature than 37°, and then test the product in some suitable host (usually a monkey or chimpanzee) before making trials in man. This involves adaptation by mutation and selection, and it has been empirically observed that, with adaptation to eggs or cultured cells, virulence for the original host is often lost.

It is possible to be more deliberate than this and produce vaccines by selecting for *ts* mutants. On theoretical grounds, and experimentally in several systems [rabbitpox virus, and the togavirus Semliki Forest virus (Fenner, unpublished results)] and with influenza virus (Mackenzie, 1969), *ts* mutants are attenuated compared with wild-type. Indeed if the cutoff temperature of the *ts* mutant is too low, it may not multiply well enough in the intact host to provoke an antibody response. This genetic approach is now being systematically and successfully used with respiratory viruses (Mills et al. 1969; Chanock, 1970), although as yet none of the *ts* mutants that have been obtained and tested in laboratory systems has been adopted for use in man.

Recombination can be used in order to facilitate the production of a viral vaccine, particularly in the special case of influenza, where antigenically novel and therefore potentially "epidemic" strains usually multiply poorly in laboratory hosts, but where it is essential to obtain large amounts of virus quickly in order to produce an inactivated (or even a live) vaccine. Influenza virus recombines with high frequency (see p. 15), and recombination has been used to obtain a virus with good growth potential combined with the required novel antigenic structure of the coat antigens (Kilbourne, 1969).

EXAMPLES OF GENETIC CHANGES IN VIRAL DISEASES

Genetic changes in viruses and genetic changes in the host animals consequent upon selection exerted by viral diseases have clearly been important in the evolution of both, but since there is no palaeontological record of viruses and since virology as a science has developed so recently, there are few examples illustrating such effects. Two examples merit a brief description here: myxomatosis, in which genetic changes have been observed in both virus and host; and human influenza, in which minor changes in the antigenicity of the viruses occur every year and major changes at irregular intervals.

MYXOMATOSIS

Myxomatosis in Australian wild rabbits provides a unique example of the interaction between a highly virulent virus and a highly susceptible mammal which has been observed since its inception and extensively studied by virologists. A detailed account has been published by Fenner and Ratcliffe (1965); in this paper attention will be directed to genetic aspects of the interaction.

Myxoma virus is a poxvirus which evolved as a parasite of rabbits in South America and California. In these *Sylvilagus* rabbits the virus produces a benign but often persistent fibroma in the skin, and it is maintained in nature by arthropods that mechanically transfer virus from one rabbit to another, after biting through the tumors. When such an infected insect bites a European rabbit *(Oryctolagus cuniculus)* a severe generalized disease ensues which is almost always fatal.

European rabbits became a major agricultural pest in Australia after they were introduced there in the middle of the nineteenth century. In 1950, after extensive investigations had established the safety of myxoma virus as far as other domestic and wild animals were concerned, myxoma virus was successfully introduced into the very large population of European rabbits that then inhabited the southern half of the Australian continent. Very extensive and very destructive epidemics occurred in the summer months, when mosquito vectors were plentiful. The virus persisted throughout the winter months, mostly at an undetectable level, and when mosquito numbers increased with the onset of hot weather explosive outbreaks occurred again. The epidemiological situation has remained much like this since then, but the impact of myxomatosis during the first few years was such that the rabbit population has been permanently reduced far below its premyxomatosis level.

Rapid transfer of a virus in a novel host, under conditions of both frequent (summer) and occasional (winter) transmission, might be expected to select for genetic changes in the virus. Conversely, lethal infection on a continental scale could, if it did not eradicate the host animal, select for genetic resistance. Both types of change in fact did occur, and their interplay has led to a modified type of disease. The end result of this process of mutual adaptation has not yet been reached.

The virulence of myxoma virus for *Oryctolagus* rabbits could be measured by the death rate in groups of laboratory rabbits inoculated intradermally with a standard dose of virus. Since the lethality of the original virus was so high (100% mortality with the virus originally introduced), some other measure was needed, and it was found that mortality rate was correlated with survival time when strains of virus which allowed a 10%, a 40%, or an 80% survival were tested in large groups of rabbits (Fenner and Marshall, 1957).

Using as the measure the mean survival time in groups of 5 rabbits that had been inoculated with a standard dose of virus, tests were made of the virulence of Australian field strains of myxoma virus recovered over a number of years (Fenner and Woodroofe, 1965). It was found that, within a year of the introduction of the South American virus (which had produced mortalities in the field, as in the laboratory, of well over 99%), strains of virus occurred which killed only 90% of rabbits and were associated with correspondingly prolonged survival times. Strains of this level of virulence became dominant by about 1953 and have remained so ever since (Table 6) in spite of the appearance of some strains of much lower virulence and the systematic annual introduction of the highly virulent virus by inoculation campaigns. Clearly, these field strains included a variety of different mutants, which were classified according to one character, their virulence, and allocated to "virulence grades." Viruses belonging to the same virulence grade came from widely separated parts of the conti-

TABLE 6.—*Changing Virulence of Naturally Occurring Strains of Myxoma Virus in Australia**

		\multicolumn{5}{c}{Virulence Grade}				
		I	II	III	IV	V
	Mean survival time, days:	≤13	14–16	17–28	29–50	—
Year	Case mortality rate, %:	>99	95–99	70–95	50–70	<50
1950–1951		100	0	0	0	0
1951–1952		33	50	17	0	0
1952–1953		4	13	74	9	0
1953–1954		16	25	50	9	0
1954–1955		16	16	42	26	0
1955–1956		0	3	55	25	17
1956–1957		0	6	55	24	15
1957–1958		3	7	54	22	14
1958–1959		0	24.6	55	14.0	6.1
1963–1964		0	0.3	60	31.0	9.0

*Modified from Fenner and Ratcliffe (1965).

nent and must have been the products of many independent processes of mutation (probably in several different genes) and selection.

In the laboratory, virologists commonly use rapid serial passage as a way of enhancing the virulence of viruses. When myxomatosis spread in Australian wild rabbits, on the other hand, serial passage repeatedly resulted in the attenuation of an originally highly virulent strain of virus. In the majority of cases, natural selection for the persistence of viruses in nature operates at the level of transmission of the virus from one animal to another. The factor militating against the indefinite survival of highly virulent myxoma virus, which killed all rabbits in about 10 days (i.e., about 5 days after they became infective), was the maintenance of serial transmission during the overwintering period. Under conditions of vector scarcity, a rabbit that survived in an infectious state for 3 or 4 weeks had a much greater chance of being the source of the virus which was transmitted to another rabbit than one which lived for only 5 days after it became infectious for mosquitoes. This selective advantage was of some importance even during epidemic spread of viruses in summer; it became of major importance for overwintering. The overwintering period thus selected viruses which allowed rabbits to live for prolonged periods in an infectious condition, i.e., viruses of reduced virulence. Having survived the winter, the attenuated viruses were in competition with virulent viruses introduced by deliberate inoculation in campaigns carried out each year by rabbit control authorities. Field experiments with virulent and attenuated viruses in natural epidemics (Fenner et al., 1957) showed that although early in a summer epidemic the virulent virus could cause a high mortality, if it had been introduced extensively, and at the right time in relation to the abundance of vectors, the attenuated virus was the only one found at the end of the epidemic and the only one that survived until the next season.

In genetically unselected Australian wild rabbits virulent myxoma virus caused a generalized disease which was almost always lethal. If neither the virus nor the rabbit had changed as a result of their interaction, the result would be the local eradication of rabbits and the consequent local disappearance of the virus, since it has no other host. On a small scale, this probably happened repeatedly and in many localities. But, as just outlined, natural selection for effective transmission, especially during the winter, led to the appearance of attenuated viruses which allowed 10 per cent or more of the infected rabbits to survive, and some of them to breed, in spite of the partial sterility found in recovered male rabbits (Sobey and Turnbull, 1956; Poole, 1960). Investigations with wild rabbits captured in the field (Marshall and Douglas, 1961), and with the progeny of recovered animals mated and tested in the laboratory (Sobey, 1969), showed that exposure of each generation of rabbits to the viruses commonly present in the field (which produce 90% mortality in genetically unselected rabbits) rapidly selected for resistance. Prior infection, passive immunity, and environmental effects were excluded as major causes for this increased resistance, which must be regarded as of genetic origin, although the physiological mechanism whereby it operates is not known. In wild rabbits exposed to epidemic myxomatosis every summer, the mortality rate after standard challenge declined from 90% to 25%, and the severity of the disease fell in parallel (Marshall and Douglas, 1961). In the laboratory experiments Sobey (1969) showed that a similar response to selection was achieved with both highly virulent and moderately attenuated strains of myxoma virus, the heritability estimate being 35-40%.

INFLUENZA

There are two common members of the myxovirus group, both important human pathogens. These are influenza type A, strains of which also exist as natural parasites of birds, swine, and horses, and influenza type B, which is a specifically human parasite. The influenza virus particle consists of a tubular ribonucleoprotein internal component, the antigenic characteristics of which are stable and determine the classification of the virus as type A or type B, enclosed within a lipoprotein envelope that contains two distinct viral protein antigens, the hemagglutinin and the neuraminidase (Laver and Valentine, 1969). These antigens differ considerably in strains of influenza A isolated from different species at any particular time, and they also differ in human strains of either type A or type B influenza virus isolated at different times (Paniker, 1968). The genome of influenza virus occurs as several (six or seven) small pieces of single-stranded RNA which are probably linked via the polypeptide of the internal antigen (Pons, 1970).

Both types of influenza virus cause frequent epidemics of respiratory disease in man, and influenza type A but not type B also causes widespread pandemics at irregular intervals (during the last century, in 1889-1890, 1918-1919 and 1957-1958). The only pandemic that has occurred since the birth of virology and the first isolation of influenza virus from man (Smith et al., 1933) was the outbreak of Asian influenza in 1957-1958. The virus recovered from this outbreak was named subtype A2, by contrast to stains of the subtype A1, which circulated between 1946 and 1957, and strains of subtype A0, which circulated between 1933 and 1946. With hindsight, it appears that subtype A1 should not have been so designated, but that Asian influenza was caused by a novel virus that merited subtype classification (see below).

As human pathogens, influenza viruses multiply only in cells lining the surfaces of the upper and lower respiratory tract. This superficial infection promotes the production of secretary immunoglobulin (IgA) in the respiratory tract, as well as circulating antibodies, the former being the more significant from the point of view of protection against reinfection (Kasel et al., 1969). Experiments in eggs (Archetti and Horsfall, 1950; Laver and Webster, 1968) and mice (Hamre et al., 1958) inoculated with influenza A viruses and antibody that reacted weakly with them showed that there was a strong selection for antigenic novelty in the hemagglutinin antigens. Laver and Webster (1968) showed that the hemagglutinin antigens of some of these antigenic variants had different peptide maps from the parental virus, suggesting that variation occurred by mutation rather than by "rearrangement" of polypeptides of constant amino acid composition, as some had postulated (Francis and Maassab, 1965). It is reasonable to assume that similar selection operates in the respiratory tract of man.

If the historical epidemiology of influenza is examined against this virological and immunological background, the vagaries of the disease can begin to be explained. The secular change in the antigenicity of both envelope antigens of human influenza type B strains ever since the virus was first isolated in 1940, and the similar changes found with influenza A between 1933 and 1956 and again between 1957 and 1970, have been called immunological drift by Burnet (1955) on the analogy with genetic drift. "Antigenic drift" is a more appropriate term, but in fact the phenomenon does not parallel genetic drift in the classic sense, i.e., random fluctuations in gene frequencies due to sampling. As pointed out below, the secular changes in antigenicity result from immunoselection. However virologists are now accustomed to use the term drift for the changes that occur every year or so, and are beginning to use the term antigenic shift for the larger changes in the hemagglutinin antigen such as occurred in 1946-1947 (A0, A1) and 1968 (A2, Hong Kong).

The situation can be represented diagrammatically, as shown in Fig. 4. Antigenic drift occurs with both of the envelope antigens of human strains (Paniker, 1968), but not with the internal antigen, and only to a trivial extent with the hemagglutinin and neuraminidase antigens of strains of swine influenza virus isolated between 1930 and 1967 (Meier-Ewert et al., 1970). Different isolates of influenza A from birds show no clear pattern of systematic antigenic drift, and avian viruses which differ considerably in their hemagglutinin antigens have been isolated from several different species of birds over the same period of time and from the same area (Pereira et al., 1967).

The presence of antigenic drift of the envelope antigens in both types of influenza virus in man, and its virtual absence in influenza A in swine and birds, can be explained by supposing that in a long-lived animal like man strains of influenza virus are always being subjected to intense natural

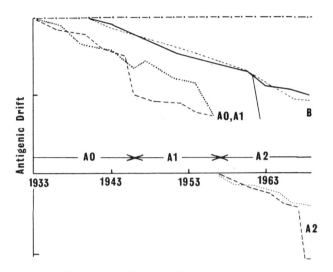

FIG. 4.—Diagram illustrating antigenic drift and the appearance of new human influenza viruses. "Antigenic drift" (ordinate) represents the serological relatedness of the antigens of influenza A virus recovered from man between 1933 and 1968 and of influenza B between 1940 and 1968. The internal (ribonucleoprotein) antigens (—·—·—) of influenza type A and type B are quite different from each other, and have not changed antigenically over the whole period. Independently of each other, both the hemagglutinin (A, - - -; B, —) and the neuraminidase (A, ····; B, - - -) have undergone changes in their antigenicity every year or so (antigenic drift). A larger change than usual in the hamagglutinin antigen of influenza A in 1946 led to the 1947 and subsequent strains being called a new subtype, A1. However, there was no parallel change in the neuraminidase in 1946. All changes from 1933 until 1957 resulted from antigenic drift among human strains of influenza A. There was a major change in the hemagglutinin of influenza B in 1962, also the result of antigenic drift, but the strain died out.

The appearance of Asian influenza virus (subtype A2) in 1957 was a major change, since both the hemagglutinin and the neuraminidase differed greatly from those of subtype A0/A1 in antigenicity and in other ways. Asian influenza was probably due to the introduction of a novel virus from an animal reservoir. Since 1957, the hemagglutinin and neuraminidase antigens of influenza A2 have themselves undergone antigenic drift. In 1968 the Hong Kong variant of A2 appeared and spread throughout the world; it differed greatly from preceding strains in the antigenicity of its hemagglutinin but not in the neuraminidase. The Hong Kong virus resulted from antigenic drift and is not a new subtype.

selection for antigenic novelty, because most individuals past infancy will have antibodies to the hemagglutinin and neuraminidase antigens of earlier strains in the secretions of their nasal and respiratory tract mucosae. This selection usually leads to the emergence of new strains each year, which differ slightly from the preexisting strain in the antigenic makeup of either or both of the envelope antigens. Their selective advantage is such that, with very few and scattered exceptions, they replace the preexisting strains. Sometimes a mutant virus is found in which a major change has occurred in one or other of the envelope antigens. This happened with influenza A in 1946-1947 and again in 1968 and with influenza B in 1962. The 1962 influenza B virus, which was recovered in Taiwan (Green et al., 1964), was not isolated elsewhere and soon disappeared in Taiwan; the 1946-1947 and 1968 influenza A isolates spread widely around the world. The 1968 Hong Kong strain caused widespread epidemics in different parts of the world in 1968, 1969, and 1970. Detailed study of this virus showed that, whereas its hemagglutinin differed greatly from that of earlier Asian (A2) strains (Dowdle et al., 1969), these differences were more like those between late A0 and early A1 serotypes than between A0-A1 antigens in general and the A2 antigens in general. The neuraminidase of Hong Kong influenza virus was almost identical, both in antigenicity and in other characteristics, with that of 1967 strains of influenza A2 (Schulman and Kilbourne, 1969). The Hong Kong virus has therefore been correctly classified as belonging to the A2 subtype.

Thus the overall picture with influenza A since its original isolation in 1933 is that there have been two subtypes. The first, called A0/A1, underwent antigenic drift with a major change in the hemagglutinin in 1946 which wrongly (on present views) led to strains recovered between 1946 and 1956 being described as subtype A1. In 1957 there was a major break, and a virus appeared and spread in pandemic fashion which differed from preexisting strains in many characters. Antigenically, both its envelope antigens showed only slight resemblances to those of A1 viruses (recovered in 1946-1956); it failed to show Burnet's O-D variation (Burnet, 1960), and the neuraminidase was much more heat-resistant than those of earlier strains. Since 1957 this new Asian (A2) virus has undergone the same sort of antigenic drift seen with the A0/A1 and B types. A larger change than usual in the antigenicity of the hemagglutinin (but not the neuraminidase) characterized the Hong Kong/1968 strain, but that virus is still a member of the A2 subtype. The fact that the Hong Kong virus, which showed a major change in the antigenicity of its hemagglutinin but none in its neuraminidase, caused widespread epidemics of human influenza, emphasizes the importance for protection of antibodies directed against the hemagglutinin and the lesser importance of those directed against the neuraminidase.

The most plausible explanation for the appearance of the A2 subtype is that it represents the adaptation to man of a virus previously circulating in some animal, most likely in swine or birds. Whether this resulted from mutation, or whether recombination played a part, is a question that cannot be answered at present. Presumably the great 1918-1919 epidemic was due to a similar event. Epidemiologists interested in influenza have noted the occurrence of antibodies to some of these "new" viruses (e.g., the 1957 A2 subtype) in very aged human beings (Mulder and Masurel, 1958). These antibodies may indicate prior circulation long ago of a virus antigenically like the "new" virus, but serological findings in aged persons who have almost invariably been subjected to repeated infections are very difficult to interpret. Serological epidemiology in influenza is inviting but deceptive; it is probably sounder to base hypotheses on the evolution of this interesting virus on studies of virus isolates than on antibody patterns occurring in human beings who have been exposed to repeated infection by constantly changing serotypes.

SUMMARY AND CONCLUSIONS

The great majority of animal viruses can be allocated to one of something under 20 groups, all members of each group having many properties in common. The differences between many of the groups are so great and of such a fundamental nature (type and arrangement of nucleic acid, mode of transcription and translation) that it is reasonable to postulate their independent evolutionary origins. Chief among the properties common to viruses of a particular group is the amount, type, base composition, and arrangement of the nucleic acid in which their genetic information is stored.

Among the deoxyriboviruses the genome is usually a single double-stranded molecule, linear in most groups but cyclic in the papovaviruses. The parvoviruses and adenovirus-associated viruses contain a single small molecule of single-standed DNA. Transcription may be due to a cellular transcriptase (demonstrably so in the papovaviruses whose DNA is infectious) or to a virus-coded enzyme which is an internal part of the virion (in poxviruses). There is some evidence that in herpesviruses the RNA molecules first transcribed in the nucleus are cleaved before they function as mRNAs in the cytoplasm, and some of the viral polypeptides of vaccinia virus undergo posttranslational cleavage.

Viruses are the only living agents whose genetic message can be encoded in RNA, a situation that gives rise to a number of interesting problems in transcription and translation which have been solved in a variety of ways, each characteristic for the group of riboviruses concerned. Data on this matter is still incomplete, but the following situations have been recognized:

(a) The genome is a single linear molecule of single-stranded RNA which is infectious and serves as the messenger RNA (picornavirus and possibly the togavirus groups). There appears to be no translational punctuation in animal cells, and this messenger RNA is translated as a giant polypeptide which is subsequently cleaved into the viral structural and nonstructural polypeptides by a process called posttranslational cleavage.

(b) The genome consists of a single large linear molecule of single-stranded RNA which is not infectious (paramyxovirus group). Complementary strands of what appear to be messenger RNA are transcribed from this in lengths shorter than the genome, but the mechanism of transcription is unknown, and there is no information about the size of the polypeptides translated from these putative mRNAs.

(c) The genome consists of several small pieces of single-stranded RNA, possibly linked together (myxovirus and rhabdovirus groups). Such genomes are not infectious. Messenger RNAs are transcribed from each piece (in the case of rhabdoviruses by a transcriptase which is part of the virion), and the viral polypeptides correspond in size to these several messenger RNAs.

(d) The genome consists of several molecules of single-stranded RNA, possibly linked in the virion. In the infected cell this is transcribed into DNA by a viral RNA-dependent DNA polymerase which is a component of the virion (leukovirus group). "Negative" strand RNA has not been found in leukovirus-infected cells; presumably the viral RNA is replicated and the messenger RNA transcribed from the DNA "provirus."

(e) The genome consists of several molecules of double-stranded RNA (reovirus group), from each of which a separate messenger RNA is transcribed by viral transcriptase which is an inner component of the virion. The viral polypeptides correspond in size with the messenger RNA molecules transcribed from the several genome fragments.

Mutation occurs in viral as in other nucleic acids; there is no evidence that viral nucleic acids are more or less mutable than those of most organisms. Increasing use is being made in virological investigations of conditional lethal (especially temperature-sensitive) mutants.

Genetic recombination occurs between deoxyriboviruses of some groups (poxvirus and probably herpesvirus) with a frequency (and probably by a mechanism) analogous to that found in the T-even bacteriophages. In cells transformed by papovaviruses the cyclic viral DNA is believed to be integrated with the cellular DNA by recombination. Recombination can occur between DNAs of viruses belonging to different groups, notably adenoviruses and papovavirus SV40.

Recombination also occurs with riboviruses of animals, although not with the ribophages. Among viral groups whose genome consists of a single linear molecule, low-frequency recombination, possibly occurring by crossing over of double-stranded replicative forms, has been recognized among the picornaviruses but not with paramyxoviruses. High frequency recombination, thought to occur by exchange or possibly addition of fragments of RNA, is found among myxoviruses, rhabdoviruses, and reoviruses, which have fragmented genomes.

Three types of gene product interaction have been recognized. Interference by the interferon mechanism involves cellular participation; other interactions occur between viral gene products. Defective viruses may complement each other in a symmetric or asymmetric manner, and some groups of viruses (e.g., adenovirus-associated viruses) only survive in nature by virtue of complementation. Viral genomes may be encapsidated or enveloped by polypeptides derived from more than one type of virus, giving rise to phenotypic mixing. Among enveloped viruses this may occur between viruses of unrelated groups, if each matures by budding through modified plasma membrane. Among nonenveloped viruses there may be completely heterologous capsidation (transcapsidation), a process by which the entire genome of one virus is enclosed within the capsid of another.

The production of disease by animal viruses involves the response of the host at cellular, organ, and organismal levels, and the host response is conditioned by both genetic and environmental factors. The susceptibility of cell and animal to infection with some viruses depends on the presence of the appropriate receptor material on the plasma membrane. Susceptibility is then dependent upon a single autosomal gene, and susceptibility (presence of receptor) is dominant to resistance. The receptor may be needed to allow the virions to attach (picornaviruses) or to penetrate (leukoviruses).

Macrophages play an important barrier function in the pathogenesis of many viral infections. In infections of certain strains of mice with togaviruses and a coronavirus, cellular and organismal susceptibility is governed by the ability of macrophages to support viral replication, the block in insusceptible macrophages occurring at some stage after viral penetration. Susceptibility depends upon a single autosomal gene, with resistance dominant in the case of coronavirus infections and susceptibility dominant in the togavirus infections.

In other cases resistance depends upon the host response at the organismal rather than the cellular level, i.e., cultured cells are susceptible, whether they come from susceptible or restraint strains of host, but the intact animals differ in resistance. This situation is found in mousepox and polyoma virus oncogenesis in C57B1 mice, whose resistance depends upon their powerful and precocious cell-mediated immunity response. Deficiency in cell-mediated immunity, found in many immunoglobulin deficiency states in man, is associated with lack of resistance to generalized viral infections.

The main practical importance of viral genetics, as distinct from its theoretical importance for understanding viral multiplication and viral oncogenesis, is the production of vaccines. In the past this has been an empirical process, but temperature-sensitive mutants provide a rational method for making live attenuated vaccines, and recombination can be used to tailor-make influenza virus vaccines of desired antigenic structure and growth potential.

Genetic changes in viruses have clearly been of major importance in their evolution. Continuing evolutionary change of two animal viruses, those causing myxomatosis and influenza, is described. In myxomatosis, selection for prolonged infectivity over the winter period led to the occurrence and dominance of strains less virulent than that originally introduced into European rabbits in Australia. The consequent survival of small numbers of rabbits allowed selection for genetic resistance of the rabbit to occur, the heritability of resistance being about 40%. Influenza differs from all other respiratory viruses of man in causing minor epidemics almost every year, with major pandemics at intervals of many years. Two different mechanisms are postulated for the emergence of viruses that cause seasonal epidemics or occasional pandemics respectively. The former are constantly being produced by the selection, by antibodies in the human respiratory tract, of minor antigenic mutation in the envelope proteins, occurring independently for the viral hemagglutinin and the neuraminidase. This process is called antigenic drift. The infrequent major pandemics occur only with one type of influenza virus (type A), which differs from the others in being a parasite of several types of animal besides man. Pandemics are thought to occur when a virus capable of spreading and causing significant disease in man is transferred to humans from an animal host. Such viruses differ from their immediate predecessors in many properties, including the antigenicity of both of their envelope antigens.

REFERENCES

Allison, A. C. 1965. Genetic factors in resistance to viral infections. Arch. Ges. Virusforsch. 17:280-294.

Alstein, A. D., and N. N. Dodonova. 1968. Interaction between human and simian adenoviruses in simian cells: complementation phenotypic mixing and function of monkey cell "adapted" virions. Virology 35:248-254.

Archetti, I., and F. L. Horsfall. 1950. Persistent antigenic variation of influenza A viruses after incomplete neutralization *in ovo* with heterologous immune serum. J. Exp. Med. 92:441-462.

Argyris, B. F. 1965. Maturation of immunological responsiveness to transplantation antigens. Transplantation 3:618-626.

Atchison, R. W., B. C. Casto, and W. McD. Hammon. 1965. Adeno-associated defective virus particles. Science 149:754-756.

Bader, J. P. 1966. Metabolis requirements for infection by Rous sarcoma virus. II. The participation of cellular DNA. Virology 29:452-461.

Baltimore, D. 1970. Viral RNA-dependent DNA polymerase in virions of RNA tumor viruses. Nature 226:1209-1211.

———, A. S. Huang, and M. Stampfer. 1970. Ribonucleic acid synthesis of vesicular stomatitis virus. II. An RNA polymerase in the virion. Proc. Nat. Acad. Sci. U.S.A. 66:572-576.

Baluda, M. A., and D. P. Nayak. DNA complementary to viral RNA in leukemic cells induced by avian myeloblastosis virus. Proc. Nat. Acad. Sci. USA. 66:329-336.

Bang, F. B., and A. Warwick. 1960. Mouse macrophages as host cells for the mouse hepatitis virus and the genetic basis of their susceptibility. Proc. Nat. Acad. Sci. U.S.A. 46:1965-1075.

Barry, R. D. 1961. The multiplication of influenza virus. II. Multiplicity reactivation of ultraviolet-irradiated virus. Virology 14:398-405.

Baum, S. G., P. R. Reich, C. J. Hybner, W. P. Rowe, and S. M. Weissman. 1966. Biophysical evidence for linkage of adenovirus and SV40 DNA's in adenovirus 7-SV40 hybrid particles. Proc. Nat. Acad. Sci. U.S.A. 56:1509-1515.

———, W. H. Wiese, and W. P. Rowe. 1970. Density differences between hybrid and non hybrid particles in two adenovirus-simian virus 40 hybrid populations J. Virol. 5:353-357.

Bedson, H. S., and K. R. Dumbell. 1964. Hybrids derived from the viruses of variola major and cowpox. J. Hyg. 62:147-158.

Béládi, I., I. Mucsi, M. Bakay, and R. Pusztai. 1970. Rescue of heat-inactivated adenovirus types 1 and 6 by ultraviolet-irradiated adenovirus type 8. J. Gen. Virol. 7:153-158.

Bellett, A. J. D. 1967a. Preliminary classification of viruses based on quantitative comparisons of viral nucleic acids. J. Virol. 1:245-259.

———, 1967b. The use of computer-based quantitative comparisons of viral nucleic acids in the taxonomy of viruses: a preliminary classification of some animal viruses. J. Gen. Virol. 1:583-585.

Benjamin, T. L. 1966. Virus-specific RNA in cells productively infected or transformed by polyoma virus. J. Molec. Biol. 16:359-373.

Berry, G. P., and H. M. Dedrick. 1936. A method for changing the virus of rabbit fibroma (Shope) into that of infectious myxomatosis (Sanarelli). J. Bact. 31:50-51.

Bishop, J. M., G. Koch, B. Evans, and M. Merriman. 1969. Poliovirus replicative intermediate: structural basis on infectivity. J. Molec. Biol. 46:235-249.

Blacklow, N. R., M. D. Hoggan, A. Z. Kapikian, J. B. Austin, and W. P. Rowe. 1968. Epidemiology of adenovirus-associated virus infection in a nursery population. Amer. J. Epidem. 88:368-378.

Blair, C. D., and W. S. Robinson. 1968. Replication of Sendai virus. I. Comparison of the viral RNA and virus-specific RNA synthesis with Newcastle disease virus. Virology 35:537-549.

Blanden, R. V. 1971. Mechanisms of recovery from mousepox. Ph.D. Thesis, Australian National University.

Bratt, M. A., and W. S. Robinson. 1967. Ribonucleic acid synthesis in cells infected with Newcastle disease virus. J. Molec. Biol. 23:1-21.

50 FRANK FENNER

Breeze, D. C., and H. Subak-Sharpe. 1967. The mutability of small plaque-forming encephalomyocarditis virus. J. Gen. Virol. 1:81-88.

Bruton, O. C. 1952. Agammaglobulinemia. Pediatrics 9:722-728.

Buchan, A., and D. H. Watson. 1969. The immunological specificity of thymidine kinases in cells infected by viruses of the herpes group. J. Gen. Virol. 4:461-463.

Burge, B. W., and E. R. Pfefferkorn. 1966. Complementation between temperature-sensitive mutants of Sindbis virus. Virology 30:214-223.

Burnet, F. M. 1955. Principles of Animal Virology, p. 382. Academic Press, New York.

———. 1960. Principles of Animal Virology, ed. 2, pp. 412-415. Academic Press, New York.

———, and P. E. Lind. 1949. Recombination of characters between two influenza virus strains. Aust. J. Sci. 12:109-110.

———, and ———. 1951. A genetic approach to variation in influenza viruses. 4. Recombination of characters between the influenza virus A strain NWS and strains of different serological subtypes. J. Gen. Microbiol. 5:67-82.

———, and ———. 1953. Influenza virus recombination: Experiments using the de-embryonated egg technique. Cold Spring Harbor Sympos. Quant. Biol. 18:21-24.

Burrell, C. J., E. M. Martin, and P. D. Cooper. 1970. Post-translational cleavage of virus polypeptides in arbovirus-infected cells. J. Gen. Virol. 6:319-324.

Carp, R. I. 1963. A study of the mutation rates of several poliovirus strains to the reproductive capacity temperature/40+ and guanidine marker characteristics. Virology 21:373-382.

Chanock, R. M. 1970. Control of acute mycoplasmal and viral respiratory tract disease. Science 169:248-256.

Choppin, P. W., and R. W. Compans. 1970. Phenotypic mixing of envelope proteins of the parainfluenza virus SV5 and vesicular stomatitis virus. J. Virol. 5:609-616.

Cinader, B., S. Dubiski, and A. C. Wardlow. 1964. Distribution, inheritance and properties of an antigen, MUB1, and its relation to hemolytic complement. J. Exp. Med. 120:897-924.

Compans, R. W., N. J. Dimmock, and H. Meier-Ewert. 1969. Effect of antibody to neuraminidase on the maturation and hemagglutinating activity of an influenza A2 virus. J. Virol. 4:528-534.

Cooper, P. D. 1965. Rescue of one phenotype in mixed infections with heat-defective mutants of type 1 poliovirus. Virology 25:431-438.

———. 1968. A genetic map of poliovirus temperature-sensitive mutants. Virology 25:584-596.

———. 1969. The genetic analysis of poliovirus. In Levy, H. B. (Ed.), The Biochemistry of Viruses, pp. 177-218. Marcel Dekker, New York.

———. 1970. Personal communication.

———, D. F. Summers, and J. V. Maizel. 1970. Evidence for ambiguity in the post-translational cleavage of poliovirus proteins. Virology 41:408-418.

Cords, C. E., and J. J. Holland. 1964a. Alteration of the species and tissue susceptibility of poliovirus by enclosure of its RNA within the protein capsid of Coxsackie B1 virus. Virology 24:492-495.

———, and ———. 1964b. Replication of poliovirus RNA induced by heterologous virus. Proc. Nat. Acad. Sci. U.S.A. 51:1080-1082.

Crittenden, L. B. 1968. Observations on the nature of a genetic cellular resistance to avian tumor viruses. J. Nat. Cancer Inst. 41:145-153.

———, H. A. Stone, R. H. Reamer, and W. Okazaki. 1967. Two loci controlling genetic cellular resistance to avian leukosis-sarcoma viruses. J. Virol. 1:898-904.

Dahlberg, J. E., and E. H. Simon. 1968. Complementation in Newcastle disease virus. Bact. Proc., p. 162.

———, and ———. 1969. Recombination in Newcastle disease virus (NDV): the problem of complementary heterozygotes. Virology 38:490-493.

Dawe, C. J. 1965. Quoted by Law et al. (1966).

Di Mayorca, G., J. Callendar, G. Marin, and R. Giordano. 1969. Temperature-sensitive mutants of polyoma virus. Virology 38:126-133.

Dowdle, W. R., M. T. Coleman, E. C. Hall, and V. Kuez. 1969. Properties of the Hong Kong influenza virus 2. Antigenic relationship of the Hong Kong virus hemagglutinin to that of other human influenza viruses. Bull. WHO 41:419-424.

Duesberg, P. H., and W. S. Robinson. 1967. On the structure and replication of influenza virus. J. Molec. Biol. 25:383-405.

Duff, R. G., and P. K. Vogt. 1969. Characteristics of two new avian tumor virus subgroups. Virology 39:18-30.

Dulbecco, R., and M. Vogt. 1958. Study of the mutability of d lines of polioviruses. Virology 5:220-235.

———, and ———. 1963. Evidence for a ring structure for polyoma virus DNA. Proc. Nat. Acad. Sci. U.S.A. 50:236-243.

Easterday, B. C., W. G. Laver, H. G. Pereira, and G. C. Schill. 1969. Antigenic composition of recombinant virus strains produced from human and avian influenza A viruses. J. Gen. Virol. 5:83-91.

Eckhart, W. 1969. Complementation and transformation by temperature-sensitive mutants of polyoma virus. Virology 38:120-125.

Ellman, L., I. Green, W. J. Martin, and B. Berracerraf. 1970. Linkage between the poly-L-lysine gene and the locus controlling the major histocompatibility antigens in strain 2 guinea pigs. Proc. Nat. Acad. Sci. U.S.A. 66:322-328.

Enders, J. F., T. H. Weller, and F. C. Robbins. 1949. Cultivation of the Lansing strain of poliomyelitis virus in cultures of various embryonic tissues. Science 109:85-87.

Fenner, F. 1959. Genetic studies with mammalian poxviruses. II. Recombination between two strains of vaccinia virus in single HeLa cells. Virology 8:499-507.

———. 1968a. The Biology of Animal Viruses, Vol. I, Molecular and Cellular Biology, pp. 1-33. Academic Press, New York.

———. 1968b. The Biology of Animal Viruses, Vol. II, The Pathogenesis and Ecology of Viral Infections, pp. 615-639. Academic Press, New York.

———. 1968c. The Biology of Animal Viruses, Vol. I, Molecular and Cellular Biology, pp. 354-360, 379-400. Academic Press, New York.

———. 1968d. The Biology of Animal Viruses, Volume II, The Pathogenesis and Ecology of Viral Infections, pp. 556-559. Academic Press, New York.

———. 1969. Conditional lethal mutants of animal viruses. Curr. Top. Microbiol. Immun. 48:1-28.

———. 1970. The genetics of animal viruses. Ann. Rev. Microbiol. 24:

———, and B. M. Comben. 1958. Genetic studies with mammalian poxviruses. I. Demonstration of recombination between two strains of vaccinia virus. Virology 5:530-548.

———, and I. D. Marshall. 1957. A comparison of the virulence for European rabbits *(Oryctolagus cuniculus)* of strains of myxoma virus recovered in the field in Australia, Europe and America. J. Hyg. 55:149-191.

———, and F. N. Ratcliffe. 1965. Myxomatosis. Cambridge University Press, London, 371 pp.

———, and J. F. Sambrook. 1966. Conditional lethal mutants of rabbitpox virus. II. Mutants (p) which fail to multiply in PK-2a cells. Virology 23:600-609.

———, and G. M. Woodroofe. 1960. The reactivation of poxviruses. II. The range of reactivating viruses. Virology 11:185-201.

———, and G. M. Woodroofe. 1965. Changes in the virulence and antigenic structure of strains of myxoma virus recovered from Australian wild rabbits between 1950 and 1964. Aust. J. Exp. Biol. Med. Sci. 43:359-370.

———, I. H. Holmes, W. K. Joklik, and G. M. Woodroofe. 1959. Reactivation of heat-inactivated poxviruses: a general phenomenon which includes the fibroma-myxoma virus transformation of Berry and Dedrick. Nature 183:1340-1341.

———, W. E. Poole, I. D. Marshall, and A. L. Dyce. 1957. Studies in the epidemiology of infectious myxomatosis of rabbits. VI. The experimental introduction of the European strain of myxoma virus into Australian wild rabbit populations. J. Hyg. 55:192-206.

Fields, D. N., and W. K. Joklik. 1969. Isolation and preliminary genetic and biochemical characterization of temperature-sensitive mutants of reovirus. Virology 37:335-342.

Francis, T., and H. F. Maassab. 1965. Influenza viruses. In Horsfall, F. L., and I. Tamm (Eds.), Viral and Rickettsial Infections of Man, pp. 689-740. J. B. Lippincott, Philadelphia.

Fraser, K. B. 1967. Immunofluorescence of abortive and complete infections by influenza A virus in hamster BHK21 cells and mouse L cells. J. Gen. Virol. 1:1-12.

Fujinaga, K., and M. Green. 1966. The mechanism of viral carcinogenesis of DNA mammalian viruses: viral-specific RNA in polyribosomes of adenovirus tumor and transformed cells. Proc. Nat. Acad. Sci. U.S. 55:1567-1574.

Fulginiti, V. A., W. E. Hathaway, D. S. Pearlman, W. R. Blackburn, C. W. Reigman, J. H. Githeus, H. N. Claman, and C. H. Kempe. 1966. Dissociation of delayed hypersensitivity and antibody-synthesizing capacities in man. Lancet 2:5-8.

———, C. H. Kempe, W. E. Hathaway, D. S. Pearlman, O. F. Sieber, J. J. Eller, J. J. Joyner, and A. Robinson. 1968. Progressive vaccinia in immunologically deficient individuals. In Good, R. A., and D. Gergsma (Eds.), Immunological Deficiency Diseases in Man: Birth Defects, Original Article Series, Vol. 4, No. 1, pp. 129-145. National Foundation, New York.

Gallily, R., A. Warwick, and F. B. Bang. 1964. Effect of cortisone on genetic resistance to mouse hepatitis virus in vivo and in vitro. Proc. Nat. Acad. Sci. U.S.A. 51:1158-1164.

Garen, A. 1968. Sense and nonsense in the genetic code. Science 160:149-159.

Gasser, D. L. 1969. Genetic control of the immune response in mice. I. Segregation data and localization to the fifth linkage group of a gene affecting antibody production. J. Immun. 103:66-70.

Gemmell, A., and F. Fenner. 1960. Genetic studies with mammalian poxviruses. III. White (u) mutants of rabbitpox virus. Virology 11:219-235.

Goodman, G. T., and H. Koprowski. 1962. Study of the mechanism of innate resistance to viral infection. J. Cell. Comp. Physiol. 59:333-373.

Granoff, A. 1962. Heterozygosis and phenotypic mixing with Newcastle disease virus. Cold Spring Harbor Sympos. Quant. Biol. 27:319-326.

———, and G. K. Hirst. 1954. Experimental production of combination forms of virus. IV. Mixed influenza A–Newcastle disease virus infections. Proc. Soc. Exp. Biol. Med. 86:84-88.

———, P. E. Came, and D. C. Breeze. 1966. Viruses and renal carcinoma of *Rana pipiens*. I. The isolation and properties of virus from normal and tumor tissue. Virology 29:133-148.

Green, I. J., S. C. Hung, P. S. Hu, G. W. Lee, and H. G. Pereira. 1964. The isolation and characterization of a new influenza type B virus on Taiwan. Amer. J. Hyg. 79:107-112.

Habel, K. 1965. Specific complement-fixing antigens in polyoma tumors and transformed cells. Virology 25:55-61.

Hamre, D., C. G. Loosli, and P. Gerber. 1958. Antigenic variants of influenza A (PR8 strain). IV. Serological characteristics of a second line of variants developed in mice given polyvalent vaccine. J. Exp. Med. 107:845-855.

Hanafusa, H., and T. Hanafusa. 1966. Determining factor in the capacity of Rous sarcoma virus to induce tumors in mammals. Proc. Nat. Acad. Sci. U.S.A. 55:532-538.

———, ———, and H. Rubin. 1963. The defectiveness of Rous sarcoma virus. Proc. Nat. Acad. Sci. U.S.A. 49:572-580.

———, ———, and ———. 1964. Analysis of the defectiveness of Rous sarcoma virus. II. Specification of RSV antigenicity by helper virus. Proc. Nat. Acad. Sci. U.S.A. 51:41-48.

———, T. Miyamoto, and T. Hanafusa. 1970. A cell-associated factor essential for formation of an infectious form of Rous sarcoma virus. Proc. Nat. Acad. Sci. U.S.A. 66:314-321.

Hanson, B. H., H. Koprowski, S. Baron, and C. E. Buckler. 1969. Interferon-mediated natural resistance of mice to arbo B virus infection. Microbios IB:51-58.

Hanson, L. 1968. Aspects of the absence of the IgA system. In Good, R. A., and D. Bergsma (Eds.), Immunological Deficiency Diseases in Man: Birth Defects, Original Article Series, Vol. 4, No. 1, pp. 2092-2097. National Foundation, New York.

Heremans, J. F., and P. A. Crabbé. 1968. IgA deficiency: general considerations and relation to human diseases. In Good, R. A., and D. Bergsma (Eds.), Immunological Deficiency Diseases in Man: Birth Defects, Original Article Series, Vol. 4, No. 1., pp. 298-307. National Foundation, New York.

Hirst, G. K. 1962. Genetic recombination with Newcastle disease virus, polioviruses and influenza. Cold Spring Harbor Sympos. Quant. Biol. 27:303-308.

Hložánek, I., I. Sovova, J. Říman, and L. Vepřek. 1970. Infection of chick embryo fibroblasts with template active RNA from avian myeloblastosis virus. J. Gen. Virol. 6:163-168.

Hoggan, M. D., A. J. Shatkin, N. R. Blacklow, F. Koczot, and J. A. Rose. 1968. Helper-dependent infectious deoxyribonucleic acid from adenovirus-associated virus. J. Virol. 2:850-851.

Holland, J. J., and C. E. Cords. 1964. Maturation of poliovirus RNA with capsid protein coded by heterologous enteroviruses. Proc. Nat. Acad. Sci. U.S.A. 51:1082-1085.

———, and E. D. Kiehn. 1968. Specific cleavage of viral proteins as steps in the

54   FRANK FENNER

synthesis and maturation of enteroviruses. Proc. Nat. Acad. Sci. U.S.A.
60:1015-1022.
————, L. C. McLaren, and J. T. Syverton. 1959. The mammalian cell virus relationship. IV. Infection of naturally insusceptible cells with enterovirus ribonucleic acid. J. Exp. Med. 110:65-80.
Hosaka, Y., H. Kitano, and S. Ikeguchi. 1966. Studies on the pleomorphism of HVJ
virions. Virology 29:205-221.
Huang, A. S., D. Baltimore, and M. Stampfer. 1970. Ribonucleic acid synthesis of
vesicular stomatitis virus. III. Multiple complementary messenger RNA molecules. Virology 42:946-957.
Huebner, R. J., and G. J. Todaro. 1969. Oncogenes of RNA tumor viruses as determinants of cancer. Proc. Nat. Acad. Sci. U.S.A. 64:1087-1094.
Huebner, R. J., J. W. Hartley, W. P. Rowe, W. T. Lane, and W. J. Capps. 1966.
Rescue of the defective genome of Moloney sarcoma virus from a noninfectious
hamster tumor and the production of pseudotype sarcoma viruses with various
murine leukemia viruses. Proc. Nat. Acad. Sci. U.S.A. 56:1164-1169.
Ichihashi, Y., and S. Matsumoto. 1968. The relationship between poxvirus and A-
type inclusion body during double infection. Virology 36:262-270.
Jacobson, M. F., and D. Baltimore. 1968. Polypeptide cleavages in the formation of
poliovirus proteins. Proc. Nat. Acad. Sci. U.S.A. 61:77-84.
————, J. Asso, and D. Baltimore. 1970. Further evidence on the formation of po-
liovirus proteins. J. Molec. Biol. 49:657-669.
Jahkola, M. 1965. Inheritance of resistance to polyoma tumorigenesis in inbred mice.
J. Nat. Cancer Inst. 35:595-601.
Joklik, W. K. 1964. The intracellular uncoating of poxvirus DNA. II. The molecular
basis of the uncoating process. J. Molec. Biol. 8:277-288.
Kantoch, M., A. Warwick, and F. B. Bang. 1963. The cellular nature of genetic sus-
ceptibility to a virus. J. Exp. Med. 117:781-798.
Kasel, J. A., R. D. Rossen, R. V. Falk, M. D. Fedson, M. D. Couch, and P. Brown.
1969. Human influenza: aspects of the immune response to vaccination. Ann.
Intern. Med. 71:369-398.
Kates, J. R., and B. R. McAuslan. 1967. Poxvirus DNA-dependent RNA polymer-
ase. Proc. Nat. Acad. Sci. U.S.A. 58:134-141.
Katz, E., and B. Moss. 1970. Formation of a vaccinia virus structural polypeptide
from a higher molecular weight precursor: inhibition by rifampicin. Proc. Nat.
Acad. Sci. U.S.A. 66:677-684.
Kiehn, E. D., and J. J. Holland. 1970. Synthesis and cleavage of enterovirus poly-
peptides in mammalian cells. J. Virol. 5:358-367.
Kilbourne, E. D. 1963. Influenza virus genetics. Progr. Med. Virol. 5:79-126.
————. 1968. Recombination of influenza viruses of human and animal origin. Sci-
ence 160:74-76.
Kilbourne, E. D. 1969. Future influenza vaccines and the use of genetic recombi-
nants. Bull. WHO 41:643-645.
Kirvaitis, J., and E. G. Simon. 1965. A radiobiological study of the development of
Newcastle disease virus. Virology 26:545-553.
Landsteiner, K., and E. Popper. 1909. Uebertragung der Poliomyelitis acuta auf
Affen. Z. Immunitätsforsch., Orig. 2:377-390.
Laver, W. G., and E. D. Kilbourne. 1966. Identification in a recombinant influenza
virus of structural proteins derived from both parents. Virology 30:493-501.

————, and R. G. Webster. 1968. Selection of antigenic mutants of influenza viruses. Isolation and peptide mapping of their hemagglutinating proteins. Virology 34:193-202.

————, and R. C. Valentine. 1969. Morphology of the isolated hemagglutinin and neuraminidase subunits of influenza virus. Virology 38:105-119.

Law, L. W., and R. C. Ting. 1965. Immunologic competence and induction of neoplasms by polyoma virus. Proc. Soc. Exp. Biol. Med. 119:823-830.

————, ————, and E. Leckband. 1966. The function of the thymus in tumour production of polyoma virus. Ciba Found. Sympos., Thymus: Experimental Clinical Studies, pp. 214-241.

Ledinko, N. 1963. Genetic recombination with poliovirus type 1. Studies of crosses between a normal horse serum-resistant mutant and several guanidine-resistant mutants of the same strain. Virology 20:107-119.

————, and G. K. Hirst. 1961. Mixed infection of cells with polioviruses types 1 and 2. Virology 14:207-219.

————, S. Hopkins, and H. Toolan. 1969. Relationship between potentiation of H-1 growth by human adenovirus 12 and inhibition of the "helper" adenovirus by H-1. J. Gen. Virol. 5:19-31.

Mackenzie, J. S. 1968. Genetic studies with influenza virus. Ph.D. Thesis, Australian National University.

————. 1969. Virulence of temperature-sensitive mutants of influenza virus. Brit. Med. J. 3:757-758.

————. 1970. Isolation of temperature-sensitive mutants and the construction of a preliminary genetic map for influenza virus. J. Gen. Virol. 6:63-75.

Marin, G., and J. W. Littlefield. 1968. Selection of morphologically normal cell lines from polyoma-transformed BHK21/13 hamster fibroblasts. J. Virol. 2:69-77.

Marshall, I. D., and G. W. Douglas. 1961. Studies in the epidemiology of infectious myxomatosis of rabbits. VIII. Further observations on changes in the innate resistance of Australian wild rabbits exposed to myxomatosis. J. Hyg. 59:117-122.

McAuslan, B. R. 1969. The biochemistry of poxvirus replication. In Levy, H. B. (Ed.), The Biochemistry of Viruses, pp. 361-413. Marcel Dekker, New York.

McBride, W. D. 1962. Cold Spring Harbor Sympos. Quant. Biol. 27:309.

McClain, M. E. 1965. The host range and plaque morphology of rabbitpox virus (RPu+) and its u mutants on chick fibroblast, PK-2a and L929 cells. Aust. J. Exp. Biol. Med. Sco. 43:31-34.

McClain, M. E., and R. M. Greenland. 1965. Recombination between rabbitpox virus mutants in permissive and non-permissive cells. Virology 25:516-522.

————, and R. S. Spendlove. 1966. Multiplicity reactivation of reovirus particles after exposure to ultraviolet light. J. Bact. 92:1422-1429.

McDevitt, H. O., and A. Chinitz. 1969. Genetic control of the antibody response: relationship between immune response and histocompatibility (H-2) typel Science 163:1207-1208.

McDonald, J., and A. J. Zuckerman. 1962. ABO blood groups and acute respiratory virus disease. Brit. Med. J. 2:89-90.

McLaren, L. C., J. J. Holland, and J. T. Syverton. 1959. The mammalian cell-virus relationship. I. Attachment of poliovirus to cultivated cells of primate and non-primate origin. J. Exp. Med. 109:475-485.

Meier, H., D. D. Myers, and R. J. Huebner, 1969. Genetic control by the hr-locus of susceptibility and resistance to leukemia. Proc. Nat. Acad. Sci. U.S.A. 63:759-766.

Meier-Ewert, H., A. J. Gibbs, and N. J. Dimmock. 1970. Studies on antigenic variations of the haemagglutinin and neuraminidase of swine influenza virus isolates. J. Gen. Virol. 6:409-419.

Mills, J., J. Van Kirk, D. A. Hill, and R. M. Chanock. 1969. Evaluation of influenza virus mutants for possible use in a live virus vaccine. Bull. WHO 41:599-606.

Millward, S., and A. F. Graham. 1970. Structural studies on reovirus: discontinuities in the genome. Proc. Nat. Acad. Sci. U.S.A. 65:422-429.

Mims, C. A. 1960. An analysis of the toxicity for mice of influenza virus. II. Intravenous toxicity. Brit. J. Exp. Pathol. 41:593-598.

———. 1964. Aspects of the pathogenesis of virus diseases. Bact. Rev. 28:30-71.

Mulder, J., and N. Masurel. 1958. Pre-epidemic antibody against 1957 strain of Asiatic influenza in serum of older people living in the Netherlands. Lancet 1:810-814.

Muschel, L. H. 1966. Bloodgroups, disease and selection. Bact. Rev. 30:427-441.

Naegele, R. F., and F. Rapp. 1967. Enhancement of the replication of human adenoviruses in simian cells by simian adenovirus SV15. J. Virol. 1:838-840.

Padgett, B. L. and J. K. N. Tomkins. 1968. Conditional lethal mutants of rabbitpox virus. III. Temperature-sensitive (ts) mutants; physiological properties, complementation and recombination. Virology 36:161-167.

Paniker, C. J. K. 1968. Serological relationships between the neuraminidases of influenza viruses. J. Gen. Virol. 2:385-394.

Payne, L. N., and P. M. Biggs. 1966. Genetic basis of cellular susceptibility to the Schmidt-Ruppin and Harris strains of Rous sarcoma virus. Virology 29:190-198.

———, and ———. 1970. Genetic resistance of fowl to MHZ reticuloendothelioma virus. J. Gen. Virol. 7:177-185.

Pereira, H. G., A. Rinaldi, and L. Nardelli. 1967. Antigenic variation among avian influenza A virus. Bull. WHO 37:553-558.

Pfefferkorn, E. R., and B. W. Burge. 1968. Morphogenetic defects in the growth of ts mutants of Sindbis virus. Perspect. Virol. 6:1-14.

Piraino, F. 1967. The mechanism of genetic resistance of chick embryo cells to infection by Rous sarcoma virus: Bryan strain (BS-RSV). Virology 32:700-707.

Pons, M. W. 1970. On the nature of the influenza virus genome. Curr. Top. Microbiol. Immun. 52:142-157.

———, and G. K. Hirst. 1969. The single- and double-stranded RNA's and the proteins of incomplete influenza virus. Virology 38:68-72.

Poole, W. E. 1960. Breeding of the wild rabbit, Oryctolagus cuniculus (L.), in relation to the environment. CSIRO Wildlife Res. 5:21-43.

Pringle, C. R. 1968. Recombination between conditional lethal mutants within a strain of foot-and-mouth disease virus. J. Gen. Virol. 2:199-202.

———. 1970. Genetic characteristics of conditional lethal mutants of vesicular stomatitis virus induced by 5-fluorouracil, 5-azaytidine, and ethyl methane sulfonate. J. Virol. 5:559-567.

Rapp, F. 1969. Defective DNA animal viruses. Ann. Rev. Microbiol. 23:293-316.

———, and M. Jerkofsky. 1967. Replication of PARA (defective SV40) adenoviruses in simian cells. J. Gen. Virol. 1:311-321.

———, and J. L. Melnick. 1966. Papovavirus SV40, adenoviruses and their "hybrids": transformation, complementation, and transcapsidation. Progr. Med. Virol. 8:349-399.

Rapp, F., L. A. Feldman, and M. Mandel. 1966. Synthesis of virus deoxyribonucleic acid during abortive infection of simian cells by human adenoviruses. J. Bact. 92:931-936.

Rechler, M. M., and R. G. Martin. 1970. The intercistronic divide: translation of an intercistronic region in the histidine operon of Salmonella typhimurium. Nature 226:908-911.

Říman, J., M. Trávníček, and L. Vepřek. 1967. Template-active RNA isolated from an oncogenic virus. Biochim. Biophys. Acta 138:204-207.

Robinson, W. S. 1967. Tumor virus RNA and the problem of its synthesis. In Colter, J. S., and W. Paranchych (Eds.), The Molecular Biology of Viruses, pp. 681-696. Academic Press, New York.

Roizman, B. 1969. The herpesviruses—a biochemical definition of the group. Curr. Top. Microbiol. Immun. 49:1-79.

Rott, R., and C. Scholtissek. 1963. Investigations about the formation of incomplete forms of fowl plague virus. J. Gen. Microbiol. 33:303-312.

Rowe, W. P. 1961. The epidemiology of mouse polyoma virus infection. Bact. Rev. 25:18-31.

Rubin, H. 1965. Genetic control of cellular susceptibility to pseudotypes of Rous sarcoma virus. Virology 26:270-276.

Sabin, A. B. 1954. Genetic factors affecting susceptibility and resistance to virus diseases of the nervous system. Ass. Res. Nerv. Ment. Dis. Proc. 33:57-66.

———. 1955. Characteristics and genetic potentialities of experimentally produced and naturally occurring variants of poliomyelitis virus. Ann. N.Y. Acad. Sci. 61:924-938.

Sambrook, J. F., B. L. Padgett, and J. K. N. Tomkins. 1966. Conditional lethal mutants of rabbitpox virus. I. Isolation of host cell-dependent and temperature-dependent mutants. Virology 28:592-599.

———, H. Westphal, P. R. Srinivasan, and R. Dulbecco. 1968. The integrated state of viral DNA in SV40-transformed cells. Proc. Nat. Acad. Sci. U.S.A. 60:1288-1295.

Schäfer, W., and R. Rott. 1962. Herstellung von Virusvaccinen mit Hydroxylamin: Verlauf der Inaktivierung und Wirkung des Hydroxylamins auf verschiedene biologische Eigenschaften einiger Viren. Z. Hyg. Infektionskrankh. 148:256-268.

Schell, K. 1960a. Studies on the innate resistance to mice to infection with mousepox. I. Resistance and antibody production. Aust. J. Exp. Biol. Med. Sci. 38:271-288.

Schell, K. 1960b. Studies on the innate resistance of mice to infection with mousepox. II. Route of inoculation and resistance; and some observations on the inheritance of resistance. Aust. J. Exp. Biol. Med. Sci. 38:289-300.

Scholtissek, C. 1969. Synthesis in vitro of RNA complementary to parental RNA by RNA polymerase induced by influenza virus. Biochim. Biophys. Acta 179:389-397.

———, and R. Rott. 1969. Hybridization studies with influenza virus RNA. Virology 39:400-407.

———, and ———. 1970. Synthesis in vivo of influenza virus plus and minus strand RNA and its preferential inhibition by antibiotics. Virology 40:989-996.

Schulman, J. L. and E. D. Kilbourne. 1969. Independent variation in nature of hemagglutinin and neuraminidase antigens of influenca virus; distinctiveness of hemagglutinin antigen of Hong Kong/68 virus. Proc. Nat. Acad. Sci. U.S.A. 63:326-333.

————, M. Khakpour, and E. D. Kilbourne. 1968. Protective effects of specific immunity to viral neuraminidase on influenza virus infection of mice. J. Virol. 2:778-786.

Scott, J. R., and N. D. Zinder. 1967. Heterozygotes of phage f1. In Colter, J. S., and W. Paranchych (Eds.), The Molecular Biology of Viruses, pp. 211-218. Academic Press, New York.

Seligmann, M., H. H. Fudenberg, and R. A. Good. 1968. A proposed classification of primary immunologic deficiencies. Amer. J. Med. 45:817-825.

Sharp, D. G. 1968. Multiplicity reactivation of animal viruses. Progr. Med. Virol. 10:64-109.

Shatkin, A. J., and J. D. Sipe. 1968. RNA polymerase activity in purified reoviruses. Proc. Nat. Acad. Sci. U.S.A. 61:1462-1469.

————, ————, and P. C. Loh. 1968. Separation of ten reovirus genome segments by polyacrylamide gel electrophoresis. J. Virol. 2:986-991.

Shif, I., and F. B. Bang. 1970a. In vitro interaction of mouse hepatitis virus and macrophages from genetically resistant mice. I. Adsorption of virus and growth curves. J. Exp. Med. 131:843-850.

————, and ————. 1970b. In vitro interaction of mouse hepatitis virus and macrophages from genetically resistant mice. II. Biological characterization of a variant virus MHV (C3H) isolated from stocks of MHV (PRI). J. Exp. Med. 131:851-862.

Simpson, R. E., and G. K. Hirst. 1968. Temperature-sensitive mutants of influenza A virus: isolation of mutants and preliminary observations on genetic recombination and complementation. Virology 35:41-49.

Sjögren, H. O. 1965. Transplantation methods as a tool for detection of tumor-specific antigens. Progr. Exp. Tumor Res. 6:289-322.

Skehel, J. J., and W. K. Joklik. 1969. Studies on the in vitro transcription of reovirus RNA catalysed by reovirus cores. Virology 39:822-831.

Smith, K. O., and W. D. Gehle. 1967. Replication of an adeno-associated virus in canine and human cells with infectious canine hepatitis virus as a "helper." J. Virol. 1:648-649.

Smith, R. E., J. J. Zweerink, and W. K. Joklik. 1969. Polypeptide components of virions, top component, and cores of reovirus type 3. Virology 39:791-810.

Smith, W., C. H. Andrewes, and P. O. Laidlaw. 1933. A virus obtained from influenza patients. Lancet 2:66-68.

Sobey, W. R. 1969. Selection for resistance to myxomatosis in domestic rabbits (Oryctolagus cuniculus). J. Hyg. 67:743-754.

————, and K. Turnbull. 1956. Fertility in rabbits recovering from myxomatosis. Aust. J. Biol. Sci. 9:455-461.

Steitz, J. A. 1969. Polypeptide chain initiation: nucleotide sequences of the three ribosomal binding sites in bacteriophage R17 RNA. Nature 224:957-964.

Subak-Sharpe, H., W. M. Shepherd, and J. Hay. 1966. Studies on sRNA coded by herpes virus. Cold Spring Harbor Sympos. Quant. Biol. 31:583-594.

Sugiura, A., and E. D. Kilbourne. 1966. Genetic studies of influenza viruses. III. Production of plaque type recombinants with A0 and A1 strains. Virology 29:84-91.

Summers, D. F., and J. V. Maizel. 1968. Evidence for large precursor proteins in poliovirus synthesis. Proc. Nat. Acad. Sci. U.S.A. 59:966-971.

Summers, D. F., J. V. Maizel, and J. E. Darnell. 1965. Evidence for virus-specific noncapsid proteins in poliovirus-infected HeLa cells. Proc. Nat. Acad. Sci. U.S.A. 54:505-513.

Takemori, N., J. L. Riggs, and C. D. Aldrich. 1969. Genetic studies with tumorigenic adenoviruses. II. Heterogeneity of *cyt* mutants of adenovirus type 12. Virology 38:8-15.

Tan, K. B., J. F. Sambrook, and A. J. D. Bellett. 1969. Semliki Forest virus temperature-sensitive mutants: isolation and characterization. Virology 38:427-439.

Temin, H. M. 1961. Mixed infection with two types of Rous sarcoma virus. Virology 38:8-15.

————. 1964a. The participation of DNA in Rous sarcoma virus production. Virology 23:486-494.

————. 1964b. The nature of the provirus of Rous sarcoma. Proc. Nat. Acad. Sci. U.S.A. 52:323-329.

————, and S. Mizutani. 1970. RNA-dependent DNA polymerase in virions of Rous sarcoma virus. Nature 226:1211-1213.

Todaro, G. J. 1968. Variable susceptibility of human cell strains to SV40 transformation. Nat. Cancer Inst. Monogr. 29:271-273.

Toyoshima, K., and P. K. Vogt. 1969. Temperature sensitive mutants of avian sarcoma virus. Virology 39:930-931.

Vainio, T. 1963. Virus and hereditary resistance *in vitro*. I. Behaviour of West Nile (E-101) virus in the cultures prepared from genetically resistant and susceptible strains of mice. Ann. Med. Exp. Fenn. 41 Suppl. 1:1-24.

————, R. Gwatkin, and H. Koprowski. 1961. Production of interferon by brains of genetically resistant and susceptible mice infected with West Nile virus. Virology 14:385-387.

Vogel, F. H., J. Pettenkofer, and W. Helmbold. 1960. Über die Populationsgenetik der ABO Blutgruppen. 2. Mitteilung. Genhäufigkeit und epidemische Erkrankungen. Acta Genet. Statist. Med. 10:267-294.

Vogt, M., and R. Dulbecco. 1962. Studies on cells rendered neoplastic by polyoma virus: the problem of the presence of virus-related materials. Virology 16:41-51.

Vogt, P. K. 1967. Phenotypic mixing in the avian tumor virus group. Virology 32:708-717.

————, and R. Ishizaki. 1965. Reciprocal pattern of genetic resistance to avian tumor viruses in two lines of chicken. Virology 26:664-672.

————, C. Moscovici, and R. Duff. 1969. Host resistance and the biological analysis of avian tumor virus infections. Canad. Cancer Conf. 8:286-312.

Wagner, E. K., and B. Roizman. 1969. RNA synthesis in cells infected with herpes simplex virus. II. Evidence that a class of viral mRNA is derived from high molecular weight precursor synthesized in the nucleus. Proc. Nat. Acad. Sci. U.S.A. 64:626-633.

Warner, J., M. J. Madden, and J. E. Darnell. 1963. The interaction of poliovirus RNA with *Escherichia coli* ribosomes. Virology 19:393-399.

Webster, R. G. 1970. Personal communication.

Weiss, M. C., B. Ephrussi, and L. J. Scaletta. 1968. Loss of T-antigen from somatic hybrids between mouse cells and SV40-transformed human cells. Proc. Nat. Acad. Sci. U.S.A. 59:1132-1135.

West, C. D., R. Hong, and N. H. Holland. 1962. Immunoglobulin levels from the newborn period to adulthood and in immunoglobulin deficiency states. J. Clin. Invest. 41:2054-2064.

Westphal, H., and R. Dulbecco. 1968. Viral DNA in polyoma- and SV40-transformed cell lines. Proc. Nat. Acad. Sci. U.S.A. 59:1158-1165.

Wildy, P. 1955. Recombination with herpes simplex virus. J. Gen. Microbiol. 13:346-360.

Woodroofe, G. M., and F. Fenner. 1960. Genetic studies with mammalian poxviruses. IV. Hybridization between several different poxviruses. Virology 12:272-282.

Zinder, N. D., D. L. Englehardt, and R. E. Webster. 1966. Punctuation in the genetic code. Cold Spring Harbor Sympos. Quant. Biol. 31:251-256.

Zweerink, H. J., and W. K. Joklik. 1970. Studies on the intracellular synthesis of reovirus-specified proteins. Virology 41:501-518.

CHAPTER 2

Genes Which Increase Chromosomal Instability in Somatic Cells and Predispose to Cancer

James German

The New York Blood Center and Cornell University Medical College, New York City.

CHROMOSOMAL ABNORMALITIES have often been observed in relation to cancer,* but their significance is unknown (Hauschka, 1961; Nowell, 1965; Levan, 1969; Turpin and Lejeune, 1969; Sandberg and Hossfeld, 1970). Some will argue that a chromosomal mutation can play an etiological role in cancer, whereas others view chromosomal changes as only one manifestation of cancer itself and of no etiological importance, though allowing some role to a shifting karyotype in the evolution of the disease once it is established. Among those who favor a chromosomal etiology are some who see the mutation itself, perhaps by duplication or deletion of a preexisting gene, as the essential change for the cell's escape from normal growth inhibition. Still others would suggest that, once the cell has undergone a certain mutation, it is susceptible to conversion to cancer by some additional oncogenic factor. An additional possibility is that, at the time a chromosomal rearrangement occurs, the disturbed mechanics permit a viral genome to combine linearly into the cell's own genome. My purpose here is to ask if new light can be thrown on the confusing question of the interrelationship of chromosomes and cancer by considering what is known about certain rare human genetic disorders in which both chromosomal instability and the expectancy of cancer are increased. It seems a

---

* The word cancer is used in this paper not in a pathological sense but to refer to both leukemias and solid tumors shown to be malignant by their behavior in vivo.

fair statement to say that the majority of oncologists today, when the degree of interest in the etiology of cancer has never been greater, do not favor the idea that chromosomal change is of fundamental importance in cancer (Rous, 1959, 1967; Braun, 1969; Sandberg and Hossfeld, 1970). However, chromosomes in cancer go in and out of fashion, and for at least some, including me, they are very much in now.

The paper will be developed to show the following:

1. Many human cancers arise from a single cell, and this cell often has one or more chromosomes that differ in morphology from any in the complement of the noncancerous cells of the affected individual.

2. Chromosomal instability, leading to an increased number of de novo chromosomal rearrangements, characterizes the cells of certain persons who have an increased risk of cancer.

3. Several rare human genetic disorders feature increased chromosomal instability, and in each there is a greatly increased expectancy for cancer to develop.

4. The genes responsible for these clinical disorders can be grouped along with other known "causes" of cancer—certain forms of radiation, certain chemicals, and certain viruses—all of which have in common the ability to produce increased numbers of cells with de novo chromosomal rearrangements.

In an epilogue, I will attempt to show that a degree of confusion over the role chromosomes play in cancer exists and will continue to exist because of the multiple aspects of the disease. Yet such confusion need not deprive us of the opportunity, little as it now may appear, to discover some special chromosomal origin for at least some cancers or classes of cancers.

Origin of Cancer in a Single Cell With a Chromosomal Mutation

Since the early 1950s, when improved cytogenetic techniques came into use, the chromosomal complements of many benign and malignant tumors and leukemias of both human and nonhuman species have been examined. Benign tumors usually show the same normal diploid complement found in nontumorous cells of the host. The well-known cancer in the mouse caused experimentally by introduction of mammary tumor virus has an apparently normal mouse chromosomal complement; this is the case both in cancer newly arisen in the mammary gland (Tjio and Ostergren, 1958) and in tumors transplanted serially for as many as 27 times by injection of intact cells into the subcutaneous tissues of normal animals (Henderson and German, 1967). However, many other cancers in animals, and most cancers in humans (Nowell, 1965), do not have a normal chromosomal complement, often having one or more chromosomes that differ in morphology from any in the complement of the host's unaffected cells (see, e.g., Fig. 1). Such marker chromosomes result from a rearrangement, either intrachromosomal or interchromosomal, and in different cancers are represented variously by apparently reciprocal translocation, unbalanced translocation, deletion, or pericentric inversion. The new chromosome has a stable configuration, permitting it to pass successfully through mitosis.

The abnormal new chromosome of any one cancer in any one patient usually appears to be unique to that patient's cancer. Additional cytogenetic abnormalities, such as missing or extra chromosomes or other morphologically abnormal chromosomes, may also be found during the examination of many cells, but the unique marker tends to be the constant finding from cell to cell, both at the primary site and in metastases (see, e.g., Spriggs et al., 1962; de Grouchy et al., 1963a, 1963b; Ford and Clarke, 1963; Makino et al., 1964; Nowell, 1965; Sasaki and Makino, 1965; Atkin and Baker, 1966; Yamada et al., 1966; Lubs and Kotler, 1967; Atkin et al., 1967; Spiers and Baikie, 1968; Turpin and Lejeune, 1969; Benedict et al., 1970).

Ford (see Ford et al., 1958; Ford and Clarke, 1963) has studied the cytogenetics of primary reticular neoplasms in the mouse and has shown that many of them represent clones of cells with one or more marker chromosomes. His careful cytogenetic observations of newly arisen marker chromosomes established the fact that a neoplastic cell population may be generated in a host by proliferation from a single ancestral cell. He also demonstrated that "variant (though related) cell-types may arise within it, and that one of these may replace another as the dominant component of the population during the course of the disease." Atkin and co-workers (Atkin and Baker, 1966; Atkin et al., 1967) have cytogenetically examined a large number of uterine cancers and found that, for any one case, there was a stemline with the same abnormal chromosomal complement from cell to cell. In the many studies such as these, in which many and often all cells of a given cancer have the same unusual, morphologically abnormal (marker) chromosome (Fig. 1), the conclusion is inescapable that the cells are descendants of a single cell which had in its chromosomal complement the same marker rearrangement. Other very recent noncytogenetic evidence leads, in effect, to the same conclusion, that the cells of certain benign tumors (Linder and Gartler, 1965) and certain leukemias (Fialkow et al., 1967; Fialkow, 1970) are the progeny of just one cell (but see also Lawler and Sanger, 1970). It would appear, then, that a chromosomal rearrangement has played some essential role in the conversion of the progenitor cell to cancer, for if it had no such role the frequency of markers in the stemlines of various cancers should be no greater

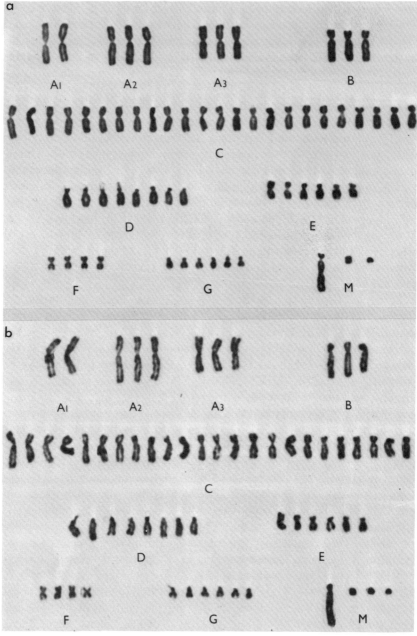

FIG. 1.—Two representative karyotypes from a seminoma of the testis (patient aged 36, uncultured material) with (*a*) 62 and (*b*) 63 chromosomes. M = marker chromosomes. The karyotypes appear identical apart from an extra minute in one. (Courtesy of Miss M. C. Baker and Dr. N. B. Atkin, Mount Vernon Hospital, Northwood, England.)

than their frequency in normal tissue cells, which is extremely low (Ford, 1964; Levan, 1969). We do not know whether the progenitor cell (i.e., the first cell that took on the features of cancer) was the cell in which the chromosomal rearrangement first occurred or whether it was but one member of a clone in which each cell contained the rearrangement. (Pseudodiploid clones of cells with no overt cancerous qualities occasionally have been detected proliferating in otherwise normal tissues, but as a rule the tissues yielding them have either been irradiated or have an unusual genetic constitution, as will be discussed subsequently.) Another possibility, but one requiring postulation of a second step in the development of the cancerous stemline, is that the first step in malignancy occurred in a cell with a normal karyotype and the chromosomal rearrangement took place in some descendant of that cell.

But under what circumstances do stable de novo chromosomal rearrangements occur in somatic cells of normal tissues, and what correlation, if any, exists between these circumstances and cancer? These questions are explored now, an unusual environmental background being considered first, and then one of genetics.

Some "Experiments" in Human Oncogenesis

Extraordinary environmental situations are known which increase for the man exposed to them the risk that he will develop cancer. Each situation can be viewed as an unplanned but nonetheless valuable experiment in human oncogenesis. For each of these unusual environments, just as for the four rare genetic disorders to be described later, it will be shown that chromosomal damage is a common denominator. Even if cytogeneticists had not already demonstrated the constancy with which a stemline with an altered and unique chromosomal complement is found in human cancer, these observations, that both (a) environmental situations which predispose to cancer as well as (b) genes which predispose to it have chromosomal instability and damage in common, would point an accusing finger at chromosomal mutation (actually, at *mutation,* because agents that break chromosomes appear also to be mutigens, and vice versa) as a factor in the etiology of human cancer. The following are some of the recognized examples of such "experiments" in human oncogenesis.

Survivors of the atomic-bomb blasts in Japan have developed leukemia in proportion to the amount of radiation they received. By 1955, about 1% of those nearest the hypocenter had developed leukemia, 0.3% of those somewhat farther away, 0.04% of those farther still, and 0.02% of those essentially removed from the range of radiation. This observation "established that ionizing radiations induce leukemia in man" (Lewis, 1957). (It should be inserted here that leukemia is not a common disease, being recognized at a yearly incidence of only 68 per million individuals. It is even rarer among the young, 24 per million of those 10-19 years old are affected each year, and only 12 per million of those 20-29 year old.) An increased number of chromosomal breaks and rearrangements have been demonstrated in the chromosomes of blood lymphocytes derived from Japanese survivors of the atomic bombings (A. D. Bloom et al., 1966; A. D. Bloom et al., 1967; Ishihara and Kumatori, 1967). Both A. D. Bloom et al. (1967) and Ishihara and Kumatori (1967) detected abnormal monocentric chromosomes in the complement of blood lymphocytes of many of those who received atomic irradiation both in Japan and

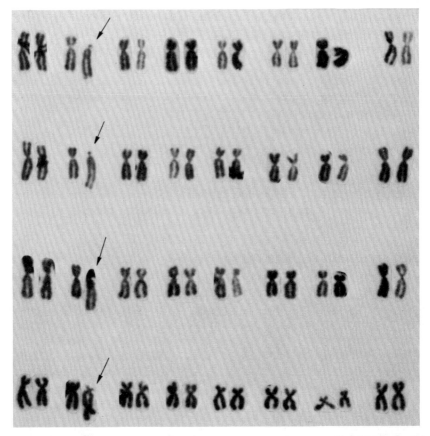

FIG. 2.—Partial karyotypes of the group C(6-X-12) chromosomes from four cells of a Hiroshima A-bomb survivor who was exposed to 403 rads of mixed gamma and neutron radiation at the time of the bombing. Each cell shows the same inversion, which implies that these cells represent a subpopulation of cytogenetically abnormal lymphocytes. These cells were obtained from the blood of this survivor in 1968 and were cultured 48 hours prior to harvesting. Unpublished study courtesy of Dr. Arthur D. Bloom, Department of Human Genetics, University of Michigan.

near Bikini. In a few of these individuals both teams of cytogeneticists discovered that multiple cells all having a similar stable chromosomal rearrangement, signifying the presence of a unique pseudodiploid clone, were proliferating among the normal diploid cells (Fig. 2). The uniqueness of each of the marker chromosomes was, in both reports, the basis for the conclusion that the several cells affected were, in a given individual, descendants of a single cell in which the rearrangement had taken place.

Arthritic individuals given X-ray therapy to the spine subsequently exhibit an increased incidence of leukemia (Court Brown and Doll, 1957), the heavier the dosage, the greater the incidence. Circulating lymphocytes from such irradiated (but not leukemic) individuals show a striking increase in chromosomal damage (Buckton et al., 1962). The nature of the chromosomal breaks and arrangements observed imply that the affected lymphocytes can circulate through the blood and other tissue for many years without undergoing a single division, although such lymphocytes do maintain their ability to divide when stimulated by phytohemagglutinin in culture. Court Brown et al. (1967) detected pseudodiploid clones of lymphocytes circulating in the blood of several individuals who had, from 11 to 25 years earlier, received X-ray therapy for ankylosing spondylitis or injections of [232]Th (in the form of Thorotrast) for cerebral angiography. The clones, in which translocations or inversions had occurred and produced abnormal marker chromosomes, comprised, on repeated sampling of the blood, no more than 5-6% of the entire lymphocyte population. There was no evidence of leukemia in the individuals in which the pseudodiploid clones were proliferating.

Engel et al. (1964) cultured fibroblasts from normal-appearing human skin which had been in the path of X-rays given to treat a lung cancer. Five different populations of cells were found, each of which had a different abnormal chromosomal complement derived through earlier chromosomal breakage and rearrangement. Because a unique marker chromosome was discovered in each of the five populations of cells, it was concluded that they represented the progeny of five distinct cells, each having had a different rearrangement. Visfeldt (1966) also recovered pseudodiploid clones from X-irradiated skin of the forearm; skin from the opposite, unirradiated forearm yielded none.

Children who during their infancy received X-ray therapy to the mid-chest region for shrinking the thymus subsequently have shown an increased incidence of leukemia (Simpson et al., 1955). Of 1400 such individuals followed for an average of 15 years, 7 or 8 developed leukemia, whereas there was no leukemia among 1795 unirradiated sibs and only 0.6 would have been expected in the general population ($p < 0.01$).

Children with cancer have been shown (Stewart and Kneale, 1970) to have received as a group more diagnostic X-radiation during their intrauterine life, especially during the early weeks, than have children without cancer. The risk of developing cancer appears to be related to the dosage of radiation received by the fetus.

Practicing radiologists, at least the older ones, appear (Seltser and Sartwell, 1965) to have had a decreased longevity when compared as a group to certain other medical specialists, owing partly to a higher incidence of leukemia and cancer. Certain other specialists who use X-ray therapy also appear to have an increased incidence of leukemia. Only a few cytogenetic studies of radiologists and radiation workers have been done. The difficulties encountered and the explanation for the small number of studies have been discussed by Visfeldt (1967).

Among those in France and Italy who have inhaled benzene occupationally for prolonged periods, leukemia has occurred on several occasions and apparently more often than in other members of the population under study (Vigliani and Saita, 1964). An increased frequency of chromosomal breaks has been found in blood lymphocytes of 20 men in Britain who in their work had been exposed to benzene for 1-20 years, even though they had not been exposed during the 2 years preceding the withdrawal of the blood sample that was studied (Tough and Court Brown, 1965).

Lacking sufficient data for human in vivo "experiments" relating viral infection to cancer, I shall discuss here the important experiments (Shein and Enders, 1962; Yerganian et al., 1962; Moorhead and Saksela, 1963; Girardi et al., 1966; Moorhead, 1970) using human fibroblasts in tissue culture infected with SV40 virus. It is known that certain nonhuman animal cells infected with SV40 while in tissue culture will be "transformed," increasing their growth rate and losing contact inhibition. Some of these "transformed" cultures, when injected back into animals, will give rise to tumors more rapidly than if this oncogenic virus alone were injected. Human cells in culture also became "transformed," altering their growth pattern, when infected with SV40 virus, but the results of reintroducing the infected cells into humans are unknown. Extensive cytogenetic analyses of these cultures before and at various times after viral infection have shown that at first no chromosomal instability is present, even though the cells are shedding virus. After several weeks, at the time, or hours after, the first evidence of altered growth patterns appears, chromosomal breakage and rearrangement become detectable. The cultures thereafter appear "transformed" and show rapid growth and striking chromosomal instability, with many obviously lethal genetic imbalances. After many weeks of this rampant and disorganized growth, a sharp decline in growth rate ("crisis") occurs, followed, after several more weeks, by the emergence of a few heteroploid cell lines capable apparently of vigorous and unlimited proliferation in culture. The emergent lines show much chromosomal variation, even after cloning, and in this and other respects resemble established cell lines, such as HeLa. Interestingly, the time required for diploid human fibroblast cultures to "transform" after infection with SV40 is shorter the nearer the culture is to Hayflick's phase III. Phase III is the time which follows the rapid proliferative period of such cultures (phase II) and is characterized by slow to absent proliferation and by chromosomal instability and production of abnormal chromosomes. Possibly related to this are the experiments of Todaro (1968) showing that the incidence of "transformation" among phase II fibroblasts is increased by X-irradiation, which also will cause chromosomal disruption.

From the foregoing examples, it appears that many of the situations from which human cancer emerges with increased frequency are also situations characterized by chromosomal instability, in which increased numbers of cells with de novo chromosomal rearrangements are emerging. In the following section of this paper are discussed additional situations that feature increased numbers of cells with chromosomal instability, breaks, and rearrangements, but these will be genetically, rather than environmentally, determined.

THE GENETICS OF CHROMOSOMES

In 1960, while searching for a possible chromosomal imbalance in a certain rare disorder of growth now referred to as Bloom's syndrome, I discovered unexpectedly that a large proportion of cultured cells from affected individuals display a strikingly abnormal cytogenetic behavior, the chromosomes frequently undergoing rearrangements (German, 1964; German et al., 1965). Subsequently, it was shown that individuals with Bloom's syndrome are homozygous for a very rare gene *(bl)* and that they are at an increased risk of developing cancer (German et al., 1965; Sawitsky et al., 1966; German, 1969). Schroeder et al. (1964) found that a high percentage of cells in a tissue culture derived from a man with Fanconi's anemia showed chromatid gaps and breaks. In addition, some cells had chromosomal rearrangements. Only later was the increased incidence of leukemia in Fanconi's anemia emphasized in medical literature. Schroeder has found that several other rare, genetically determined hematological disorders are also characterized by chromosomal instability (Schroeder, 1966; Schroeder and Kurth, 1971), and individuals with those disorders often develop leukemia as well. When we found these examples of genetically determined chromosomal instability, neither Schroeder nor I was aware of the relation of cancer to the genetic disorder we were studying. Hecht et al. (1966) found an increased degree of chromosomal breakage in lymphocytes from patients with another rare genetic disorder which often eventuates in cancer, the Louis-Bar syndrome. Finally, we (German et al., 1970) detected in cultured skin fibroblasts a different type of cytogenetic disturbance, a tendency toward formation of pseudodiploid clones, in xeroderma pigmentosum, another human disorder with an exceptionally high incidence of cancer. In the next section of this paper I shall present a clinical and cytogenetic summary of each of these four rare disorders, but first I shall show that other genes, both human and nonhuman, are known to have an effect on the chromosomes. They, along with the genes responsible for Bloom's syndrome, Fanconi's anemia, the Louis-Bar syndrome, and xeroderma pigmentosum, may be viewed as genes which affect the phenotype of the chromosome.

The chromosome's phenotype (Lima de Faria and Sarvella, 1962; German, 1966) derives not only from its morphological appearance but also from its behavior. It varies at different times in the cell cycle and with different normal or experimental conditions. The phenotype of the chromosome can be shown at times to be under genetic control, i.e., either its morphology or its behavior can be influenced by its own genetic constitution or by that of other chromosomes in the cell, and its phenotype can be said to be genetically variable. Sometimes this genetically determined variability in morphology or function affects just certain chromosomes or chromosomal regions; at other times all chromosomes of the complement may be affected.

Examples of the genetic determination of abnormal or unusual chromosomal behavior, only a few of which need be mentioned here, are known in both plant and nonhuman animal species (Bridges, 1923; Lesley and Frost, 1927; Blakeslee, 1930; Clausen, 1931; Stern, 1936; Lima de Faria and Sarvella, 1962). Chaganti (1965) tabulated and discussed more than 20 genetic determinants in plants and animals which exert an effect on meiotic chromosomal behavior. Beadle (1933) described the effects of the gene *st* in maize; when homozygous, *st* has a profound effect on meiotic (though less on mitotic) chromosomes, causing aberrant clumping of chromatin at metaphase, followed by chromatin bridging at anaphase, fragmentation of chromosomes, and formation of micronuclei at interphase. McClintock (1956) showed that the *Ds* (dissociator) element in maize causes an increased frequency of chromosomal breakage in chromatin it may adjoin (*Ds* moves to various chromosomal regions) and also exerts an effect on the genetic activity of its neighboring genes; another element, *Ac* (activator) located elsewhere in the complement, regulates the frequency with which *Ds* will break chromosomes. Erickson (1965) studied the RD line of *Drosophila,* in which an X-borne genetic determinant, when present in a male, causes the Y chromosome to undergo various types of breakage, mainly at the second meiotic division. Sandler et al. (1968) are studying mutant genes in *Drosophila* that affect meiotic chromosomal behavior, such as the pairing and the disjunctional processes, and these genes probably should be included here. In the mouse, Van Valen (1966) has studied a gene that, when homozygous, results in fragmentation of chromatin and the formation of abnormal nuclei at a specific time early in embryogenesis.

In man as well, several examples have been found in which a single genetic determinant, inherited in Mendelian fashion, exerts an effect on the phenotype of chromosomes. In some individuals the proximal segment of the long arm of chromosome 1 appears attenuated at metaphase; the genetic determinant for this trait, which has been named *Un* 1 (uncoiler), segregates as a dominant and is linked to the locus determining the Duffy blood group (Donohue et al., 1968; Ying and Ives, 1968). A similar variation in the phenotype of the proximal segment of the long arm of chromosome 16 segregates in some families (German, 1966). Also transmitted in dominant fashion is a determinant which evokes a prominent secondary constriction in the distal segment of the short arm of chromosome 17 (German, 1966) (Fig. 3). Another, reported to be linked to the haptoglobin locus (Magenis et al., 1970), produces a similar effect in the distal segment of the long arm of chromosome 16. Emerit et al. (1968) observed two families in which there was a tendency, segregating as a dominant, for an isochromatid gap or break to appear in the distal segment of the long arm of one chromosome of group C, and other laboratories (e.g., Kunze-Mühl et al., 1970) have detected similar families.

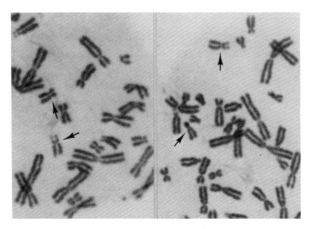

FIG. 3.—Chromosomes 17 (arrows) from two cells from one man. A proportion of his and his sister's cells showed a prominent constriction near the end of the short arm of one chromosome 17, giving it a satellite.

Schmid and Vischer (1969) reported a father and son whose chromosomal complements revealed an exceptionally long, late-DNA-synthesizing juxtacentromeric constriction in the proximal segment of the long arm of one autosome of group C; in the son, this region often was disrupted, with loss of the distal acentric segment. Lejeune et al. (1966) discovered a peculiar abnormal behavior of human chromosomes in which one segment of one chromosome duplicates itself twice while the remainder of the affected chromosome and all other chromosomes in the cell duplicate themselves once. The tendency for this *endoréduplication sélective* to affect chromosome 2 specifically has been shown to be transmitted in several families as a dominant, whereas the same phenomenon has been seen sporadically and infrequently affecting segments of chromosomes other than number 2 (Fig. 4a). These examples suffice to show that unusual morphological features and also unusual functioning of human chromosomes can be under genetic control. Some of these may be examples of genetic regulation of chromosomal behavior in the wider sense (e.g., like that of *Ac* on *Ds* in corn), whereas others may simply be transmission of a mutant chromosome region. The biological significance, if any, of the examples of genetically determined variation in the chromosomal phenotype just mentioned is still unknown.

FOUR HUMAN GENES; CLINICAL AND CYTOGENETIC ASPECTS

Four genes are discussed now, however, that not only determine unusual chromosomal behavior but also have severe clinical consequences, among which is an increased risk of cancer. For three of these genes, direct cytogenetic observation has shown that, when the gene is homozygous, the chromosomes of cells in tissue culture exhibit an unusual instability and tend to undergo disruption and rearrangements, with the result that many cells are present in the culture at any one time with variously rearranged chromosomal complements. For the fourth gene, that for xeroderma pigmentosum, although an increased tendency for chromosomal disruption and rearrangements has not been observed directly, clones of skin fibroblasts with pseudodiploid complements have been detected growing amid normal diploid fibroblasts in tissue cultures; because this is an unusual finding in other cell lines, it suggests that at some time earlier, either in vitro or in vivo, a tendency for chromosomal rearrangement existed, probably when the cells had received exposure to ultraviolet light.

Bloom's Syndrome

The syndrome (D. Bloom, 1966; German, 1969) results from homozygosity for the rare autosomal gene *bl*. The predominating clinical features

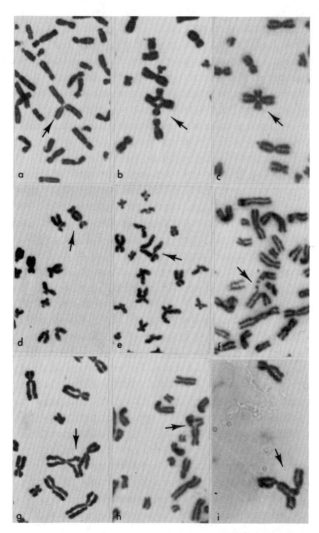

Fig. 4.—Chromosomal abnormalities observed at metaphase, orcein stain, 2000×. (a) *Endoréduplication sélective* affecting the long arm of a chromosome 2, blood lymphocyte. (b) *and* (c) Quadriradials, Bloom's syndrome, blood lymphocytes. (d) *and* (e) Dicentric chromosome and triradial configuration, Bloom's syndrome, bone marrow. (f), (g), *and* (h) Chromatid disruption, complex interchanges, and triradial configuration, Fanconi's anemia, blood lymphocytes. (i) Triradial configuration, Louis-Bar syndrome, blood lymphocyte.

of Bloom's syndrome are small body size and a sun-sensitive telangiectatic skin lesion in a butterfly distribution over the face. Growth retardation, both intrauterine and postnatal, is severe, the average full-term birth weight being around 4 lb, 6 oz (2000 g). The average height of affected individuals who have passed the age of 20 is 4 ft, 9 in. (142 cm), and only one individual is known whose height exceeds 5 ft. The well-proportioned minuteness of the affected individual is the most striking clinical feature of the syndrome, but also impressive is a characteristic facial appearance (see German, 1969, for numerous photographs); café-au-lait spots almost always are present, and minor anatomical defects often can be detected.

The immunity system is disturbed in Bloom's syndrome. Plasma concentrations of IgA or IgM or both are below normal. Many affected children have serious infections more often than normal children, which probably explains why the condition went unrecognized before the antibiotic era. Consequently, the 33 known individuals with the syndrome now alive constitute a young group, with an average age of 13 in 1971.

An important observation concerns the cause of death in the only 5 recognized affected individuals who have died. One very small infant failed to thrive and died with an infection at 3 months of age. Two of the three individuals Dr. David Bloom originally reported have since died of acute leukemia, one at age 13 and the other at 25; and then a more recently recognized affected woman died at 23, also of acute leukemia (Sawitsky et al., 1966). Finally, an affected 32-year-old man died of a carcinoma that originated near the base of his tongue. The remaining affected individuals are under the surveillance of our laboratory, and no death from cancer (or other causes) has occurred since 1966. A child of 4 currently has leukemia. The oldest person with this syndrome yet recognized has developed at age 39 two primary cancers, a squamous cell carcinoma of the upper esophagus and an adenocarcinoma of the sigmoid colon; the excised adenocarcinoma was heteroploid, with 65-75 chromosomes per cell, and each cell contained several morphologically similar abnormal (marker) chromosomes (German and Chaganti, unpublished data). A man of 38 has developed adenocarcinoma of the sigmoid. Thus, by our surveillance program it has been determined that of the first 5 cases of Bloom's syndrome to have been recognized (see German, 1969, for sequential numbering of the known cases), 4 individuals have developed cancer. All 3 individuals with the syndrome who have passed the age of 30 have developed at least one cancer of the gastrointestinal tract.

I have examined dividing lymphocytes, sometimes fibroblasts, from 21 of the 33 living known affected individuals and from 2 of the 5 who are now dead of cancer. The lymphocytes apparently respond normally to phytohemagglutinin, so that in most cases many cells in metaphase displaying excellent chromosomal morphology have been available for study, a requirement for estimating the frequency of breaks and rearrangements. Skin cells from homozygous affected individuals (*bl/bl*) do not develop into a vigorous tissue-culture cell line as readily as do those from normal (+/+) individuals, but seven lines from five different *bl/bl* homozygotes have been developed. Fibroblasts show abnormal chromosomal behavior similar to that of blood lymphocytes.

The most characteristic abnormal finding in both lymphocytes and fibroblasts at metaphase is a quadriradial configuration (Qr) (Figs. 4*b*, 4*c*). In one culture a Qr was present in one of every 10 dividing lymphocytes. A Qr is a figure derived from two chromosomes and has four arms, each arm consisting of the sister chromatids of one of the two chromosomes. The Qr characteristic of Bloom's syndrome is composed of two homologous chromosomes, for example, both homologs of chromosome pair 1 or both of pair 17. This figure is strikingly symmetrical, with the two centromeres in opposite arms and equidistant from the point of crossing; opposite arms of the figure have similar lengths. Usually, the centromeres are very near the crossing in the Qr (Fig. 4*b*), and not uncommonly they appear right at the crossing (Fig. 4*c*). Qr formation in Bloom's syndrome shows a strong predilection for certain autosomes (German and Crippa, unpublished data), most commonly involving chromosome pair 1 and members of group F(19-20), least often involving pair 2. The Qr as seen at metaphase is the result of an exchange of chromatids between two chromosomes, one chromatid from each chromosome having been affected. (The equal and symmetrical Qr (Figs. 4*b*, 4*c*) may be regarded (German, 1964) as cytogenetic evidence that a process which is the same as or genetically equivalent to crossing over occurs in human somatic cells.) The exchange would have occurred at some time before the onset of metaphase, at a time when the affected regions of each of the two chromosomes were effectively doubled or in the process of doubling; a reasonable prediction would place this at the time the two affected points on both chromosomes were duplicating themselves and when an opening existed in the replicons at corresponding regions along the DNA strands of each chromatid involved.

Also to be found in *bl/bl* cells at a frequency far greater than that in control cultures or cultures from most individuals with various other genetic and cytogenetic abnormalities are Qr's that are nonsymmetrical, dicentric chromosomes (Fig. 4*d*), triradial formations (Fig. 4*e*), and abnormal new monocentric chromosomes. In addition, somewhat increased numbers of cells usually but not always contain chromatid or isochromatid breaks, acentric fragments, or apparently telocentric chromosomal fragments.

Monolayers of *bl/bl* skin fibroblasts, when compared with +/+ cells, show increased numbers of cells in anaphase with chromatin bridges or lagging chromatin fragments and many more interphase cells with distorted nuclei or micronuclei (German and Crippa, 1966), further evidence of the drastic rearrangements observed in greater detail at metaphase. Such observations leave no doubt that many cells which have undergone profound change in their genetic constitution, in the form of both rearranged chromosomal segments and deleted or duplicated chromosomal segments, are capable of survival following a cellular division in vitro. Rauh and Soukup (1968) detected a pseudodiploid subpopulation of cells proliferating in one of two separate skin fibroblast cultures derived from their patient. Needless to say, however, the prospects are poor for long-term survival of those cells with the more drastic disturbances, and actually the high mortality among abnormal proliferating cells, if it occurs in vivo, provides a ready explanation (though possibly not the correct one) for the severely stunted intra- and extrauterine growth that is the most striking clinical feature of this syndrome. Strongly favoring the occurrence of chromosomal instability in vivo are the results of an examination of 364 cells in metaphase aspirated directly from the bone marrow of an affected 7-year-old boy (German and Crippa, unpublished data). Most of the cells displayed no abnormality, but seven or eight showed dicentric chromosomes, triradial configurations, or other complex exchange figures (Figs. 4d, 4e).

The biochemical defect in Bloom's syndrome remains to be elucidated, but one can surmise that the enzyme affected probably is intimately concerned with chromosomal metabolism. My cytogenetic observations suggest that the affected enzymatic reaction, rather than being absent or severely deficient, simply proceeds somewhat more slowly than normal, because all of the manifestations of chromosomal instability I have observed in bl/bl lymphocytes and skin fibroblasts I have also observed in cell cultures derived from heterozygous (bl/+) and from normal (+/+) individuals: viz., chromosomal breaks and rearrangements in metaphase figures, lagging and bridged chromatin at anaphase and telophase, and distorted nuclei and formation of micronuclei at telophase and interphase. In the heterozygote, for example, Qr's are seen less frequently than in the homozygote (bl/bl) but more frequently than in the normal individual. In other words, Qr's, dicentric chromosomes, and frankly abnormal chromosomes may be found in many persons' cells in culture provided enough cells are examined, but they are more frequently found among cells derived from persons carrying the gene bl. The enzymatic defect might either increase the frequency with which openings appear in the DNA strand or decrease the speed with which normally or spontaneously appearing openings are closed ("healed"). As a first approach to this question, and because of the sun sensity in Bloom's syndrome, we submitted bl/bl cells to the same experiments we used (Setlow et al., 1969) to demonstrate the ultraviolet-specific endonuclease deficiency in xeroderma pigmentosum and have shown that this enzyme, which is responsible for the first step in the repair of ultraviolet-induced damage to DNA, functions normally in bl/bl cells (Regan et al., in press). Examination of the other enzymes which act in the repair of breakage induced by radiation is currently in progress.

Fanconi's Anemia

Descriptions of fewer than 200 affected persons with this syndrome have appeared in the literature since its recognition as a clinical entity by Fanconi in 1927 (Fanconi, 1967). Gmyrek and Syllm-Rapoport (1964) made a valuable review of the first 129 cases to be reported. This rare disorder is characterized by a hematological abnormality consisting of pancytopenia and bone-marrow hypoplasia, symptoms of which usually appear between the fourth and twelfth years of life. The course of the disease is chronic and progressive, death usually occurring in childhood as result of hemorrhage or some other manifestation of failure of the marrow. Anatomical defects are prominent in the syndrome and may include skeletal deformities, especially of the thumb and radius, renal anomalies, strabismus, hypogenitalism, deafness, and anomalies of the ear and heart. Intrauterine growth retardation as well as stunted postnatal growth and microcephaly also are characteristic but not invariably present. Mental retardation often occurs. Brownish pigmentation of the skin is prominent, but it has a different distribution and is much more extensive than the café-au-lait spots characteristic of Bloom's syndrome. Thus, in Fanconi's anemia we observe an unusual combination of (a) a functional defect in a relatively unstructured cellular system, the bone marrow—and all elements of the marrow are affected, a decrease in the platelets, the erythrocytes, or the granulocytes possibly being responsible for the initial clinical manifestations—with (b) major anomalies of solid structures such as the skeleton, kidney, and heart.

The syndrome often affects sibs, and this, along with an increased incidence of parental consanguinity, provides evidence for its being genetic in origin and transmitted as an autosomal recessive. However, family members other than sibs are sometimes affected, and certain other observations (e.g., a preponderance of affected males) are not so characteristic of recessive transmission. The possibility clearly exists that this clinical entity, which presents variability in both anatomical features and age of onset of symptoms of the failing bone marrow, is genetically heterogeneous, as discussed by Fanconi (1967). The demonstration of a hexokinase deficiency in some patients (Löhr et al., 1965; Schroeder, 1966a) but not in others

(Schroeder, 1966b; Schroeder and Kurth, 1971) provides some further support for this possibility.

The view that there is an increased risk for individuals with this syndrome to develop leukemia now seems to be generally accepted. (It is curious, however, that the most extensive clinical reviews (Gmyrek and Syllm-Rapoport, 1964; Fanconi, 1967) have not emphasized this.) Silver et al. (1952) described a girl who developed a leukocytosis during the last few months of life. Cowdell et al. (1955) described two brothers, both of whom probably had Fanconi's anemia; one brother died at 22 of severe bone marrow hypoplasia, the other at 27 of acute leukemia. G. E. Bloom et al. (1966) mentioned that 2 of their patients had died of acute monocytic leukemia but presented no details other than that one was 8 years old and that each had had pancytopenia. Gmyrek et al. (1967) made a detailed study of one patient. These few cases are probably enough, in view of the infrequency of occurrence both of leukemia and of the syndrome itself, to indicate an increased association of the two, but a careful collection and analysis of data pertaining to the intriguing clinical, cytogenetic, genetic, and oncological questions in Fanconi's anemia would be a welcome addition to the scientific literature. One observation is that, regardless of the increased propensity to develop leukemia, few persons with Fanconi's anemia survive the panmyelopathy which usually makes its symptomatic appearance in early childhood. If a neoplastic cell line is to emerge and replenish the marrow, it must do so before the patient dies, say, by cerebral hemorrhage or overwhelming infection. (Gmyrek et al. (1967) have actually observed and documented the supervention of leukemia in their patient.) An additional point of interest in relation to neoplasia and Fanconi's anemia, and one which has attracted the attention of clinical investigators for over 15 years (Cowdell et al., 1955; Garriga and Crosby, 1959; G. E. Bloom et al., 1966; Fanconi, 1967; Gmyrek et al., 1967), is that the heterozygote may also have an increased risk for leukemia; Swift (1971) has presented evidence supporting this possibility.

The cytogenetics of most cases of Fanconi's anemia is similar on first inspection to that of Bloom's syndrome, but closer scrutiny shows this to be inexact (Schroeder and Kurth, 1971; Schroeder and German, unpublished data). Schroeder et al. (1964) were the first to report the important fact that blood lymphocytes dividing in vitro display an increased frequency of various types of chromosomal breakage (Figs. 4f, 4g, 4h). Only a few patients have been reported not to show it (G. E. Bloom et al., 1966; see also Schroeder and Kurth, 1971). Skin fibroblasts in culture also display the chromosomal instability (German and Crippa, 1966). Although the equal and symmetrical Qr sometimes is found in the metaphase figures, it can be concluded from published reports that this configuration is not nearly as common a finding as it is in Bloom's syndrome. Also, rearrangements, such as dicentric chromosomes and frankly abnormal monocentrics, are said (Schroeder, 1966a; Schmid, 1967) to be uncommon, although in my experience they certainly are found more often than in normal subjects. A great proportion (38-74%) of lymphocyte mitoses in Fanconi's anemia display breaks and gaps in the chromatids (Schmid et al., 1965; Schroeder, 1966a, 1966b; Hirschman et al., 1969), many more than are seen in Bloom's syndrome (German and Crippa, unpublished data). Although a comparison of the pattern of breaks and rearrangements in the two disorders must be made in a single laboratory under the same culture conditions, published descriptions by those who have studied larger numbers of patients than we have indicate that the cytogenetic phenomenon in Fanconi's anemia is different from that in Bloom's syndrome, the most characteristic lesion in the former being a chromatid gap or break (Figs. 4f, 4g) rather than an equal and symmetrical Qr, as in the latter (Figs. 4b, 4c). The genes certainly have a different effect clinically, and a difference in the pattern of chromosomal breakage would not be unexpected. On the other hand, the primary enzymatic disturbances in both Bloom's syndrome and Fanconi's anemia, though quite dissimilar, could, finally, lead to a disturbance of some common pathway affecting the chromosomes, which would be manifested by similar cytogenetic alterations in metaphase cells. As to the cause of the breakage here, Schroeder et al. (1964; Schroeder, 1966a) related it to the hexokinase deficiency reported by Löhr et al. (1965) to be characteristic of Fanconi's anemia; some patients' cells, however, have no such deficiency but still have breaks (Schroeder, 1966a, 1966b). Thus the role of this deficiency, if any, in the pathogenesis of Fanconi's anemia remains obscure. The fundamental biochemical defect in Fanconi's anemia—or defects, if the clinical entity turns out to be heterogeneous genetically—remains to be elucidated.

Here, as in Bloom's syndrome, the degree to which the chromosomal peculiarity so readily demonstrable in cells in culture actually occurs and is of importance in the patient's tissues in vivo must be determined. And, as in Bloom's syndrome, the methods by which this might be detected and studied are distinctly limited, direct examination of aspirated bone marrow being essentially our only means for examining a cell which has been through its cell division cycle and entered metaphase in its normal habitat. Schroeder (1966a) has made such observations and found increased numbers of nuclear and mitotic aberrations, including anaphase bridges, fragments, and micronuclei, in the bone marrow of patients with Fanconi's anemia.

Todaro et al. (1966), because of the association of leukemia with Fanconi's anemia, have used the SV40 virus to infect diploid fibroblastic cell lines (as discussed earlier in this paper) which were either homozygous or heterozygous for the gene(s) of Fanconi's anemia and have shown that such cell lines, in comparison with control lines, develop greater numbers of areas of "transformation," localized areas in the monolayer composed of cells undergoing rapid and disarrayed proliferation. In control cultures, 1.6-5.1 areas of "transformation" appeared for every 10,000 cells planted on the surface of the culture dish, in contrast to 20.1-28.2/10,000 cells containing in their genome one gene for Fanconi's anemia and 41.4-79.7/10,000 cells containing two genes. It must be admitted that just what the significance is of a "transformed" area of a monolayer of fibroblasts is far from clear, much less the increased incidence of "transformation" in cells carrying the gene(s) for Fanconi's anemia. In the context of the present paper, however, it may be observed that the three situations which have given rise to the most striking increase in the number of areas of "transformation"—X-irradiation of the fibroblasts, the use of normal fibroblasts approaching or in Hayflick's phase III, and the use of fibroblasts with the gene(s) for Fanconi's anemia—are all situations associated with chromosomal breakage and instability.

The Louis-Bar Syndrome (Ataxia Telangiectasia)

This syndrome (Boder and Sedgwick, 1963; Karpati et al., 1965; Peterson and Good, 1969), which also is transmitted as an autosomal recessive, was well described by Madame Louis-Bar in 1941, but only in 1957 (Wells and Shy; Biemond; Boder and Sedgwick) did other reports of additional cases begin to appear and its genetic etiology become apparent. Between 100 and 200 patients have been referred to in the scientific literature, and hence it may be classified as a rare condition. A review of the clinical features in the first 101 cases to be recognized was made by Boder and Sedgwick (1963).

Affected individuals appear normal at birth but exhibit cerebellar ataxia after a few months of life or after a few years, often when they begin to walk. Either about the same time or somewhat later, telangiectases appear in the bulbar conjunctivae. These two features, which are responsible for the descriptive name also given to this syndrome—ataxia telangiectasia—are progressive. Over a period of several years, neurological deterioration and general debility eventuate in the patient's confinement to a wheel chair and bed and not uncommonly are accompanied by mental deterioration. At autopsy, loss and regressive changes in the Purkinje cells and, to a lesser degree, in the basket cells and granular layer of the cerebellar cortex can be demonstrated; occasionally, lesions elsewhere in the brain have been noted. The bilaterally symmetrical telangiectasia may remain mild but usually becomes more widespread and prominent and may progressively involve other areas, such as the skin of the face, ears, neck, antecubital fossae, wrists, hands, and knees. Because telangiectasia usually appears later than does the cerebellar ataxia, the diagnosis may be delayed until age 4 to 6. Ovarian hypoplasia and probably also testicular hypoplasia are commonly present, and general stunting of growth often occurs. Café-au-lait spots are said to be common (Boder and Sedgwick, 1957). The pathogenesis of all of these manifestations, and particularly the relation of the vascular and neuronal lesions, is obscure.

Increased numbers of infections of the sinuses and lungs often occur in this syndrome, bronchiectasis may develop, and pneumonia in adolescence is a common cause of death. Most, but possibly not all, affected individuals exhibit disturbed immunity (Peterson et al., 1966; Strober et al., 1968) characterized by "a decreased capacity to manifest cellular immunity plus various abnormalities in serum immunoglobulin levels, the most common being a low IgA" (Peterson and Good, 1969) and IgE (Biggar et al., 1970). The majority of those affected show no delayed hypersensivity and fail to reject skin homografts with normal vigor. The histology of both the thymus and the lymph nodes is severely abnormal, both being characteristically deficient in lymphoid elements, and the similarity between the Louis-Bar syndrome and neonatally thymectomized animals has been emphasized. Among recognized cases of the Louis-Bar syndrome, malignant neoplasia has occurred much more frequently than in the general population; the cancers have often originated in lymphoid reticular tissues (Peterson et al., 1966). (Here, as with Fanconi's anemia, a welcome addition to the literature would be an extensive documentation and commentary on known cases of the syndrome with and without cancer.)

The karyotype in the Louis-Bar syndrome is normal (as it is in Bloom's syndrome, Fanconi's anemia, and xeroderma pigmentosum). That some cytogenetic disturbance exists, however, was first mentioned by Hecht et al. (1966), who reported "a high frequency (20-30%) of chromosome breakage in vitro" but gave no details as to the number of cells or the types of aberrations observed. An inadequate number of cytogenetic studies of this rare condition have been reported, but the few reports available (Hecht et al., 1966; Gropp and Flatz, 1967; Hecht and Case, 1969; Pfeiffer, 1970) appear to indicate that blood lymphocytes display in vitro an increased number of breaks and abnormal chromosomes. My experience with one case is compatible with this observation (Fig. 4i) and agrees also with an impression of others, that the explanation for there being so few reports of cytogenetic studies of this syndrome is the difficulty in obtaining adequate numbers of blood lymphocytes in metaphase. Not only do the patients tend to have an absolute lymphopenia but also only an unusually small proportion of their circulating lymphocytes will divide in response to phytohemagglutinin (Naspitz et al., 1968; Peterson and Good, 1969). Gropp and Flatz (1967), after repeated attempts at culturing blood lymphocytes from 2 affected sibs, succeeded in obtaining from each sib a dozen mitoses suitable for analysis; these showed many breaks and a few rearrangements. Pfeiffer (1970) has summarized, in an abbreviated fashion, what must be considered until now the most extensive cytogenetic study of the Louis-Bar syndrome, the analysis of cells from 6 individuals. In contrast to the experience of others, he observed a normal mitotic rate in phytohemagglutinin-stimulated lymphocytes in cultures from 4 of the 6 individuals. In 2 brothers who had received much diagnostic X-irradiation he did find some breaks and exchanges, but after a comparison with his X-irradiated controls he concluded that "a specific breakage effect due to the basic disorder seems to be unlikely." In 2 other individuals he found no evidence of chromosomal instability. In each of the 2 oldest patients he obtained evidence for the proliferation in vivo of a clone with an abnormal chromosomal complement. Hecht and Case (1969), studying one affected individual, observed over a period of months the ascendency among circulating blood lymphocytes of members of a pseudodiploid clone with the complement 46,XY,t(13q+;14q−) (Fig. 5a). When first detected, the abnormal clone represented only 1-3% of the dividing lymphocytes, but the proportion progressively increased to 46% after 32 months (Fig. 5b). Bone marrow cells and fibroblasts from the same patient had the complement 46,XY. Because of the absence of clinical evidence for cancer in the patient, the authors believe their findings signify the presence of "a non-malignant clone of lymphocytes with a proliferative advantage."

Thus, for the Louis-Bar syndrome, data from a sufficiently large number of patients are not available to give us a clear picture of the chromosomal behavior in dividing lymphocytes, although there emerges fairly strongly the suggestion that an aberrant pattern does indeed exist in at least some cases. Questions which are prominent among those unanswered are the following: Does the tendency to breakage and rearrangements expressed at metaphase resemble that in either Bloom's syndrome or Fanconi's anemia? Is it expressed only in lymphoid cells? Do lymphoid cells from all patients show the abnormality or is there heterogeneity? Will pseudodiploid clone formation, already observed by some (Hecht and Case, 1969; Pfeiffer, 1970), be detected in additional affected individuals? And are the lymphoid neoplasms which so often emerge in persons with this genetic constitution characterized by a chromosomal rearrangement?

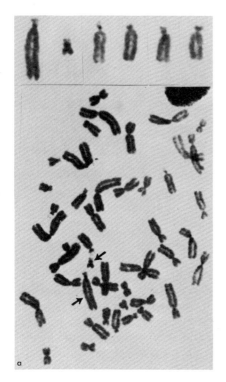

FIG. 5.—A cell (*a*) from a pseudo-diploid clone (note translocation between two of the long acrocentric chromosomes mounted above the metaphase) discovered in a patient with the Louis-Bar syndrome (Hecht and Case, 1969). (*b*) Increase with time in the frequency with which the abnormal cells were detected among dividing blood lymphocytes. Unpublished data of Dr. Frederick Hecht, University of Oregon Medical School, Portland.

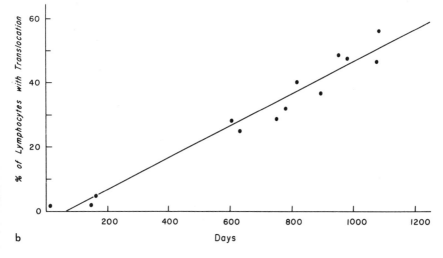

Xeroderma Pigmentosum

In this rare disorder, the skin of the homozygous affected individual appears normal at birth, but usually before age 3 severe changes consequent to sun exposure appear and progress relentlessly. Freckles, varying in size and depth of color, appear and are accompanied by increasing dryness of the skin, telangiectasia, atrophy, and numbers of keratoses. Histopathologically, there is a combination of hyperkeratosis, marked atrophy of the dermis with irregular proliferation of certain layers, edema, dilatation of vessels, and a greatly increased accumulation of pigment. The eyes are affected, and photophobia may be intense; scarring of the eyelids, ulceration of the cornea, and blindness may occur. Cancers of the skin, sometimes of multiple types, occur and often cause death before age 30. Basal cell and squamous cell epitheliomata may appear in such large numbers over the course of years that the surprising thing is not that the patient eventually succumbs to one of them but that he is able to survive so many for so long. Various other forms of benign and malignant tumors of ectodermal and mesodermal origin also occur with a much increased frequency in affected individuals. The major manifestations appear to be the consequence of exposure to sunlight. In addition to the skin lesions, there may be stunting of growth and poor physical development. Genetic heterogeneity of xeroderma pigmentosum, though not yet verified, is suggested by the observation that most individuals with the classic form of the disorder have normal intelligence, whereas a small number have severe neurological abnormalities and mental deficiency in addition to the skin condition; the term "De Sanctis–Cacchione syndrome" is sometimes applied to this unusual group. Little has been written concerning the heterozygous carrier of the gene for xeroderma pigmentosum, although increased freckling has been noted in some carriers. No increased risk of cancer has been described, but I am aware of no surveys.

There is little to summarize concerning the cytogenetics of xeroderma pigmentosum, but certain preliminary findings in our laboratory seem interesting enough to justify the inclusion of a discussion of the disorder in this paper. I derived a diploid skin-fibroblast cell line (Setlow, et al, 1969) from a tiny fragment of non-neoplastic-appearing skin from the arm of a 20-year-old affected man. This line was derived for use in biochemical studies (which I will summarize below), but at its fourth subculture generation a flask of cells was used for a routine cytogenetic characterization of the line and to search for any possible increased chromosomal instability (German et al., 1970). Two hundred and eleven cells were examined, and all but nine appeared to have the same normal human diploid chromosomal complement 46,XY we had already demonstrated in this patient's dividing blood lymphocytes. In neither the lympho-cytes nor the fibroblasts was there any evidence of an increased tendency for chromosomal breakage or rearrangement similar to that characteristic of Bloom's syndrome or Fanconi's anemia. The nine abnormal fibroblasts fell into three distinct classes: (a) one cell with a long abnormal subacro-centric chromosome, but detailed analysis was impossible since the cell had been ruptured; (b) two cells with the abnormal complement 46,XY,t(Cp+;Cq−), apparently the consequence of a reciprocal translo-cation between two members of group C; and, (c) six cells (Fig. 6) with the abnormal complement 46,XY,t(1q−;Dq+), apparently the conse-quence of a reciprocal translocation between a chromosome 1 and a mem-ber of group D. Although the number of abnormal cells was small, their abnormalities were so unusual and yet so similar among the cells of classes b and c that we concluded that two pseudodiploid subpopulations of cells, or clones, each composed of cells with a uniquely abnormal chro-mosomal complement, were proliferating in the predominantly diploid cul-ture. Three biopsies from the man have been taken subsequently, and five new cell lines were derived from them; in two of these five evidence for the presence of distinctively aberrant pseudodiploid clones is being accu-mulated.

We believe the ease with which we have detected pseudodiploid clones in cells homozygous for the xeroderma pigmentosum gene signifies a pre-disposition for their formation either in vitro or in the patient's skin. How-ever, the observations require controls, and extensive studies of other cell lines derived and maintained in our laboratory are now in progress and must be completed before the discovery in the xeroderma pigmentosum cell cultures can be interpreted further. (Controls in one sense are avail-able; during 10 years of intensive study in many laboratories of the chro-mosomal complement of human cells, the detection of such clones in un-treated tissues has been reported but rarely.) So far they have been grown in the dark in glass vessels and have not shown a tendency to breakage and rearrangements, but the discovery of so many pseudodiploid clones suggests that at some earlier time, possibly before the cells were excised from the man's skin, rearrangements were occurring at an increased rate. Both the clinical observations of sun-sensitivity and the cellular biochemi-cal abnormality to be described now would argue for this having had oc-curred at a time when the cell had received ultraviolet exposure. Experi-ments must be performed to determine whether the xeroderma pigmen-tosum fibroblasts actually will respond to ultraviolet irradiation with a much greater number of chromosomal breaks and rearrangements than control cells.

In the DNA of microorganisms and various other cell types, dimeriza-

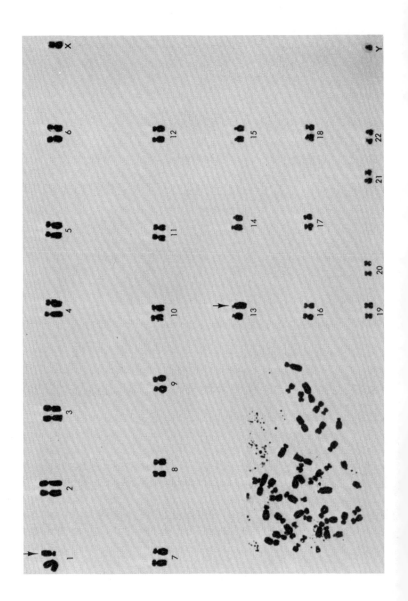

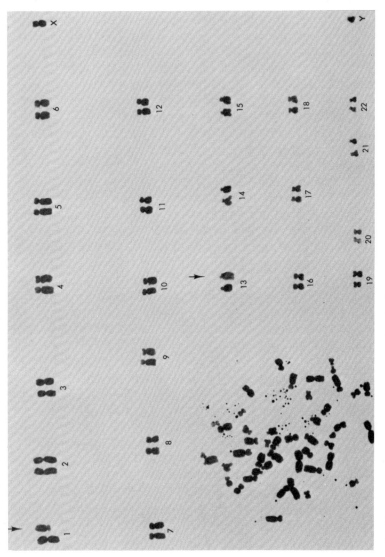

FIG. 6.—Two fibroblasts found in division at the fourth subculture generation of a predominantly diploid (46,XY) tissue culture cell line derived from the skin of a man with xeroderma pigmentosum. They were two of six cells each with a similarly abnormal pseudo-diploid karyotype (46,XY,t(1q−;Dq+), interpreted to be members of an abnormal subpopulation of cells (a clone) derived from a single cell in which the translocation occurred (German et al., 1970).

tion of adjacent pyrimidine residues is the biologically important lesion induced by ultraviolet irradiation (Setlow, 1967). These lesions may be repaired in the dark by a process that involves excision of dimers from cellular DNA, repair replication, and rejoining of DNA strands. In 1968, Regan et al. presented evidence that excision repair occurs in normal human cells; further experiments have shown that the sequence of events in excision of dimers is similar if not identical to that in bacteria. After considering the significance of ultraviolet damage and its repair in microorganisms, the dimer excision repair system in normal human cells, and the extreme reaction of xeroderma pigmentosum skin to ultraviolet, we developed the cell line mentioned above and investigated excision repair in the cells to obtain evidence regarding the fate of ultraviolet-induced pyrimidine dimers.

The four steps in the pyrimidine dimer excision repair system of ultraviolet-damaged DNA can be summarized in the following way: step 1, breakage in a single strand next to a dimer, the action of ultraviolet-specific endonuclease; step 2, excision of the dimerized pyrimidine, the action of exonuclease; step 3, filling of the gap with new, undamaged bases by the action of a DNA polymerase; step 4, closure of the broken strand, the action of ligase. It is implied in the scheme that a given step will not take place if the one before it has not been completed. Thus, if the ultraviolet-specific endonuclease is nonfunctional, the subsequent steps in repair will not follow. Cleaver (1968) first called attention to the possibility that the gene of xeroderma pigmentosum results in deficient repair. He found that xeroderma pigmentosum cells do not exhibit "repair replication," i.e., synthesis of DNA at times other than the S period of the cell division cycle, indicating absence of step 3 of the repair system. We (Setlow et al., 1969) examined xeroderma pigmentosum and normal skin fibroblasts for step 2, the excision of dimers. Xeroderma pigmentosum cells were found to excise essentially no measurable number of dimers after ultraviolet irradiation, whereas normal skin cells in comparable experiments removed a majority of their dimers within 24 hours after irradiation. We also examined xeroderma pigmentosum cells for the first step in excision repair and found them unable to perform the first critical step in repair, presumably because they do not have a functional form of the ultraviolet-specific endonuclease.

The various clinical and biochemical observations, taken together, suggest that the molecular basis of xeroderma pigmentosum is the lack of a functional ultraviolet-specific endonuclease. They also suggest that accumulation of dimers in the DNA of skin cells results in the extreme reaction seen in these cells to ultraviolet irradiation. Furthermore, the multiple skin cancers which regularly occur in xeroderma pigmentosum may be the direct or indirect result of dimer accumulation in the DNA. This leads me to enquire whether the tendency for dimer accumulation in the DNA chain predisposes to chromosomal rearrangements. If the molecular events accompanying chromosomal rearrangements and the structure of a mammalian chromosome were known with certainty, the answer might be obvious. On the other hand, an uncorrected aberrant bonding of adjacent bases in a DNA strand would appear to be a perfectly reasonable starting point for trouble at the time the chromosome begins to duplicate itself.

CONCLUSION

The observations just reviewed appear to shed some light on the question raised at the outset of this paper concerning the significance of chromosomal mutation in cancer. From the literature it was shown that many human cancers have a demonstrable stemline that includes in its chromosomal complement one or more marker chromosomes, new chromosomes different from any in the normal human complement but derived from normal chromosomes through breakage and rearrangement. The marker tends to be present from cell to cell, whether or not these cells have additional numerical or structural chromosomal variations. The uniqueness and constancy of the markers in cancers demand an explanation and are at the core of the problem. The simplest explanation, and one with which available information does not conflict, is that the particular cell which had first undergone conversion to a cancerous cell and became the progenitor of all the cells of the cancer itself contained the mutated chromosome. Whether the mutated chromosome appeared for the first time in that original cancer cell or was present in a minor cell line beforehand is unknown. Furthermore, if the former were true, it is unknown whether the chromosomal rearrangement occurred simultaneously with, preceded, or followed the cellular event that constituted conversion. And if the chromosomal mutation occurred simultaneously with the conversion to cancer, it is unknown whether they are one and the same, a view favored by some, or are mutually dependent but separate events, e.g., a rearrangement that would permit, during its formation, incorporation into the linear structure of the cell's own chromatin of a length of DNA from a virus. The exact events are not known; the point essential to this argument would be just that a chromosomal mutation is often present in the single cell from which all the cells one can sample in an established cancer have been derived. The great paucity of cells with chromosomal mutations among the cells of normal tissues dramatizes the association of structurally rearranged marker chromosomes and stemlines of cancers.

However, this plausible conclusion just elaborated upon cannot be validly deduced at present. Alternatively, the cell converting to cancer might have had a normal karyotype, in which case the chromosomal rearrangement producing the marker(s) would have to have arisen in one of the descendants of that first cell and to have had, by virtue of the mutated karyotype, a proliferative advantage over both normal cells and all the other (nonmutated) cancer cells. This second possibility, which also cannot be eliminated at present, is intrinsically less attractive because it requires the additional *ad hoc* hypothesis that the karyotypically normal cell once converted to cancer must undergo a second change, a chromosomal rearrangement, and that the already cancerous cell in which the appropriate new karyotype finally occurs will then have a proliferative advantage and become the cell from which the entire tumor will be derived. Ford et al. stated this fundamental problem in 1958 by asking "whether the neoplastic process began in a cataclysmic * event involving major rearrangements of genetic material or in a gradual accumulation of a series of changes, each small in itself." Do the data derived from the study of Bloom's syndrome, Fanconi's anemia, the Louis-Bar syndrome, and xeroderma pigmentosum allow us to favor one of these possibilities over the other?

It was shown that increased chromosomal instability is characteristic of cells taken from many persons who fall into groups with a high risk for cancer by virtue of their exposure to some unusual environment, irradiated persons and certain chemical workers being the best examples known. In addition to the generally increased numbers of broken and rearranged chromosomes in the lymphocytes of irradiated persons, in a number of instances clones of cells with unique marker chromosomes have been detected circulating in the blood. These clones, though clearly showing an aberrant chromosomal complement, exhibit no malignant characteristics; the important thing is that such clones are found in increased frequency in populations in which cancer also is found in increased frequency and that both they and stemlines of cancers are characterized by an origin from a single cell that contained a stable chromosomal rearrangement. Pseudodiploid clones have been detected only occasionally in the skin or blood of normal or malformed persons, even though large numbers of such populations now have been examined in detail for possible mosaicism. (However, see Court Brown et al. (1967) for a discussion of the experimental difficulties involved in detection of a clone with a chromosomal mutation.)

Chromosomal instability in human cells has been detected in some indi-

---

* Dr. Ford used the word catastrophic in 1958 but, in retrospect, prefers cataclysmic (personal communication).

viduals who have not been exposed to radiation or chemicals but who are homozygous for one of several rare genes. Those whose chromosomes have been studied most extensively have had Bloom's syndrome or Fanconi's anemia. Less extensive studies have been made in patients with the Louis-Bar syndrome, xeroderma pigmentosum, and certain very rare anemias. In each of these rare genetic disorders a moderately to greatly increased risk of cancer exists. Although in each disorder chromosomal instability has been demonstrated mainly in vitro, evidence for its occurrence in vivo in both Bloom's syndrome and Fanconi's anemia was cited. Pseudodiploid clones have been detected among circulating lymphocytes in the Louis-Bar syndrome and among bone marrow cells in Fanconi's anemia. In cultures of fibroblasts from the apparently noncancerous skin of a man with xeroderma pigmentosum, several distinctively different pseudodiploid clones have been detected growing amid the predominating normal diploid cells.

Although the possibility exists that in each of the rare genetic disorders just referred to a different biochemical mechanism predisposes conversion of a normal cell to a cancerous one, the simplest view at present is that they, as a group, represent but another means by which increased numbers of cells with mutations obtain, thereby increasing the opportunity for a specific one to occur which will either itself be cancer or will make the cell susceptible to conversion by an additional oncogenic factor. In this way, individuals with genetic constitutions predisposing to chromosomal breakage join those irradiated, those exposed to certain chromosome-breaking chemicals, and possibly those with certain viral infections as members of our population who are at an increased risk of developing cancer. In any one of the genetic disorders, if cells of a certain tissue manifest the tendency to form new chromosomal rearrangements more than do others, e.g., skin cells exposed to sunlight in xeroderma pigmentosum or lymphoid cells in the Louis-Bar syndrome, then that tissue would be the one from which the cancer would probably emerge. Thus, to answer the question asked three paragraphs earlier, the observations in these rare genetic disorders make me strongly in favor of the first of the two possible explanations for the presence of marker chromosomes in the stemlines of cancers, i.e., that chromosomal rearrangement occurred in the cell which originally converted to cancer; and furthermore that the mutation is an integral part of the conversion.

Such a view does not necessarily detract from the interest these rare human genes hold in relation to the cancer problem. It may suggest, however, that elucidation of the specific enzymatic defect associated with each gene will not contribute particularly to our understanding of cancer, i.e., to the explanation for either the change in the cellular surface or the failure at restriction of the cell's entry into the division cycle which results in uncontrolled proliferation. Their potential usefulness in molecular genetics and cell biology may be greater. The gene causing xeroderma pigmentosum has already been shown to be an abnormal allele at a locus that codes for one of the most important enzymes concerned with the metabolism of the chromosome itself. It can be assumed that the other three genes, those causing Bloom's syndrome, Fanconi's anemia, and the Louis-Bar syndrome, will also be abnormal alleles for similarly important genes whose products are concerned with the physiology and metabolism of the nucleus and maintenance of the genetic apparatus. Any or all, when elucidated completely, should be useful tools for the cell biologist and will enlarge our understanding of nuclear biochemistry.

EPILOGUE: MAKING SENSE FROM THE CONFUSION OVER CHROMOSOMES IN CANCER?

If the chromosomal basis for mongolism had not already been discovered and if a mongol with leukemia had been given X-ray treatments, the finding of (a) an extra chromosome 21 in all his cells, (b) a different aneuploid subpopulation of cells in his bone marrow and blood, and (c) many chromatid breaks and abnormal chromosomes in his lymphocytes in culture would certainly present a problem in interpretation, particularly for those intent on finding a single explanation for all the cytogenetic abnormalities. Actually, three separate explanations are required, although all three cytogenetic abnormalities are in a sense interrelated. But what is important is that all the chromosomal changes not be disregarded completely and considered meaningless simply because they are too numerous and too different and because their significance might not be clearly understood at first, the tack taken by some students of cancer today (Rous, 1967; Braun, 1969).

Just as in the case of this imaginary mongol, chromosomes appear to enter the cancer picture in too many places. Three different points for their entry are suggested: 2, 3, and 4 below. Consideration of each individually not only makes their contradictions less formidable but also opens up different possible experimental approaches to the general problem of understanding exactly what is occurring at the cellular level before the cancer emerges, as conversion to cancer occurs, and during its progression and evolution. The possibility that two classes of cancer exist only serves to introduce even more confusion into the cytogenetics of cancer and, consequently, will be discussed first.

1. Many human cancers have a stemline with an abnormal chromosomal complement, whereas some of the most extensively studied animal

cancers, particularly the MTV-associated mammary carcinoma in mice, are diploid. Confusion will be inevitable if two classes of cancer exist, one arising from an infection of cells with an unaltered chromosomal complement by some RNA-containing virus and another in which chromosomal rearrangement plays a role, while the disease itself would, regardless of its class, exhibit similar pathological progression and clinical manifestations. In both classes the cancer cells would have lost, possibly by different mechanisms, the ability to respond to the cease-division signals from neighboring cells and humoral factors. One might ask whether the cytogenetical findings, so normal in some cancers and so neatly abnormal in others, are not pointing to these two classes.

2. In those cancers characterized by a stemline with a marker chromosome, the marker differs in morphology from case to case of the same cancer. For example, the marker in one woman's squamous cell carcinoma of the uterine cervix will look different from that in the next woman's, yet both women will have stemlines with a marker chromosome. The one definite exception is chronic myelogenous leukemia, in which the same marker, the Ph[1] chromosome, is present in the neoplastic stemline in more than 80% of the affected persons. It must be remembered, however, that the techniques of mammalian cytogenetics do not permit great resolution, and in the case of marker chromosomes the actual nature of the rearrangement, and often even the identification of exactly which chromosomes were involved, virtually always defies analysis. The abnormality in chronic myelogenous leukemia, affecting the long arm of the tiny chromosome 22, is suitably located for microscopic recognition. The point is that in other cancer stemlines the chromosomal site of mutation might be more specific than is presently recognized, even though the marker chromosomes themselves differ in morphology from case to case. The constancy of the Ph[1] chromosome, even though it is exceptional, suggests that judgment should be reserved.

3. Chromosomal instability appears characteristic of cellular systems from which cancer is likely to emerge, as discussed throughout the present paper. Although the degree of chromosomal disruption and rearrangement in such systems may be impressive, it is probable that the instability alone has nothing to do directly with cancer other than to provide a predisposing background. For example, in a patient with Bloom's syndrome who developed acute leukemia, the high proportion of dividing lymphocytes showing chromosomal rearrangements was the same after the appearance of the leukemia as it had been during the previous 3 years (Sawitsky et al., 1966).

On occasion, chromosomal mutations arise in an individual's tissues without this high background of chromosomal instability, and, in fact, increased instability is not detected, as far as I am aware, in the nonmalignant cells of most cancer patients. (It might prove interesting to search for it in persons developing multiple primary cancers or in members of families demonstrating a predisposition to cancer, seemingly on a multigenic basis.)

4. Cancer is characterized pathologically by aberrant mitoses and nuclear pleomorphism (Kirkland et al., 1967; Levan, 1969). These abnormalities appear as an integral part of rampant, uncontrolled growth and are of the nature of cancer. Examination of cells in established cancers, as in established tissue-culture cell lines (Fig. 7), shows wide fluctuations in

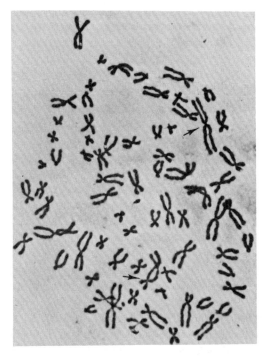

Fig. 7.—This metaphase from a human cell is abnormal because of both aneuploidy (72 chromosomes) and morphologically abnormal chromosomes (*arrows*). It is from an established tissue culture cell line (NCTC 3075) which was derived by Dr. V. J. Evans in 1953 from the skin of a normal man. Established cell lines, i.e., those capable of continuous growth in vitro, characteristically share many features in common with established cancers: the capacity for vigorous and continuous proliferation; aneuploidy; abnormal divisions with resulting variation in chromosome number from cell to cell; and marker chromosomes, derived through rearrangements, which characteristically are stable from generation to generation (*arrows*). Cell lines which have been derived from explants of normal tissue of experimental animals and which have become "established" in vitro have, in many cases, been shown to be malignant when transplanted back into the animal.

the number of chromosomes per cell (Spriggs et al., 1962; Yamada et al., 1966; Sandberg and Hossfeld, 1970), with occasional new chromosomal rearrangements as well. Ordinarily, cancers at this stage have acquired numerous extra chromosomes, and this, along with their newly achieved freedom from normal curbs on proliferation, permits the establishment of many different viable karyotypes. The confusing array of cytogenetic disturbances at this stage, although unrelated to any chromosomal mutation which may have been present or come into existence at the time of the original conversion to cancer, probably plays a role in its progression (Hauschka, 1961) and the evolution of "sidelines" (Grouchy, 1968; Levan, 1969; Turpin and Lejeune, 1969). Amid such a profusion of various karyotypes, a marker chromosome—common to all of the cells—might readily escape detection. (It is noteworthy that such changes in established cancers are the ones that have received the most attention from cytogeneticists from the time of Hansemann, 1890, down to the present.)

As with the imaginary mongol mentioned above, in whom it would have been a mistake to ignore chromosomal change as of etiological importance just because of the existence of complexity and confusion resulting from too many cytogenetic findings, it very well may be a serious mistake to ignore chromosomal mutation as of possible etiological importance in cancer simply because the problem is complex and as yet unclarified. If this attitude toward the cytogenetics of cancer is even nearly correct, the chromosomes will not only be restored to favor among professional oncologists but will also be studied with even greater diligence.

ACKNOWLEDGMENTS

I acknowledge with gratitude the financial support of the American Cancer Society (Grant E-461) and the National Institutes of Health (Grants HD 04134 and HE 09011). I also thank Mr. Edwin S. Geffner for helpful discussions and criticism of the manuscript.

REFERENCES

Atkin, N. B., and M. C. Baker. 1966. Chromosome abnormalities as primary events in human malignant disease: evidence from marker chromosome. J. Nat. Cancer Inst. 36:539-557.

Atkin, N. B., M. C. Baker, and S. Wilson. 1967. Stem-line karyotypes of 4 carcinomas of the cervix uteri. Amer. J. Obstet. Gynec. 99:506-514.

Beadle, G. W. 1933. A gene for sticky chromosomes in Zea mays. Z. Induktive Abstammungs- Vererbungslehre. 63:195-217.

Benedict, W. F., I. H. Porter, C. D. Brown, and R. A. Florentin. 1970. Cytogenetic diagnosis of malignancy in recurrent meningioma. Lancet 1:971-973.

Biemond, A. 1957. Paleocerebellar atrophy with extrapyramidal manifestations in association with bronchiectases and telangiectases of the conjunctiva bulbi as a familial syndrome. In van Bogaert, L., and J. Radermacker (Eds.), Proceedings of the First International Congress of Neurological Sciences, Vol. IV, pp. 206-208. New York, Pergamon Press.

Biggar, D., N. Lapointe, K. Ishizaka, H. Meuwissen, R. A. Good, and D. Frommel. 1970. IgE in ataxia-telangiectasia and family members. Lancet 2:1089.

Blakeslee, A. F. 1930. Quoted in Carnegie Inst. Yearbook, Vol. 29, p. 39.

Bloom, A. D., S. Neriishi, A. A. Awa, T. Honda, and P. G. Archer. 1967. Chromosome aberrations in leucocytes of older survivors of the atomic bombings of Hiroshima and Nagasaki. Lancet 2:802-805.

————, ————, N. Kamada, T. Iseki, and R. J. Keehn. 1966. Cytogenetic investigation of survivors of the atomic bombings of Hiroshima and Nagasaki. Lancet 2:672-674.

Bloom, D. 1966. The syndrome of congenital telangiectatic erythema and stunted growth: observations and studies. J. Pediat. 68:103-113.

Bloom, G. E., S. Warner, P. S. Gerald, and L. K. Diamond. 1966. Chromosome abnormalities in constitutional aplastic anemia. New Eng. J. Med. 274:8-14.

Boder, E., and R. P. Sedgwick. 1957. Ataxia-telangiectasia. A familial syndrome of progressive cerebellar ataxia, oculo-cutaneous telangiectasia and frequent pulmonary infection. Univ. Southern Calif. Med. Bull. 9:15-27, 51.

————, and ————. 1963. Ataxia-telangiectasia. A review of 101 cases. Little Club Clin. Develop. Med. 8:110-118.

Braun, A. C. 1969. The Cancer Problem. New York, Columbia University Press.

Bridges, C. B. 1923. Elimination of a chromosome due to a mutant (Minute-n) in Drosophila melanogaster. Proc. Nat. Acad. Sci. U.S.A. 11:701-706.

Buckton, K. E., P. A. Jacobs, W. M. Court Brown, and R. Doll. 1962. A study of the chromosome damage persisting after X-ray therapy for ankylosing spondylitis. Lancet 2:676-682.

Chaganti, R. S. K. 1965. Cytogenetic Studies of Maize-Tripsicum Hybrids and Their Derivatives, pp. i-iii, 93. Boston, Bussey Institution of Harvard University.

Clausen, R. E. 1931. Inheritance in Nicotiana tobaccum. XI. The fluted assemblage. Amer. Naturalist 65:316-331.

Cleaver, J. E. 1968. Defective repair replication of DNA in xeroderma pigmentosum. Nature 218:652-656.

Court Brown, W. M., and R. Doll. 1957. Leukemia and aplastic anemia in patients irradiated for spondylitis. Med. Res. Counc. Rep. no. 295.

————, K. E. Buckton, and A. O. Langlands. 1967. The identification of lymphocyte clones, with chromosome structural aberrations, in irradiated men and women. Int. J. Radiat. Biol. 13:155-168.

Cowdell, R. H., P. J. R. Phizackerley, and D. A. Pyke. 1955. Constitutional anemia (Fanconi's syndrome) and leukemia in two brothers. Blood. 10:788-801.

Donahue, R. P., W. B. Bias, J. H. Renwick, and V. A. McKusick. 1968. Probable assignment of the Duffy blood group locus to chromosome 1 in man. Proc. Nat. Acad. Sci. U.S.A. 61:949-955.

Emerit, I., J. de Grouchy, and P. Vernant. 1968. Deux observations de cassures identiques d'un même chromosome du groupe C. Ann. Genet. 11:22-27.

Engel, E., J. M. Flexner, M. L. Engel-de Montmollin, and H. E. Frank. 1964. Blood and skin chromosomal alterations of a clonal type in a leukemic man previously irradiated for lung carcinoma. Cytogenetics 3:228-251.

Erickson, J. 1965. Meiotic drive in Drosophila involving chromosome breakage. Genetics 51:555-571.

Fanconi, G. 1927. Familiäre infantile perniziosaartige Anämie (perniziöses Blutbild und Konstitution). Jahrb. Kinderheilk. 117:257-280.

———. 1967. Familial constitutional panmyelocytopathy, Fanconi's anemia (F. A.). I. Clinical aspects. Seminars Hemat. 4:233-240.

Fialkow, P. J. 1970. Genetic marker studies in neoplasia. In Genetic Concepts and Neoplasia, Baltimore, Williams & Wilkins, pp. 112-137.

———, S. M. Gartler, and A. Yoshida. 1967. Clonal origin of chronic myelocytic leukemia in man. Proc. Nat. Acad. Sci. U.S.A. 58:1468-1471.

Fitzgerald, P. H. 1967. The life-span and role of the small lymphocyte. In Evans, H. J., W. M. Court Brown, and A. S. McLean (Eds.), Human Radiation Cytogenetics, pp. 94-98. Amsterdam, North-Holland.

Ford, C. E. 1964. Selection pressure in mammalian cell populations. Sympos. Int. Soc. Cell Biol. 3:27-45.

———, and C. M. Clarke. 1963. Cytogenetic evidence of clonal proliferation in primary reticular neoplasms. Canad. Cancer Conf. 5:129-146.

———, J. L. Hamerton, and R. H. Mole. 1958. Chromosomal changes in primary and transplanted reticular neoplasms of the mouse. J. Cell. Comp. Physiol. 52 (Suppl. 1):235-269.

Garriga, S., and W. H. Crosby. 1959. The incidence of leukemia in families with hypoplasia of the marrow. Blood 14:1008-1014.

German, J. 1964. Cytological evidence for crossing-over in vitro in human lymphoid cells. Science 144:298-301.

———. 1966. The chromosomal structural load. Texas Rep. Biol. Med. 24 (Suppl.):347-364.

———. 1969. Bloom's syndrome. I. Genetical and clinical observations in the first twenty-seven patients. Amer. J. Hum. Genet. 21:196-227.

———, and R. S. K. Chaganti. Unpublished data.

———, and L. P. Crippa. 1966. Chromosomal breakage in diploid cell lines from Bloom's syndrome and Fanconi's anemia. Ann. Genet. 9:143-154.

———, and L. P. Crippa. Unpublished data.

———, R. Archibald, and D. Bloom. 1965. Chromosomal breakage in a rare and probably genetically determined syndrome of man. Science 148:506-507.

———, T. Gilleran, J. La Rock, and J. D. Regan. 1970. Mutant clones amid normal cells in cultures of xeroderma pigmentosum cells. Amer. J. Hum. Genet. 22:10a.

Girardi, A. J., D. Weinstein, and P. S. Moorhead. 1966. SV40 transformation of human diploid cells. Ann. Med. Exp. Fenn. 44:242-254.

Gmyrek, D., and I. Syllm-Rapoport. 1964. Zur Fanconi-Anämie. Analyse von 129 beschriebenen Fällen. Z. Kinderheilk. 91:297-337.

———, R. Witkowski, I. Syllm-Rapoport, and G. Jacobasch. 1967. Chromosomenaberrationen und Stoffwechselstörungen der Blutzellen bei Fanconi-Anämie vor und nach Übergang in Leukose am Beispiel einer Patientin. Deutsch. Med. Wschr. 92:1701-1707.

Gowen, M. S., and G. W. Gowen. 1922. Complete linkage in Drosophila melanogaster. Amer. Naturalist. 56:286-288.

Gropp, A., and G. Flatz. 1967. Chromosome breakage and blastic transformation of lymphocytes in ataxia-telangiectasia. Humangenetik 5:77-79.

Grouchy, J. de, 1968. A chromosomal theory of carcinogenesis. Ann. Int. Med. 69:381-391.

———, G. Vallée, and M. Lamy. 1963a. Analyse chromosomique de cellules cancéreuses et de cellules médullaires et sanguines irradiées "in vitro." Ann. Genet. 6:9-20.

———, ———, and ———. 1963b. Analyse chromosomique directe de deux tumeurs malignes. C. R. Acad. Sci. 256:2046-2048.

Hansemann, D. V. 1890. Über asymmetrische Zellteilung in Epithelkrebsen und der Biologische Bedeutung. Virchow Arch. [Path. Anat.] 119:299-326.

Hauschka, T. S. 1961. The chromosomes in ontogeny and oncogeny. Cancer Res. 21:957-974.

Hecht, F., and M. Case. 1969. Emergence of a clone of lymphocytes in ataxia-telangiectasia. Program of the annual meeting, American Society of Human Genetics, San Francisco (abstract), and personally communicated information.

———, R. D. Koler, D. A. Rigas, G. S. Dahnke, M. P. Case, V. Tisdale, and R. W. Miller. 1966. Leukaemia and lymphocytes in ataxia-telangiectasis. Lancet 2:1193.

Henderson, J. S., and J. German. 1967. Unpublished cytogenetic data. See footnote in J. Exp. Med. 125:71-90.

Hirschman, R. J., N. R. Shulman, J. G. Abuelo, and J. Whang-Peng. 1969. Chromosomal aberrations in two cases of inherited aplastic anemia with unusual clinical features. Ann. Int. Med. 71:107-117.

Ishihara, T., and T. Kumatori. 1967. Chromosome studies on Japanese exposed to radiation resulting from nuclear bomb explosions. In Evans, H. J., W. M. Court Brown, and A. S. McLean (Eds.), Human Radiation Cytogenetics, pp. 144-166. Amsterdam, North-Holland.

Jordan, N., and J. McGuire. Dyskeratosis congenita: a report of two cases. In preparation.

Karpati, G., A. H. Eisen, F. Andermann, H. L. Bacal, and P. Robb. 1965. Ataxia-telangiectasia. Amer. J. Dis. Child. 110:51-63.

Kirkland, J. A., M. A. Stanley, and K. M. Cellier. 1967. Comparative study of histologic and chromosomal abnormalities in cervical neoplasia. Cancer 20:1934-1952.

Kunze-Mühl, E., P. Fischer, and E. Golob. 1970. Spezifische Aberration eines Chromosoms der C-Gruppe bei mehreren Mitgliedern einer Sippe. Humangenetik 9:91-96.

Lawler, S. D., and R. Sanger. 1970. Xg blood-groups and clonal-origin theory of chronic myeloid leukaemia. Lancet 1:584-585.

Lejeune, J., R. Berger, and M. O. Rethore. 1966. Sur l'endoreduplication sélective de certains segments du génome. C. R. Acad. Sci. Paris. 263:1880-1882.

———, B. Dutrillaux, J. Lafourcade, R. Berger, D. Abonyi, and M. D. Rethore. 1968. Endoreduplication sélective du bras long du chromosome 2 chez une femme et sa fille. C. R. Acad. Sci. 266:24-26.

Lesley, M. M., and H. B. Frost. 1927. Mendelian inheritance of chromosome shape in Matthiola. Genetics 12:449-460.

Levan, A. 1969. Chromosome abnormalities and carcinogenesis. In Lima de Faria, A., (Ed.), Handbook of Molecular Cytology, pp. 716-731. New York, Wiley.

———, and J. J. Biesele. 1958. Role of chromosomes in cancerogenesis, as studied in serial tissue culture of mammalian cells. Ann. N.Y. Acad. Sci. 71:1022-1053.

Lewis, E. B. 1957. Leukemia and ionizing radiation. Science 125:965-972.

Lima de Faria, A., and P. Sarvella. 1962. Variation of the chromosome phenotype in *Zea, Solanum* and *Salvia.* Chromosoma 13:300-314.

Linder, D., and S. M. Gartler. 1965. Glucose-6-phosphate dehydrogenase mosaicism: utilization as a cell marker in the study of leiomyomas. Science 150:67-69.

Löhr, G. W., H. D. Waller, F. Anschütz, and A. Knopp. 1965. Hexokinasemangel in Blutzellen bei einer Sippe mit familiärer Panmyelopathie (Typ Fanconi) Klin. Wschr. 43:870-875.

Louis-Bar, Madame. 1941. Sur un syndrome progressif comprenant des télangiectasies capillaires cutanées et conjonctivales symétriques, à disposition naevoïde et des troubles cérébelleux. Confin. Neurol. 4:32-42.

Lubs, H. A., and S. Kotler. 1967. The prognostic significance of chromosome abnormalities in colon tumors. Ann. Int. Med. 67:328-336.

Magenis, E. R., F. Hecht, and E. W. Lovrien. 1970. Heritable fragile site on chromosome 16: probable localization of haptoglobin locus in man. Science 170:85-87.

Makino, S., M. S. Sasaki, and A. Tonomura. 1964. Cytological studies of tumors. XL. Chromosome studies in fifty-two tumors. J. Nat. Cancer Inst. 32:741-777.

McClintock, B. 1956. Controlling elements and the gene. Cold Spring Harbor Sympos. Quant. Biol. 21:197-216.

Moorhead, P. S. 1970. Virus effects on host chromosomes. In Genetics: Concepts and Neoplasia, pp. 281-306. Baltimore, Williams & Wilkins.

———, and E. Saksela. 1963. Non-random chromosomal aberrations in SV40-transformed human cells. J. Cell. Comp. Physiol. 62:57-72.

Naspitz, C. K., A. H. Eisen, and M. Richter. 1968. DNA synthesis in vitro in leukocytes from patients with ataxia telangiectasia. Int. Arch. Allerg. 33:217-226.

Nowell, P. C., 1965. Chromosome changes in primary tumors. Progr. Exp. Tumor Res. 7:83-103.

Peterson, R. D. A., M. D. Cooper, and R. A. Good. 1966. Lymphoid tissue abnormalities associated with ataxia-telangiectasia. Amer. J. Med. 41:342-359.

———, and R. A. Good. 1969. Ataxia-telangiectasia. Birth Defects: Orig. Art. Ser. 4(1):370-377.

Pfeiffer, R. A. 1970. Chromosomal abnormalities in ataxia-telangiectasia (Louis-Bar's syndrome). Humangenetik 8:302-306.

Pomerat, C. M., A. Awa, and Y. Ohnuki. 1961. Some comparative effects of smoked paper, tobacco and cigarettes on chromosomes in vitro. Texas Rep. Biol. Med. 19:518-528.

———, Y. H. Nakanishi, and M. Mizutani. 1959. Smoke condensates on lung cells in tissue culture with special reference to chromosomal changes. Texas Rep. Biol. Med. 17:542-590.

Rauh, J. L., and S. W. Soukup. 1968. Bloom's syndrome. Amer. J. Dis. Child. 116:409-413.

Regan, J. D., J. E. Trosko, W. L. Carrier. 1968. Evidence for excision of ultraviolet-induced pyrimidine dimers from the DNA of human cells in vitro. Biophys. J. 8:319-325.

Regan, J. D., R. B. Setlow, W. L. Carrier, and W. H. Lee. Molecular events following the ultraviolet irradiation of human cells from ultraviolet-sensitive individuals. Proc. 4th Int. Congr. Radiat. Res. In press.

Rous, P. 1959. Surmise and fact on the nature of cancer. Nature 183:1357-1361.

———. 1967. The challenge to man of the neoplastic cell. Cancer Res. 27:1919-1924.

Sandberg, A. A., and D. K. Hossfeld. 1970. Chromosomal abnormalities in human neoplasia. Ann. Rev. Med. 21:379-408.

Sandler, L., D. L. Lindsley, B. Nicoletti, and G. Trippa. 1968. Mutants affecting meiosis in natural populations of Drosophila melanogaster. Genetics. 60:525-558.

Sasaki, M. S., and S. Makino. 1965. Cytological studies of tumors. XLII. Chromosome abnormalities in malignant lymphomas in man. Cancer 18:1007-1013.

Sawitsky, A., D. Bloom, and J. German. 1966. Chromosomal breakage and acute leukemia in congenital telangiectatic erythema and stunted growth. Ann. Int. Med. 65:487-495.

Schmid, W. 1967. Familial constitutional panmyelocytopathy, Fanconi's anemia (F.A.). II. A discussion of the cytogenetic findings in Fanconi's anemia. Seminars Hemat. 4:241-249.

———, and D. Vischer. 1969. Spontaneous fragility of an abnormally wide secondary constriction in a human chromosome No. 9. Humangenetik 7:22-27.

———, K. Schärer, Th. Baumann, and G. Fanconi. 1965. Chromosomenbrüchigkeit bei der familiären Panmyelopathie (Typus Fanconi). Schweiz. Med. Wschr. 95:1461-1464.

Schroeder, T. M. 1966a. Cytogenetische und cytologische Befunde bei enzymopenischen Panmyelopathien und Pancytopenien. Familiäre Panmyelopathie Typ Fanconi, Glutathionreduktasemangel-Anämie und megaloblastare Vitamin B12-Mangel-Anämie. Humangenetik 2:287-316.

———. 1966b. Cytogenetischer Befund und Ätiologie bei Fanconi-Anämie. Ein Fall von Fanconi-Anämie ohne Hexokinasedefekt. Humangenetik 3:76-81.

———, and J. German. Unpublished data.

———, and R. Kurth. 1971. Spontaneous chromosomal breakage and high incidence of leukemia in inherited disease. Blood 37:96-112.

———, F. Anschütz, and A. Knopp. 1964. Spontane Chromosomenaberrationen bei familiärer Panmyelopathie. Humangenetik 1:194-196.

Seltser, R., and P. E. Sartwell. 1965. The influence of occupational exposure to radiation on the mortality of American radiologists and other medical specialists. Amer. J. Epidem. 81:2-22.

Setlow, J. K. 1967. The effects of ultraviolet radiation and photoreactivation. In Florkin, M., and E. H. Stotz (Eds.), Comprehensive Biochemistry, Vol. 27, pp. 157-209. Amsterdam, Elsevier.

Setlow, R. B., J. D. Regan, J. German, and W. L. Carrier. 1969. Evidence that xerodermapigmentosum cells do not perform the first step in the repair of ultraviolet damage to their DNA. Proc. Nat. Acad. Sci. U.S.A. 64:1035-1041.

Shaw, M. W., and M. M. Cohen. 1965. Chromosome exchanges in human leukocytes induced by mitomycin C. Genetics 51:181-190.

Shein, H. M., and J. F. Enders. 1962. Transformation induced by simian virus 40 in human renal cell cultures. I. Morphology and growth characteristics. Proc. Nat. Acad. Sci. U.S.A. 48:1164-1172.

Silver, H. K., W. C. Blair, and C. H. Kempe. 1952. Fanconi syndrome; multiple congenital anomalies with hypoplastic anemia. Amer. J. Dis. Child. 83:14-25.

Simpson, C. L., L. H. Hempelmann, and L. M. Fuller. 1955. Neoplasia in children treated with X-rays in infancy for thymic enlargement. Radiology 64:840-845.

Spiers, A. S. D., and A. G. Baikie. 1968. Cytogenetic studies in the malignant lymphomas and related neoplasms. Cancer 22:193-217.

Spriggs, A. I., M. M. Boddington, and C. M. Clarke. 1962. Chromosomes of human cancer cells. Brit. Med. J. 2:1431-1435.

Stern, C. 1936. Somatic crossing over and segregation in *Drosophila melanogaster.* Genetics 21:625-730.

Stewart, A., and G. W. Kneale. 1970. Radiation dose effects in relation to obstetric X-rays and childhood cancers. Lancet 1:1185-1188.

Strober, W., R. D. Wochner, M. H. Barlow, D. E. McFarlin, and T. A. Waldmann. 1968. Immunoglobulin metabolism in ataxia telangiectasia. J. Clin. Invest. 47:1905-1915.

Swift, M. 1971. Fanconi's anaemia in the genetics of neoplasia. Nature 230:370-373.

Tjio, J. H., and G. Ostergren. 1958. The chromosomes of primary mammary carcinomas in milk virus strains of the mouse. Hereditas 44:451-465.

Todaro, G. J. 1968. Radiation enhancement of SV40 transformation in 3T3 and human cells. Nature 219:520-521.

————, H. Green, and M. R. Swift. 1966. Susceptibility of human diploid fibroblast strains to transformation by SV40 virus. Science 153:1252-1254.

Tough, I. M., and W. M. Court Brown. 1965. Chromosome aberrations and exposure to ambient benzene. Lancet 1:684.

Turpin, R., and J. Lejeune. 1969. Leukemia and cancer. Human Afflictions and Chromosomal Aberrations, pp. 134-158. New York, Pergamon Press.

Van Valen, P. 1966. Oligiosyndactylism, an early embryonic lethal in the mouse. J. Embryol. Exp. Morph. 15:119-124.

Vigliani, E. C., and G. Saita. 1964. Benzene and leukemia. New Eng. J. Med. 271:872-876.

Visfeldt, J. 1966. Clone formation in tissue culture. Experience from long-term cultures of irradiated human skin. Acta Path. Microbiol. Scand. 68:305-312.

————. 1967. Chromosome aberrations in occupationally exposed personnel in a radiotherapy department. In Evans, H. J., W. M. Court Brown, and A. S. McLean (Eds.), Human Radiation Cytogenetics, pp. 167-173. Amsterdam, North Holland.

Wells, C. E., and G. M. Shy. 1957. Progressive familial choreoathetosis with cutaneous telangiectasia. J. Neurol. Neurosurg. Psychiat. 20:98-104.

Yamada, K., N. Takagi, and A. A. Sandberg. 1966. Chromosomes and causation of human cancer and leukemia. II. Karyotypes of human solid tumors. Cancer 19:1879-1890.

Yerganian, G., H. M. Shein, and J. F. Enders. 1962. Chromosomal disturbances observed in human fetal renal cells transformed in vitro by simian virus 40 and carried in culture. Cytogenetics 1:314-324.

Ying, K. L., and E. J. Ives. 1968. Asymmetry of chromosome number 1 pair in three generations of a phenotypically normal family. Canad. J. Genet. Cytol. 10:575-589.

CHAPTER 3

The Future of Human Population Genetics

Newton E. Morton

Population Genetics Laboratory, University of Hawaii, Honolulu, Hawaii.

ONE OF THE CHARMS OF MOLECULAR GENETICS is that its senior practitioners, when they tire of the laboratory bench, can be sure of reverent attention if they philosophize about human populations. Such sport is ordinarily closed to the population geneticist, whose qualifications are quite properly suspect. Therefore when I was invited to write this paper, I welcomed the opportunity as one that will not soon recur, only to discover that the three terms *human, population genetics,* and *future* are loaded and obscure.

To begin with the superficially innocuous attribute of humanity, this restricts me to the genus *Homo,* of which Mayr (1950) has written: "There is no conclusive evidence that more than one species of hominids has ever existed at a given time." Surely not a disturbing conclusion, until one considers the opinion of Lewontin (1967) that "population genetics is really evolutionary genetics. . . . The major unsolved problem of descriptive population genetics is an adequate specification of the genetic difference between two closely related species as compared to the genetic difference between two populations of the same species." While biochemical and serological polymorphisms and the fixation of amino acid substitutions make possible many comparisons between the related genera *Homo* and *Pongo* (to which the chimpanzee and gorilla belong), man is not an especially favorable organism for population genetics if we accept Lewontin's definition.

Is it true that "population genetics is really evolutionary genetics"? Suppose we agree with Dobzhansky (1951) that "evolution is a change in the genetic composition of populations." Then genetic equilibria due to balance between opposing forces of selection, mutation, or migration are not an aspect of evolution. Or suppose we agree with Mayr (1942) that "the

---

PGL paper 86.

systematist who studies the factors of evolution wants to find out how species originate, how they are related, and what this relationship means." This orientation made it natural for Mayr (1959) to write that Fisher, Wright, and Haldane "have worked out an impressive mathematical theory of genetical variation and evolutionary change. But what, precisely, has been the contribution of this mathematical school to evolutionary theory?"

Both survivors of the great triumvirate of population genetics rose to the question. Wright (1960) argued that "The role of the mathematical theory is that of an intermediary between the bodies of factual knowledge discovered at two levels, that of the individual and that of the population. It must deduce from the postulates at the level of the individual and from models of population structure what is to be expected in populations, and then modify its postulates and models on the basis of any discrepancies with observation and so on." Haldane (1964) characteristically preferred counterattack to defense. What, he asked, have been the contributions of the nonmathematical "newer population genetics" which Mayr so greatly admired? The last decade has provided the answer. Such vague concepts as "the coadapted harmony of the gene pool," "genetic cohesion," and "the genetics of integrated gene complexes," while eminently suitable for biological philosophers, have not proved heuristic guides to experimentation or mathematical deduction. Haldane (1964) put the matter succinctly when he wrote, "I hope I have given enough examples to justify my complete mistrust of verbal arguments when algebraic arguments are possible, and my skepticism when not enough facts are known to permit of algebraic arguments."

This discussion has made it perfectly clear to me that population genetics is mathematical genetics, of which evolutionary genetics is a subspeciality. Mathematical genetics may undertake from established properties of individuals to determine the properties of populations, or (as is often more interesting in nonexperimental material) to infer from the manifestation of a phenotype in a population its inheritance in individuals. To a geneticist the forward solution is no more basic than the backward solution. It may sometimes be meaningful to distinguish studies which lead to novel mathematical deductions as "theoretical population genetics," in opposition to "inductive population genetics," which uses familiar mathematical results, but such a distinction is more relevant to mathematicians than to geneticists, who judge research not in terms of its mathematical sophistication but the richness of its biological implications.

Having attempted to clarify the scope of human population genetics, the definition of *future* need not long concern us. I believe that the remarks of this paper will hold true for the next decade. After that, prophecy becomes more dangerous, but I think that Haldane's opinion will be justified for a much longer time: "beanbag genetics, so far from being obsolete, has hardly begun its triumphant career."

PHENOTYPE SYSTEMS

The formal correspondence between genotypes and phenotypes is an example of mathematical genetics with a wealth of applications in populations (Cotterman, 1953). Recently emphasis has shifted to the subset called *factor-union systems,* in which it is possible to assign to each allele a set of binary properties, called *factors,* in such a way that the phenotypes of all genotypes are specified by Boolean unions of alleles. Thus each factor is dominant to its absence. The formal properties of factor-union systems give simple parentage-exclusion rules and are the basis of general computer programs for determining gene frequencies and segregation patterns (Cotterman, 1969). Factors subject to diagnostic errors may be omitted or redefined to improve classification of phenotypes (Morton, 1969), or a set of factors may be used to define a sublocus (Bodmer et al., 1969), the common alleles in a population, or the allelic associations of a new factor with previously recognized ones (Morton and Miki, 1968). In an antigenic system each factor ideally corresponds to one antiserum, the value of which for various types of genetic study may be readily ascertained by comparing the information in the system when the factor is included or excluded. Such comparison should be a routine part of large population studies, where too inclusive a choice of factors can lead to enormous cost with little yield.

Leukocyte antigens, with their great significance for tissue transplantation, provide a fertile field for factor-union concepts. Many of the reagents are weak or multispecific. Therefore various methods of cluster analysis have been applied to define antigenic specificities (Bodmer et al., 1969; Elston, 1967). To test whether a specificity defined in this way belongs to a factor-union system, we must show that there is negligible overlap between phenotypes with and without the factor. A simple test is by stepwise least-squares regression of a preliminary dichotomy of antigenic specificity on reagent scores, the resulting discriminant being trichotomized into 0,1, and ?. Rejecting the doubtful group, a second stepwise regression gives an improved discriminant which should be sharply bimodal and may be used to classify individuals with respect to the factor. Segregation analysis and estimation of allele frequencies in association with previously defined factors complete the evidence. If fully penetrant, such factors defined on multivariate scores can be treated just as any other components of a factor-union system. Diagnosis of factors in host and prospective donors is the major problem of histocompatibility in man, and its solution should greatly increase the success of tissue transplantation.

ESTIMATION AND TESTS OF HYPOTHESES

While population genetics is mathematical, it is not entirely deductive (just as cytogenetics is not entirely microscopical, or molecular genetics entirely biochemical). Predictions must be "checked against observed proportions to see whether the theory that has been developed is sufficient to explain the facts. If prediction and observation are not in agreement, new phenomena, not previously considered, must be sought and, indeed, are sometimes found. It is this testing of prediction against observation and the subsequent resolution of contradictions that provides the only constructive method for the discovery of new phenomena in population genetics" (Lewontin, 1967).

Classical methods of estimation depend on taking partial derivatives of the logarithmic likelihood when this is specified, or of a sum of squares otherwise. Roots of such equations are readily found by iteration unless the likelihood surface departs too markedly from a multinormal form. Evaluation of derivatives as finite differences makes it feasible to study mathematically complex hypotheses, such as arise in multifactorial inheritance. Various hill-climbing methods to explore an ill-conditioned likelihood surface have been proposed, but seldom used (Elston, 1969). Failure of iteration to converge poses problems in numerical analysis which are still not satisfactorily solved.

Population genetics provides examples of completely specified prior probabilities suitable for Bayesian methods of estimation. These have been explored in the case of linkage, where typically only a single parameter has to be determined (e.g., Renwick, 1969). However, the prior probability is only known approximately, so that some investigators have preferred not to introduce it into tests of significance (Morton, 1962). The power of Bayesian and probability ratio methods under various prior probabilities remains to be studied.

In many areas of population genetics recurrence equations arise which defy explicit solution. Too often an asymptotic approximation is accepted, when numerical solution by a computer is easy and much more accurate. For example, in the limit for large distance the decline of kinship depends on dimensionality of migration (Malécot, 1959; Kimura and Weiss, 1964), whereas direct numerical evaluation shows that at distances small enough for kinship to be measurable, dimensionality is unimportant (Imaizumi et al., 1970).

Development of high-speed computers has made possible a novel kind of hypothesis-testing through stochastic (Monte Carlo) simulation, in which pseudorandom numbers are introduced to represent effects of assortative mating, differential fertility, and segregation. Such simulation is enormously expensive compared to deterministic processes, and there is general agreement that algebraic solutions be used as much as possible (Levin, 1969; Bodmer, 1969). Whether there will remain stochastic elements intractable to analytic formulation remains to be seen, but I share Haldane's "skepticism when not enough facts are known to permit of algebraic arguments."

Through emphasis on tests of hypotheses, population genetics has much to contribute to genetic anthropology. For many years the *Annals of Eugenics* bore on its cover a quotation from Francis Galton beginning: "General impressions are never to be trusted. Unfortunately when they are of long standing they become fixed rules of life, and assume a prescriptive right not to be questioned. Consequently those who are not accustomed to original inquiry entertain a hatred and a horror of statistics." It is likely that any anthropology journal imprudent enough to place such a passage on its cover would have lost its subscribers. A respected handbook of the Royal Anthropological Institution (*Notes and Queries on Anthropology,* 1967) advises: "It should be stated whether the clans are exogamous," as if all marriages followed a rule. Actually, in most societies the frequencies of mating patterns are not clearly perceived either by the members or by qualitative observers, and are not accurately described by rules except those derived from a statistical analysis of the matings themselves. It is a remarkable fact that the hundreds of references of kinship contain little information on the frequencies of mating patterns, raising the question whether the intricate subsections and circulating connubia of kinship theory have ever existed at any time in any population (Morton et al., 1970a). Fusion of population genetics with anthropology should help to disseminate quantitative methods in the human sciences.

SEGREGATION ANALYSIS

In the period B.C. (before computers) ingenious methods were devised to study homogeneous segregation patterns, but it was not until the introduction of maximum likelihood scoring by high-speed computers that analysis of complex segregation patterns became feasible. Early results were for families that could and could not segregate and for a mixture of sporadic and high-risk cases (Morton, 1959). These have now been generalized to a mixture of many segregation patterns, as with multifactorial inheritance or incomplete penetrance at a single locus (Elandt-Johnson,

1970). Smith (1970) introduced the polychotomized normal distribution to compute probabilities by summation instead of multiple integration, making it possible to test the hypothesis of quasicontinuity, under which a normal distribution of genetic liability is acted on by a cumulative normal environmental risk function. It remains to be determined whether this model is tenable for traits of complex etiology, like clubfoot and cleft lip, and whether it can be discriminated from other complex models, such as the generalized single locus with incomplete penetrance.

This question is far from academic, since genetic counseling and the long-term consequences of improved treatment and carrier detection differ markedly among genetic hypotheses. Statements of recurrence risk as a function of normal and affected relatives have been remarkably imprecise. Many counselors are content to know the magnitude of risk for a large class of families. This is analogous to a life insurance company assigning premiums independent of age and physical condition. A minimum standard for genetic counseling is to determine the risks associated simultaneously with 0, 1, or 2 parents affected and s sibs of whom r are affected. Such statements can be made and the risks tabulated for any genetic hypothesis which fits the segregation data. Very limited experience supports the expectation that two hypotheses which fit a substantial body of data necessarily predict closely similar risks for all the commonly observed segregation patterns.

While it may not be important for genetic counseling to discriminate between two *well-fitting* hypotheses, the long-term effects of treatment and carrier detection depend critically on the genetic basis of affection. The prevention of disease due to a single locus with manifest carriers is relatively easy, whereas multifactorial systems offer less opportunity for carrier detection and respond poorly to selection on a rare phenotype. Even collection of large bodies of data suitable for complex segregation analysis may not resolve the basis of affection, although providing reliable risks for genetic counseling.

Special challenges are posed by chromosomal anomalies, which may segregate differently among families. Analysis must test for and describe this heterogeneity. A possible approach is through the hypergeometric Gini-Skellam distribution, which arises through binomial trials from risks which vary as a beta distribution among families (Morton, 1969).

KINSHIP

Human biologists often make statements about the relationship of two populations, say I and J. Such a statement can take several forms, for example:

1. I is more related to J than to a third population K.

2. I and J are descended from the same ancestral population K some t generations (or fissions) ago.

3. The probability that a random gene in I be identical by descent with a random allele in J is ϕ_{ij}.

The first of these statements is inherently vague. We are not told what "related" means, although it presumably implies common ancestry, and so we cannot demand whether I is twice as related to J as to K, or 10% more related, or in general enquire what the relationship is. The usual approach is to maximize a sum of squares, although this confers the undesirable property of increasing with the number of variables, and the object of these studies is not to discriminate among populations. In this misapplication of discriminant functions no estimation problem is raised, and each investigator is free to define his own "index of biological distance" without the slightest risk that it be dismissed as irrelevant or inefficient (Balakrishnan and Sangvhi, 1968).

The second statement seems by comparison delightfully precise, since it purports to measure the time span back to an ancestral population. This is, in fact, a classical approach to major taxonomic categories. It is informative to deduce from the fossil record that hominids diverged from the great apes about 10 million years ago; while the estimate is inexact, there is no doubt that the two reproductively isolated phylogenies did indeed separate at roughly that time. Unfortunately, once we turn out attention to the subspecific level, and especially to microtaxonomic differences, a model of population fusion without hybridization becomes unacceptable, especially when applied to a migratory species like man (Kurcyznski, 1969). If we suspend, for the moment, any reservations about the assumptions underlying recent exercises in microtaxonomy (Edwards, 1969), what meaning are we to attach to the inference that Guaymi Indians are separated by one fission from Yanomama and by five fissions from Jivaro (Fitch and Neel, 1969), when the fissions are entirely hypothetical and ignore the population movement and hybridizations which are an essential part of microevolution? One is discouraged from a more detailed consideration of this approach, requiring as it does the hypothesis of uniform rates of change of angularly transformed gene frequencies, together with empirical approximations to the apparently intractable maximum likelihood estimation of tree form and node times (Edwards, 1968).

As a geneticist, therefore, I favor statements of the third type, invoking the concept of identity by descent. Admittedly this approach requires that a sample of loci determining selected traits be considered a random sample of all loci. This assumption, which underlies all other approaches, does not seem a major objection, and in any case can be satisfied asymptotically by increasing the number of loci sampled. The advantage of this formulation is that ϕ_{ij}, unlike other measures of biological distance, is a clearly defined genetic parameter (the coefficient of kinship, or more briefly, *kinship*) and has a simple interpretation in terms of the expected phenotype frequencies in a cross between populations. No transformation of gene frequencies is necessary or desirable, and there is no need to determine the latent roots of a matrix. Estimates of kinship may be averaged over loci simply by weighting with the amounts of information. Microtaxonomy can only hope to recognize phenotypic similarity, without being able to impose on plausible assumptions any nonreticulate branching process. Kinship summarizes all of the taxonomic information, and the next decade should see complete abandonment of less genetic ways to measure biological distance.

Undoubtedly the slowness of investigators to adopt kinship to measure biological distance is due to difficulty in its estimation. The direct approach through gene frequency variance includes errors of estimation from dominance and incomplete sampling (Workman and Niswander, 1970). Random pairing of phenotypes avoids this, but is valid only if ϕ_{ij} is less than all gene frequencies (Yasuda, 1969). Simple dominant systems give no information, and ABO-like systems negligible information, if kinship and gene frequencies are estimated simultaneously.

Recently an alternative procedure has been advanced, which estimates the frequency of homozygosis

$$\sum_k q_{ki}^2$$

for a locus with frequency q_{ki} of the kth allele in the ith panmictic subpopulation (Morton et al., 1970b). Kinship is a simple function of these quantities. Frequencies of genes not known to be present in the subpopulation are set to zero. No assumption is made about the relative magnitudes of kinship and gene frequencies. Information is extracted even from dominant and ABO-like systems. An analogous procedure estimates kinship from clan or surname concordance (isonymy) and from quantitative traits (assuming known heritability and a homogeneous environment among subpopulations). Therefore uniformity of kinship estimates can be tested among genetic systems, with the possibility of pooling estimates or recognizing meaningful heterogeneity among systems due to differences in selection or other systematic pressures.

Kinship bioassay is now at the stage of linkage detection and gene frequency estimation of a generation ago. A succession of workers (Bernstein, Wiener, Haldane, and Fisher) developed appropriate methods of increasing efficiency. However, it was not until Fisher examined the likelihood that fully efficient estimation became feasible. The likelihood for kinship depends on the distribution of gene frequencies among populations. If all populations were of the same size and subject to the same systematic pressure, gene frequency variation would approximate the multivariate beta density, with suitable modification for populations in which a gene has temporarily been lost (Crow and Kimura, 1970). However, the assumption of uniform population structure is not generally valid. This is unfortunate, not only because it forces us to use eclectic estimators of unknown efficiency instead of maximum likelihood theory, but also because one would like to find some use for the gene frequency distributions to which theoretical population geneticists have devoted so much effort.

Bioassay contrasts with deduction of kinship from genealogy and migration. The genealogical method has the unique property of predicting kinship not only as a mean between groups of individuals, but primarily as a relation between pairs of individuals. In practice random pairs are usually substituted for all possible pairs, so that ϕ_{ij} is estimated rather than deduced precisely. The estimate of ϕ_{ii} is usually found to agree closely with α_i, the inbreeding in population i averaged over all marital pairs, since avoidance of incest tends to be balanced by an excess of more remote consanguinity. The main limitation of the genealogical method is that it assumes complete knowledge of the pedigree for indefinitely many generations.

This assumption is avoided both in bioassay and the method of migration matrices (Malécot, 1950; Imaizumi et al., 1970), which therefore provide a measure of the importance of systematic pressures and of relationship so remote that it is not given in the pedigree. The main disadvantage of migration matrices is that the input parameters must be estimated, usually over a small number of generations, and so estimates of ϕ_{ij} may have large errors. Bioassay therefore provides the ultimate test of predictions derived from genealogy and migration. The number of studies which have used all three or even any two of these methods to estimate kinship is still small, so that our knowledge of kinship in human populations is scanty. Interest in this area is high, and suitable data are already available or not difficult to collect. It seems likely that many studies will soon be directed to this problem, especially in populations at demographic extremes of isolation, small size, low density, and preferential exogamy or consanguineous marriage. Especially in southern India populations have been reported with strongly preferential consanguineous marriage. There remains some doubt whether the alleged relationships are biological or classificatory. If the former, these populations may provide an opportunity to observe the effects of high levels of inbreeding and simultaneously to determine the consequences of clan exogamy and caste endogamy.

POPULATION STRUCTURE

A large body of theory, treating closed populations of effective size N, is inapplicable to real populations, which are never closed. Therefore Wright (1931) and Malécot (1948) introduced the concept of linearized systematic pressure,

$$m = -\frac{\partial \Delta}{\partial q} \Big| Q$$

where

$$\Delta = -m(q - Q) + O(q - Q)^2$$

is the rate of change of gene frequency q per generation and Q is the equilibrium value of q. The effects of mutation and migration on Δ are exactly linear in q, whereas selection is in general a quadratic function of q, but the linear part dominates unless Nm is small.

Population geneticists have tended to underestimate the contribution of migration to m. Kimura et al. (1963) found that genetic loads increase as population size decreases, but their mathematical results hold only for closed populations. MacCluer and Schull (1970) considered that crude immigration rates of 8.4% for males and 13.5% for females (mostly from nearby populations) made negligible contributions to m in a Japanese isolate, which they simulated by a closed artificial population of small size. Naturally inbreeding in the artificial population increased asymptotically to unity, whereas the observed value was only 0.011. While this is an underestimate because it omits remote relationship, the true value is certainly closer to 0.011 than to 1, since genetic variability is about as great in isolates as in large populations (Neel and Salzano, 1967).

Because of the great biological importance of m, and the likelihood that it is dominated by migration, it seems interesting to define an effective value m_e which describes the evolution of kinship with time. The basic equation for kinship in the tth generation is

$$\phi^{(t)} \doteq \Phi(1 - e^{-t/2N_e\Phi})$$

$$\Phi \equiv \phi^{(\infty)} = \frac{1}{4N_e m_e + 1}$$

Here the effective size is denoted by N_e to symbolize the fact that it also is estimated from the evolution of kinship. A complex migration pattern described by a migration matrix, a vector of effective population sizes, and a linearized systematic pressure m (usually ignoring mutation and selection) predicts $\phi^{(t)}$, successive values of which may be fitted by the above equation, estimating N_e and m_e simultaneously (Morton et al., 1970a). We find that short-range migration within the matrix contributes to m_e, and N_e is larger than estimated from census size and fertility of the local population because of contributions from neighboring gene pools. Formally this equation can be fitted to off-diagonal elements of the kinship matrix, in which case N_e may be much larger than local population size, testifying to the slowness with which such kinship approaches equilibrium. Estimates of $\phi^{(t)}$ from genealogies also permit calculations of N_e and m_e. Since m_e is nearly constant when the vector of population sizes is multiplied by a constant, the best procedure in either natural or artificial populations is to estimate N_e and m_e simultaneously from a preliminary vector of population sizes (N), the pressure m, and a migration matrix, and then use this value of m_e to obtain an improved estimate of N_e from genealogies, which need not extend for many generations (Morton et al., 1970b). In this way the relevant demographic variables and the genealogy are condensed into the two parameters m_e and N_e for each population and pair of populations, and the future state of a system with these parameters can be predicted. If N_e and m_e are not constant and there is enough knowledge to estimate $N_e^{(t)}$ and $m_e^{(t)}$, we may use the recurrence

$$\phi^{(t)} = [1 - m_e^{(t)}]^2 \{1/2N_e^{(t)} + [1 - 1/2N_e^{(t)}]\phi^{(t-1)}\}$$

but usually this refinement is neither feasible nor necessary.

The central problem of population structure was posed by Lewontin (1967): "It is unavoidable that effective population sizes and migration rates will be very difficult to estimate except for rare cases of completely isolated populations living in well-defined areas. For more continuous distribution, it may be that N and m are simply inappropriate parameters and that some other way of describing the breeding structure is preferable." We see that N_e and m_e are appropriate parameters for any population or pair of populations. It is no accident that the solution of Lewontin's problem was provided by human material, since no other organism yet furnishes comparable data on migration and genealogy.

As the number of populations in an array increases, we lose interest in the specific values of kinship and look for a more succinct description of population structure. This was provided by the theory of Malécot (1959), which depends on the Euclidean distance d between pairs of populations. In practice it seems to make little difference, and may sometimes be more appropriate, if we take d as the shortest road distance (Cavalli-Sforza, 1969).

As originally derived, in the limit for large distances, there was an annoying effect of dimensionality of migration. Fortunately, at the smaller distances where kinship is significantly positive, observations on real populations and study of artificial populations have shown that

$$\phi(d) \doteq ae^{-bd}$$

where

$$a \doteq \frac{1}{1 + 4N\sqrt{m(m + 2 - 2H)}}$$

$$b \doteq \sqrt{2m/\sigma^2}$$

regardless of dimensionality (Imaizumi et al., 1970). Here σ^2 is defined somewhat ambiguously as the expected value of the square of the distance between birth places of parent and child, excluding long-range migration which enters only into systematic pressure m, and H is the proportion of parents born in a population who reproduce there.

Kinship studies are concerned not as much with the approximation for a and b as with the wide validity of the exponential form $\phi(d)$. Earlier work concentrated on this relationship, whose parameters a, b vary widely among populations (Morton, 1969). Large values of a (0.03 or more) have been found in island and primitive populations, while large values of b are characteristic of continental isolates but not oceanic islands or wide-ranging hunters and gatherers (Roisenberg and Morton, 1969; Imaizumi et al., 1970). Clearly b is inversely related to migration.

Whereas only predictive approaches are applicable to the evolution of kinship in time, both bioassay and deduction may be used for isolation by distance, which therefore is applicable to large extant bodies of data on phenotypes, metrics, and isonymy in man, and to phenotypes and metrics in other organisms. In this way we can determine $a, b,$ and σ^2, which are the basis parameters of complex population structure, just as m_e and N_e are the fundamental parameters when considering a local population.

The relation between these two sets of parameters is an important problem in mathematical genetics, depending for its solution on the leptokurtic distribution of marital distances, $m(d)$. As a first approximation, consider the exponental distribution,

$$m(d) = ze - dz \qquad (d > 0)$$

in which the mean distance D is $1/z$ and $E(d^2) = 2/z^2 = 4\sigma^2$, where σ^2 is the variance of parent-offspring distances along a fixed axis. If we take

$$a \doteq \frac{1}{4N_e m_e + 1}$$

$$b \doteq \sqrt{2m_e/\sigma^2} \doteq 2\sqrt{m_e}/D$$

then

$$m_e \doteq D^2b^2/4$$

$$N_e \doteq (1 - a)/aD^2b^2$$

where m_e, N_e relate to a typical local population. This may be only a poor approximation. It would be worth considerable effort by a mathematician to find a better one and strenuous exertion by geneticists to collect data for a critical test.

POLYMORPHS

The genetic locus in man often cannot with certainty be homologized with the cistron, operon, or other recognized unit of molecular biology. This is partly because of the limited power of recombination tests to discriminate closely linked loci from alleles. We are therefore led to avoid the term locus in favor of the more general concept of *system,* defined as *the unit of closely linked genetic information whose phenotypic factors are nonrandomly associated in panmictic populations of higher organisms.* The alternative genetic forms of a system may without ambiguity be called alleles. They are distinguished by binary attributes called factors, which if completely penetrant and dominant yield a factor-union system. Allelic frequencies are grouped into three broad classes: rare idiomorphs, with gene frequencies less than 0.01; common polymorphs, with gene frequencies between 0.01 and 0.99; and very common monomorphs, with gene frequencies greater than 0.99. Nothing is implied in these definitions about the forces (mutation, selection, migration, or drift) which established or may maintain the three classes of gene frequencies.

A polymorphic system, or polymorphism, has two or more polymorphic alleles in a given population, and a monomorphic system, or monomorphism, has no polymorphic alleles. Idomorphic alleles occur in both systems.

Progress in molecular genetics has revealed that a substantial proportion of all systems in man are polymorphic (Lewontin and Hubby, 1966). The dynamics of this diversity are poorly understood, partly because of four properties of polymorphism. *Specificity* signifies that selection acts on a polymorphism at particular developmental stages and by particular agents; at other stages of the life cycle selection may be reversed or negligible. *Intermittence* implies that selection acts strongly in some generations, in response to a specific environmental agent or genetic background. If the intermittence is not cyclic, or if the cycle is long, the polymorphism may be nearly neutral for many generations. *Plasticity* connotes the change in selective forces and genetic modifiers under different environments and gene frequencies. Yasuda (1965) and Morton et al. (1967) found that genetic differentiation of ethnic groups, measured by mean kinship, is greatest for polymorphisms with gene frequencies near one-half and decreases as the gene becomes rarer or more common. This parabolic regression of kinship on gene frequency is more pronounced for major races than for minor ethnic groups, and is absent within an ethnic group. Cavalli-Sforza (1969) showed that these results, while inexplicable if ethnic divergence is through genetic drift, are predictable if selection varies among geographic regions. (An alternative hypothesis is that selection is uniform among regions, but less for genes of intermediate frequency.) Environmental changes and accumulation of genetic modifiers may make a balanced polymorphism degenerate into a transient polymorphism, leading to *diminution* of the segregation load.

These attributes of specificity, intermittence, plasticity, and diminution suggest that many polymorphisms are virtually noncontributory to the genetic load. Also, the increasing tempo of discovery of polymorphisms, forcing the conclusion that many loci are polymorphic, must signify that the average selective effect is small. Perhaps this is partly because of intense epistasis (Sved et al., 1967), although there is no evidence that this is the case, and small effects might be expected to act nearly additively on fitness.

Finally, studies of population structure have revealed that the systematic pressure due to migration is more than 1% even for Pacific atolls, and is therefore presumably sufficient to maintain polymorphism in the absence of local mutation or selection, providing selection is balanced in the region from which migrants are drawn or varies among geographic regions.

The above considerations have led to some division among population geneticists. One group continues to emphasize the study of selection by one of nine methods:

1. Association between genotype and a specific type of morbidity or response to a specific agent.

2. Identification of the relevant environmental differences between populations with high and low gene frequencies.

3. Detection of systematic departures of genotype frequencies from Hardy-Weinberg equilibrium.

4. Analysis of adaptive trends in genotype frequency with age or among successive generations.

5. Detection of different genotype frequencies in the two sexes.

6. Measurement of fertility and mortality differentials among genotypes.

7. Analysis of departures from Mendelian segregation frequencies.

8. Detection of significant deviations of gene frequencies in hybrid populations from expectations based on admixture frequencies.

9. Computer simulation of genetic models.

The first two methods have been successful for hemoglobin S and G-6-PD deficiency. Methods 6 and 7 have been useful to study ABO incompatibility (Chung and Morton, 1961; Levene and Rosenfield, 1961). Recently the complication of meiotic drive has been suggested (Hiraizumi and Grove, 1969). Method 8 might be pursued with profit in Afro-Americans, especially in the Caribbean, but present results are inconclusive because evidence about ancestral populations has been insufficient to compute reliable admixture frequencies. Method 9 is an exercise in solipsism which has so far been unrewarding.

Because progress in studying selection has been slow, and the number of inexplicable claims is exceeded only by the unrepeatable ones, many population geneticists have preferred to regard polymorphisms as nearly neutral markers for study of formal genetics and population structure. This tendency is most pronounced in those who argue that amino acid substitutions in phylogenetic trees are due to fixation of neutral mutations by random genetic drift (non-Darwinian evolution). The argument is basically as follows: Let m be the linearized systematic pressure per codon per generation, which may be considered the probability that a gene be substituted by mutation or selection into the chain from ancestral to descendant gene. Then after t generations the probability of no substitution is $(1 - m)^t \doteq e^{-mt}$ with respect to a particular codon, and $\prod(1 - m)^t \doteq e^{-Mt}$ per protein, where $M = \sum m$ is the linearized systematic pressure per cistron and the summation is over all codons. Studies of various proteins have suggested that m is less than 10^{-6} and perhaps less than 10^{-8}. This indicates that selection has been so weak as to be easily confused with mutation. Since, however, the parabolic relation discussed above between kinship and gene frequency among racial groups is unequivocal evidence of variable selection, either among regions or among polymorphic alleles, the hypothesis of non-Darwinian evolution appears untenable for fixation of polymorphs.

A generation ago some biologists supposed that marker genes were essentially different from the "polygenes" determining quantitative inheritance. This controversy is not dead, and a part of quantitative inheritance may be due to different reaction rates of equivalent transfer RNAs, rates of synthesis of ribosomal RNA, and cryptic mutation which may affect rate of protein synthesis by altering a base pair without changing the encoded aminoacid. However, none of these mechanisms has yet proved amenable to study, and the principle of parsimony suggests that quantitative effects should be attributed to the same genes which by other techniques of observation are recognized as major. Support for this hypothesis is found in the enormous genetic variability revealed as polymorphism, and in studies of population structure which find the same effect of geographic distance on anthropometrics and polymorphs (Azevedo et al., 1969). Thus the systematic pressures on polymorphs and the genes of quantitative genetics are the same, and the two classes may well be identical. It seems likely that this equivalence of polymorphs and polygenes will become increasingly popular, but proof requires direct experimental evidence that both idiomorphs and genes not revealed by aminoacid substitution are negligible sources of quantitative variability.

IDIOMORPHS

Rare alleles are divisible into the broad classes of markedly deleterious and quasineutral. If dominant or sex-linked, the former give evidence of sporadic cases due to mutation, and the frequency of sporadic cases is sufficient to explain the gene frequency by balance between mutation and adverse selection. For autosomal recessives the evidence of mutation is indirect, and a few lethals such as cystic fibrosis may have reached polymorphic frequencies in some populations through heterozygous advantage. However, because of quantitative agreement between gene frequencies and the hypothesis of mutation-selection balance, and because of the rarity of heterotic lethals in other organisms, most population geneticists suppose that the typical recessive lethal idiomorph is not heterotic.

In all organisms the estimation of mutation rates is based on recognition of a particular phenotype. Since only a small proportion of mutants at a locus may produce the given phenotype, there are great hazards in extrapolating to a mutation rate per codon. For example, only about 1% of single amino acid substitutions in the beta chain of human hemoglobin produce methemoglobinemia. Only one "porcupine" mutation (ichthyosis histrix gravior) is known in the history of mankind, other mutations of the same gene presumably giving rise to other phenotypes. Ignoring short-lived mutable alleles, such as may be induced by nitrogen mustard, and considering that each cistron is typically composed of at least 100 codons, the law of large numbers should guarantee a rather homogeneous mutation rate per cistron. On this argument it seems likely that the higher mutation rates in man (say 10^{-5} per cistron per generation) are at loci where a large proportion of mutations give rise to a recognized phenotype, whereas the low rates (say 10^{-7} per cistron) are at loci where only a small proportion of mutants give rise to a recognized phenotype. Bodmer and Cavalli-Sforza (1970), on the other hand, assume that the proportion of mutants giving rise to a recognized phenotype is rather homogeneous among loci, and therefore conclude that the low mutation rates are typical. Not only does their assumption appear implausible, but as Sewall Wright (1950) showed many years ago, a mutation rate of 10^{-7} per cistron leads to a prediction of a doubling dose of about 3 rads. If their conclusion were true, it would be terrifying. Fortunately the evidence from Hiroshima and Nagasaki and from mammalian experiments suggests that the doubling dose of acute radiation is probably at least 30 rads, so that a mean mutation rate of less than 10^{-6} per cistron (10^{-8} per codon) seems unlikely. However, this question is of such great importance for the establishment of radiation tolerances that great effort should, and probably will, be expended to determine the spontaneous mutation rate per codon in systems such as structural proteins and isozymes where a known fraction of mutants at a given codon can be detected electrophoretically. Unfortunately, the result in human mating is necessarily an overestimate because of parentage errors, even when all marker systems are applied to detect such errors, whose frequency among apparent mutations increases with the gene frequency in the population.

Since many idiomorphs produce phenotypes which have not been differentially diagnosed, it has seemed important to devise a technique for revealing effects of idiomorphs not individually discriminated. This is provided by consanguinity analysis, which is applicable both to broad classes of morbidity and mortality and to more specific attributes such as severe mental defect, limb-girdle muscular dystrophy, and deaf-mutism. Segregation analysis reveals that most of the inbred load at low levels of inbreeding is due to single genes of high penetrance. In *Drosophila* the same result has been obtained for genes affecting morbidity and mortality, but epistatic effects with low penetrance become apparent at high levels of inbreeding. In both man and *Drosophila* there is quantitative agreement between the inbred load due to major genes and the mutation rate on the hypothesis that this load is due to a balance between mutation and selection.

Evidence in favor of a mutation-selection balance weakens progressively as the phenotype approaches neutrality. For most of the numerous rare variants in antigenic systems and isozymes (so-called private factors) there is at present no evidence of any departure from normalcy. Are these quasineutral idiomorphs really neutral, or maintained by a balance between low mutation rates and slightly adverse selection, or are they adaptive polymorphs *in status nascendi,* or former polymorphs slowly being eliminated by selection? Obviously all these mechanisms are possible, so we must ask which is most important.

It may be helpful to reconsider, in terms of periodic selection, the model of linearized systematic pressure which was introduced for polymorphs. Atwood et al. (1951) found that *Escherichia coli* auxotrophs maintained in a supplemented media under constant growth rates in a chemostat did not show a monotonic increase of prototrophic mutants, as expected on the simplest hypothesis of mutational balance. Instead, an initial increase was followed by rapid decline, and this irregular cycle was repeated many times during their experiment. They were able to show that the anomalous declines were due to advantageous mutants which spread through the population, eliminating the previous clone with its accumulated mutants. The same process must occur in protein evolution. Following the spread of an advantageous allele, or by chance at periods of low population size, a polymorphic system may become monomorphic. Gradually neutral mutants of the monomorph will increase under a systematic pressure m, the expected frequency of neutral mutant alleles before back-mutation becomes important being $1 - e^{-mt}$, where t is the number of generations after monomorphism was established. Neutral amino acid substitutions in a given cistron should have a modal frequency determined by the number of generations since the system was last monomorphic. Let us assume a generation of 20 years for hominids and consider the expected effect of systematic pressure on neutral alleles. Table 1 shows that a monomorphism established at the origin of *Homo sapiens* would have a mutant frequency of only 0.000025 if m is less than 10^{-8} per codon per generation. Even if the monomorphism were established as long ago as the origin of hominids, the mutant frequency would be only 0.005. Examination of idiomorph frequencies for structural proteins and isozymes may throw light on both the frequency of neutral mutations and the rate of protein evolution. Meanwhile, although it may tentatively be suggested that few polymorphs attained their present frequencies without selection, the proportion of idiomorphs which are neutral remains unknown.

It is interesting to consider Table 1 from the standpoint of neutral mu-

TABLE 1.—*Benchmarks in Human Evolution*

Event	No. of generations, t	Mutant frequency per codon, $1 - \exp(-10^{-8}t)$	Mutant frequency per cistron, $1 - \exp(-10^{-6}t)$
Origin of hominids (*Oreopithecus*)	500,000	0.005	0.393
Origin of *Australopithecus* (*Homo transvaalensis*)	100,000	0.001	0.095
Origin of *Sinanthropus* (*Homo erectus*)	20,000	0.0002	0.020
Origin of *Homo sapiens*	2,500	0.000025	0.0025

tation rates per cistron. Suppose that the rate is 10^{-8} per codon, and that there are 100 codons per cistron at which mutations are neutral. Then from the last column of Table 1 we see that neutral idiomorphs would be rare in the aggregate for a monomorphism established some 2500 generations ago, but common for a monomorphism established 500,000 generations ago. No locus is known in man to approach the diversity expected for an old monomorphism. Evidently the rate of adaptive protein evolution is higher, or the frequency of neutral mutations lower, than we have assumed for this example. In the future, the complexities introduced by periodic selection should be considered in studies of protein evolution.

Envoi

In these few pages I have been able to touch on only a few aspects of population genetics. Inevitably these were chosen from the topics in which I am most interested. They seem to me important, and likely to be important in the future, but they may not be the most significant aspects of population genetics.

The population geneticist of today has good reason to fear, if he is a biologist, that his mathematical skill will prove inadequate in the future or, if he is a mathematician, that his biological insight will prove superficial. Success in science, as on any journey, is problematical. Of one thing we can be sure, however. Genetics has led the biological sciences in applying mathematics and statistics, and the great leaders in this field have felt a certain anthropocentrism, the sentiment that the science of genetics is deficient if it can be applied to man only by extrapolation, that unusual effort is justified in overcoming the technical difficulties of human material, and that, in some degree, the proper study of mankind is man. Conjoined with this is a purely intellectual interest in realizing the potentialities of nonexperimental genetics. Every science, as it becomes more exact, becomes more mathematical. However significant the developments of molecular genetics and cytogenetics may be, the role of mathematics in genetics, and especially human genetics, will certainly increase.

References

Atwood, K. C., L. K. Schneider, and J. Ryan. 1951. Periodic selection in *Escherichia coli*. Proc. Nat. Acad. Sci. U.S.A. 37:146-155.

Azevedo, E., N. E. Morton, C. Miki, and S. Yee. 1969. Distance and kinship in northeastern Brazil. Amer. J. Hum. Genet. 21:1-22.

Balakrishnan, V., and L. D. Sanghvi. 1968. Distance between populations on the basis of attribute data. Biometrics 24:859-865.

Bodmer, W. R. 1969. Discussion on population structure. In Morton, N. E. (Ed.),

Computer Applications in Genetics, pp. 69-70. Honolulu, University of Hawaii Press.

————, and L. L. Cavalli-Sforza. 1970. Genetics of Human Populations. San Francisco, Freeman.

————, J. Bodmer, D. Ihde, and S. Adler. 1969. Genetic and serological association analysis of the HL-A leukocyte system. In Morton, N. E. (Ed.), Computer Applications in Genetics, pp. 117-127. Honolulu, University of Hawaii Press.

Cavalli-Sforza, L. L. 1969. Human diversity. Proc. XII Intern. Congr. Genet. 2:405-416.

Chung, C. S., and N. E. Morton. 1961. Selection at the ABO locus. Amer. J. Hum. Genet. 13:9-27.

Cotterman, C. W. 1953. Regular two-allele and three-allele phenotype systems. Amer. J. Hum. Genet. 5:193-235.

Crow, J., and M. Kimura. 1970. An Introduction to Population Genetics Theory. New York, Harper.

Dobzhansky, T. 1951. Genetics and the Origin of Species, Ed. 3. New York, Columbia University Press.

Edwards, A. W. F. 1968. Likelihood estimation of the branch points of a Brownian-motion/Yule process. Submitted to J. Roy Stat. Soc.

————. 1969. Genetic taxonomy. In Morton, N. E. (Ed.), Computer Applications in Genetics, pp. 14-142. Honolulu, University of Hawaii Press.

Elandt-Johnson, R. C. 1970. Segregation analysis for complex modes of inheritance. Amer. J. Hum. Genet. 22:129-144.

Elston, R. C. 1967. Genetic analysis of white cell blood groups. Amer. J. Hum. Genet. 19:258-264.

————. 1969. Iteration problems. In Morton, N. E. (Ed.), Computer Applications in Genetics, pp. 30-34. Honolulu, University of Hawaii Press.

Fitch, W. M., and J. V. Neel. 1969. The phylogenic relationships of some Indian tribes of Central and South America. Amer. J. Hum. Genet. 21:384-397.

Haldane, J. B. S. 1964. A defense of beanbag genetics. Persp. Biol. Med. 7:343-359.

Hiraizumi, Y., and J. S. Grove. 1969. Personal communication.

Imaizumi, Y., N. E. Morton, and D. E. Harris. 1970. Isolation by distance in artificial populations. Genetics 66:569-582.

Kimura, M., and G. H. Weiss. 1964. The steppingstone model of population structure and the decrease of genetic correlation with distance. Genetics 49:461-576.

————, T. Maruyama, and J. F. Crow. 1963. The mutational load in small populations. Genetics 48:1303-1312.

Kurczynski, T. W. 1969. Discussion of estimation of gene frequencies and inbreeding. In Morton, N. E. (Ed.), Computer Applications in Genetics, pp. 97-98. Honolulu, University of Hawaii Press.

Levene, H., and R. E. Rosenfield. 1961. ABO incompatibility. In Steinberg, A. G., and A. G. Bearn (Eds.), Progress in Medical Genetics, Vol. I, pp. 120-157. New York, Grune & Stratton.

Levin, B. R. 1969. Simulation of genetic systems. In Morton, N. E. (Ed.), Computer Applications in Genetics, pp. 36-46. Honolulu, University of Hawaii Press.

Lewontin, R. C. 1967. Population genetics. Ann. Rev. Genet. 1:37-70.

————, and J. L. Hubby. 1966. A molecular approach to the study of genetic heterozygosity in natural populations. II. Amount of variation and degree of heterozygosity in natural populations of *Drosophila pseudoobscura*. Genetics 54:595-609.

MacCluer, J. W., and W. J. Schull. 1970. Frequencies of consanguineous marriage and accumulation of inbreeding in an artificial population. Amer. J. Hum. Genet. 22:160-175.

Malécot, G. 1948. Les mathématiques de l'hérédité. Paris, Masson.

——. 1950. Quelques schemas probabilistes sur la variabilité des populations naturelles. Ann. Univ. Lyon, Sec. A. 13

——. 1959. Les modèles stochastiques en génétique de population. Publ. Inst. Statist. Univ. Paris. 8:173-210.

Mayr, E. 1942. Systematics and the Origin of Species. Columbia University Press, N. Y.

——. 1950. Taxonomic categories in fossil hominids. Cold Spring Harbor Symposia on Quantitative Biology. 15:109-118.

——. 1959. Where are we? Cold Spring Harbor Symposia on Quantitative Biology. 24:1-14.

Morton, N. E. 1959. Genetic tests under incomplete ascertainment. Amer. J. Hum. Genet. 11:1-16.

——. 1962. Segregation and linkage. In Burdette, W. J. (Ed.), Methodology in Human Genetics, pp. 17-52. San Francisco, Holden-Day.

——. 1969. Human population structure. In Roman, H. L. (Ed.), Annual Review of Genetics, Vol. 3, pp. 53-73. Palo Alto, Annual Reviews.

——, and C. Miki. 1968. Estimation of gene frequencies in the MN system. Vox Sang. 15:15-24.

——, C. S. Chung, and M. P. Mi. 1967. Genetics of Interracial Crosses in Hawaii. Basel, Karger.

——, Y. Imaizumi, and D. E. Harris. 1970a. Clans as genetic barriers. Amer. Anthrop. In press.

——, S. Yee, and R. Lew. 1970b. Bioassay of kinship. Theoret. Pop. Biol. In press.

Neel, J. V., and F. M. Salzano. 1967. Further studies on the Xavante Indians. X. Some hypotheses-generalizations resulting from these studies. Amer. J. Hum. Genet. 4:554-574.

Renwick, J. H. 1969. Genetic linkage in man. In Morton, N. E. (Ed.), Computer Applications in Genetics, pp. 103-111. Honolulu, University of Hawaii Press.

Roisenberg, I., and N. E. Morton. 1970. Population structure of blood groups in Central and South American Indians. Amer. J. Phys. Anthrop. 32:373-376.

A Committee of the Royal Anthropological Institute of Great Britain and Ireland. 1967. Notes and Queries on Anthropology, ed. 6. London, Routledge and Kegan Paul.

Smith, C. 1970. Heritability of liability and concordance in monozygous twins. Ann. Hum. Genet. (Lond.) 34:85-91.

Sved, J. A., T. E. Reed, and W. F. Bodmer. 1967, The number of balanced polymorphisms that can be maintained in a natural population. Genetics 55:469-481.

Workman, P. L. and J. D. Niswander. 1970. Population studies on southwestern Indian tribes. II. Local genetic differentiation in the Papago. Amer. J. Hum. Genet. 22:24-49.

Wright, S. 1931. Evolution in Mendelian populations. Genetics 16: 97-159.

——. 1950. Discussion on population genetics and radiation. J. Cell Comp. Physiol. 35:187-210.

————. 1960. "Genetics and twentieth century Darwinism": A review and discussion. Amer. J. Hum. Genet. 12:365-372.

Yasuda, N. 1965. The genetical structure of northeastern Brazil. Thesis, University of Hawaii, Honolulu.

————. 1969. Estimation of the inbreeding coefficient and gene frequency from mating type frequency. In Morton, N. E. (Ed.), Computer Applications in Genetics, pp. 87-96. Honolulu, University of Hawaii Press.

CHAPTER 4

Enzyme Defects

Henry N. Kirkman

Department of Pediatrics, University of North Carolina School of
Medicine, Chapel Hill, North Carolina

Supported by U. S. Public Health Service research grants AM-11065 and HD-03110 from the National Institutes of Health.

THE PAST FEW YEARS have brought major changes in concepts and research opportunities concerning enzyme defects of man. An appreciation of these changes seems to require a brief statement of the thinking and approaches that prevailed until recently. The first, direct evidence that human metabolic disease can result from deficiency in activity of a specific enzyme, came from the investigations of type I glycogen storage disease by Dr. G. T. Cori and her husband (1952). This evidence came nearly a half century after the first propositions of Sir Archibald Garrod, and nearly a decade after the demonstration by Sawin and Glick (1943) of genetically determined differences in activity of atropinesterase in rabbits. Despite this gradual start, the discovery of other human enzymic defects has proceeded at an increasing pace, until even the most diligent student of biochemical genetics now has difficulty following developments in the field. Genetically determined abnormalities would seem to exist for each of the many human enzymes, if consideration is given to both the nature of the genetic code and the types of known enzyme defects. Also impressive, but equally predictable from the genetic code, is the variety of ways in which an enzyme is capable of being affected. Genetic heterogeneity is found so often as to lead to the suspicion that it underlies most hereditary metabolic defects, even those with a uniform clinical expression.

Other concepts have become familiar to students of medical genetics. Of the hereditary metabolic disorders for which an understanding of the basic mechanism exists, most represent deficiencies in activity of a specific enzyme, and most are recessive in their clinical expression. When enzymic activities have been measured carefully in relatives and in normal people, these measurements usually reveal activities in heterozygous subjects that are intermediate between those of normal individuals and fully affected subjects. Full deficiencies in activity of a specific enzyme sometimes lead to deficiency of an essential product. Often they lead to toxic levels of a substrate or metabolic side product of substrate. These findings, in turn, prompted efforts to offset metabolic defects by either providing an essential product or reducing exposure of the affected individual to substances proximal to the metabolic obstruction. As such treatment for certain metabolic errors became possible, attention was appropriately given to the early diagnosis of those disorders with preventable complications.

Human metabolic defects focused early attention on enzymes, as products of individual genes, but they failed to provide clues to the molecular mechanisms of genetic control. Human hemoglobins and microbial proteins, not human enzymes, offered the abundant examples of amino acid substitution with which modern geneticists are familiar. Similarly, complexities of mammalian chromosomes and limitations in laboratory approaches have hampered efforts to understand mechanisms of metabolic regulation in mammalian cells. Until recently, the mechanism of human enzymic defects could only be inferred from well-defined examples both of structural changes in human hemoglobin and microbial proteins and of regulatory mechanisms in microorganisms.

Findings over the past few years have served to reinforce some of these generalizations while refuting others. Many additional examples of genetic heterogeneity have been uncovered, and heterozygotes for even some of the more recently discovered inborn errors of metabolism have been found to have levels of enzymic activity intermediate between those of normal and fully affected subjects. On the other hand, sufficient data are available to suggest that the mechanisms of enzymic deficiency in man differ significantly from those which receive emphasis in studies of microorganisms, and they differ in ways which have profound diagnostic and therapeutic significance. Not only have new principles for treating inborn errors of metabolism begun to emerge but also the recent development of methods for antenatal diagnosis now makes diagnosis of untreatable disease as important as the diagnosis of treatable disorders. Moreover, methods for the culture, manipulation, and hybridization of mamalian cells represent new techniques for unraveling the regulatory mechanisms that have been refractory to study in mammals before now. It is toward these recent developments that the present review is directed.

PARTIAL ENZYMIC DEFICIENCIES

For those who survey the many hereditary enzymic deficiencies of man, one of the most recurring observations is that deficiencies in activity are seldom complete: between 0.1 and 20% of the normal amount of activity often remains. Some exceptions exist. Even the use of ^{14}C-labeled galactose fails to reveal activity of galactose-1-phosphate uridyl transferase in the red cells of subjects with galactosemia. Essentially no activity of affected enzyme is encountered in the "silent" type of pseudocholinesterase deficiency or in the Japanese type of catalase deficiency. But even among these classes of enzymic defects, partial deficiencies are encountered. Segal et al. (1971) point out that significant levels of transferase can be found in intestinal mucosal and hepatic cells of certain Negro subjects with galactosemia.The relatively prevalent Duarte variant of the same enzyme is accompanied by approximately half-normal levels of activity of the enzyme (Beutler et al., 1966). Appreciable catalase activity is seen in the Swiss type of acatalasia (Aebi et al., 1968), and subjects with the most common type of pseudocholinesterase defect seem to have nearly normal serum levels of this enzyme when precautions are not taken to measure the function of the enzyme under physiological conditions (Davies et al., 1960).

Seemingly significant levels of activity of the affected enzyme are encountered among many of the sphingolipidoses and among the deficiencies of red cell enzymes that lead to chronic hemolytic disease. Indeed, among several of these defects, the level of activity is so high as to cause the diagnosis to be missed in a standard assay. Deficiencies of glucose-6-phosphate dehydrogenase (G-6-PD), which affect over 100 million of the human population, serve as examples of incomplete deficiencies. Nearly 70 apparently distinct, qualitatively different variants of this enzyme have been reported (Yoshida et al., 1971; Kirkman, 1971). Approximately half of these are accompanied by reduced levels of activity of the enzyme in red cells. That qualitative characteristics of this enzyme can be studied is testimony to the fact that these deficiencies are incomplete. None of the many hundreds of samples of G-6-PD-deficient blood examined in the laboratory of this reviewer over the past 12 years has been fully deficient. Admittedly some have had levels of activity too low to be perceptible in assays utilizing hemolyzates. Activity could be measured, however, when hemoglobin was removed during purification of the enzyme. Moreover, levels of G-6-PD activity of white cells have been measured in many types of red cell G-6-PD deficiency. In each case, the deficiency has been found to be even less severe in white cells than in red cells. Whenever the red cell G-6-PD is observed to be electrophoretically abnormal, the white cell enzyme is similarly affected, so it would seem unlikely that the two are structurally and genetically distinct enzymes (Kirkman, 1971).

Partial deficiencies of enzymic activity not only exist in microorganisms but also provide some of the earliest examples of genetic influences on the qualitative characteristics of proteins (Maas and Davis, 1952; Horowitz and Fling, 1956). Recent work with microbial mutants, however, has served to emphasize the existence of complete deficiencies in activity of enzymes. Thus, the microbial and human systems seem to stand in sharp contrast to one another on the matter of level of residual activity. Part of this difference is a matter of ascertainment: partially deficient strains of bacteria are less useful for many investigations in microbial genetics, and these strains tend to be disregarded. Natural processes, on the other hand, may tend to favor the existence of partial deficiencies in man. One is led to wonder if complete deficiencies might not be incompatible with life in utero or difficult to achieve in the face of multiple isozymes. Whatever the cause of this difference between microorganisms and man, the partial deficiencies of human enzymes hold diagnostic and, in some instances, therapeutic significance. They also provide hints that the mechanisms of regulation and enzymic deficiency in microorganisms may not be representative of those seen in mammals. The nature of these partial deficiencies, therefore, deserves review.

Residual Activity from Enzymes Determined at Other Genetic Loci

Studies of deficiencies and electrophoretic patterns of mammalian enzymes have emphasized the frequency with which similar catalytic functions may be exhibited by two or more enzymes with structures which seem to be determined by different genetic loci. Occasionally, the two proteins share a common subunit, in a manner analogous to the way in which hemoglobins A_2, A, and F share a common (α) subunit. Such enzymes may or may not coexist in developmental time or in anatomical or subcellular location. The extent to which they do coexist in time and place has serious diagnostic significance. Although galactose-1-phosphate uridyl transferase is largely a hepatic enzyme, it is present in human red cells also. This is a fortunate circumstance for the diagnosis of deficiencies in activity of this enzyme in patients with galactosemia. Similarly, an enzymic assay for type VI glycogen storage disease is based on the fact that the phosphorylase activities of human liver and white cells seem to arise from the same enzyme (Williams and Field, 1961). Conversely, the structural and genetic distinctiveness of phosphorylase from liver and muscle renders white cells inappropriate for efforts to diagnose muscle phosphorylase deficiency.

The distinctiveness of enzymes catalyzing the same reaction in two type of cells poses a particular problem in the diagnosis of red cell pyruvate kinase deficiency. White cells have a pyruvate kinase which seems to be qualitatively and genetically distinct from that in red cells (Koler et al., 1968). Although white cells form only 1% of the packed cell volume of whole blood, they are very active in pyruvate kinase. Their contribution to the total pyruvate kinase activity of blood can mask a deficiency of red cell pyruvate kinase, if precautions are not taken to remove white cells from the sample. Recent efforts to diagnose inborn errors of metabolism in the fetus have also attracted attention to the question of whether or not an enzyme in one tissue is the same as that in another tissue. Such efforts at antenatal diagnosis are directed at providing a diagnosis on the fetus of parents who are at risk for having an abnormal child, and providing the diagnosis early enough to allow a therapeutic abortion if the fetus is affected. The diagnosis is usually made on fetal cells cultured from 5 to 20 ml of amniotic fluid, which can be obtained with relative safety by transabdominal amniocentesis after the fourteenth week of pregnancy. For certain couples, this approach offers an acceptable means of being assured the birth of an infant who is free of the disease in question. Despite desirable features of antenatal diagnosis, however, certain limitations and pitfalls exist. It is difficult to conceive of a diagnostic approach which must be made under greater "blind" conditions: an opportunity does not exist to check the laboratory diagnosis with the physical examination and clinical course of the patient. An interpretation is impossible if the enzyme in question is not present in amniotic cells, as in type I glycogen storage disease and phenylketonuria, if it does not reflect the activity of the enzyme in the primary organ of involvement, or if it is not the same enzyme that is affected later in life. Salafsky and Nadler (1971) have observed that amniotic fluid and fetal kidney reflect poorly the deficiency of α-1,4-glucosidase in liver cells and amniotic cells, and Taylor et al. (1971) have observed that a fetal form of thymidine kinase seems to be present in utero. The complications introduced by the presence of a fetal form of a protein are well illustrated by efforts to diagnose sickle cell disease early in life. The amino acid substitution of sickle hemoglobin involves the β chain of adult hemoglobin, but synthesis of the β chain does not occur readily until late in fetal development. The fetal counterpart of adult hemoglobin, fetal hemoglobin, has the γ chain, instead of the β chain. The two polypeptide chains are determined by different genetic loci.

Special precautions are necessary for the detection of an enzymic defect when the same biochemical reaction is catalyzed by two different enzymes in the same cell. This situation became apparent during studies of Tay-Sachs disease, an infantile, neurodegenerative disorder characterized by excessive accumulation of GM_2 ganglioside in brain and, to a lesser extent, other organs. The degradation of GM_2 ganglioside seems to require removal of N-acetylgalactosamine, which is accomplished by hexosaminidase (Fig. 1). Okada and O'Brien (1969) found that this enzyme has two components, an electrophoretically fast fraction (hexosaminidase A) and

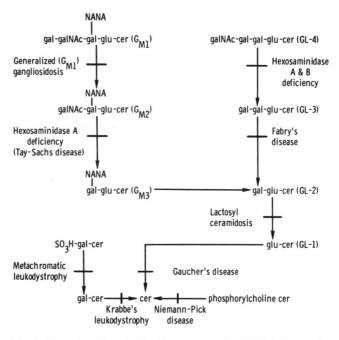

FIG. 1.—Metabolism of sphingolipids. Cer = ceramide. NANA N-acetylneuraminic acid. (Modified from Dawson and Stein, 1970.)

an electrophoretically slow component (hexosaminidase B). Activities of the two components are nearly equal in serum and fibroblasts of normal people. In contrast, infants with Tay-Sachs disease have an amount of hexosaminidase A in serum and fibroblasts equal to only a small percentage of the total hexosaminidase activity. The diagnosis would be scarcely apparent from a determination of the total hexosaminidase activity of either serum or fibroblasts, for the decrease in activity of hexosaminidase A is accompanied by an increase in activity of hexosaminidase B (Okada et al., 1971). Okada et al. (1970) have observed a similar relationship in a milder type of hexosaminidase A deficiency, juvenile GM_2 gangliosidosis.

A comparable situation exists for the enzymic diagnosis of metachromatic leukodystrophy, another infantile neurodegenerative disorder in the group of sphingolipidoses (Fig. 1). This disease is characterized by excessive amounts of cerebroside sulphate in brain and kidney and is accompanied by a deficiency of arylsulfatase in brain, urine, leukocytes, and fibroblasts (Kaback and Howell, 1970). There are two major types of the enzyme: arylsulfase A, which is themolabile and is inhibited by barium acetate, and arylsulfase B, which is inhibited by sodium pyrophosphate. Austin et al. (1965) have shown that, of the two enzymes, it is arylsulfatase A which is decidedly diminished in activity in samples from infants with metachromatic leukodystrophy. As with Tay-Sachs disease, accurate enzymic diagnosis requires that an effort be made to determine how much of the activity is arising from only one of the two components.

Similarly, the excessive deposition of neutral fats and cholesterol in viscera of infants with Wolman's disease is accompanied by a deficiency of acid lipase (esterase), but not of neutral lipase (Patrick and Lake, 1969). Altay et al. (1970) have observed a comparable relationship in deficiencies of hexokinase from human red cells. Absence of one of the four electrophoretic bands of red cell hexokinase does not seem to be deleterious, but deficiency of the other three bands is accompanied by hemolytic disease.

A question immediately suggests itself when one considers that disease can result from deficiency of only one of two enzymes catalyzing the same reaction within a cell. Why is not the activity of the other enzyme sufficient to meet metabolic needs? The answer to this question is not always known, although several possible explanations can be formulated. In some instances the two enzymes lie in different subcellular compartments, where comparable metabolic steps occur independently. The α-1,4 linkages of glycogen, for example, can be broken either by hydrolysis, through the action of lysosomal α-1,4-glucosidase, or by phosphorolysis, through the action of phosphorylase. Phosphorylase is present in the soluble fraction of cells. It is noteworthy that deficiency of α-1,4-glucosidase in Pompe's disease (type II glycogen storage disease) results in accumulation of glycogen in and about the lysosomes. A comparable situation may exist in Wolman's disease, resulting from deficiency of lysosomal acid esterase.

Nevertheless, other enzymic diseases occur even when both enzymes are present in the same subcellular compartment. Some other explanation must be sought for the failure of one enzyme to compensate for the deficiency in activity of the other. It is quite possible that the conditions of enzymic assay do not correspond to conditions in vivo sufficiently to allow a fair evaluation of the relative contribution of two enzymes catalyzing the same reaction. If an artificial substrate is used, the two enzymes may not use the substrate in the same manner in which they use the natural substrate. Mehl and Jatzkewitz (1968) observe that arylsulfatase A utilizes cerebroside sulfate readily as a substrate, but arylsulfatase B is only slightly active toward this natural substrate. Suzuki and Suzuki (1971) find that the diagnosis of Krabbe's globoid cell leukodystrophy would be missed if one attempted to measure activity of galactocerebrosidase with the substrate 4-methylumbelliferyl β-galactoside. Activities and deficiencies of this enzyme are best determined through the use of the natural substrate, galactocerebroside (Fig. 1). Moreover, the pH, ionic conditions, and concentration of substrate or inhibitors are usually not the same in an enzymic assay as in a cell. These differences also may lead to a false appraisal of the physiological contribution of two enzymes catalyzing the same reaction. As will become apparent, the same uncertainties arise in using a standard enzymic assay to estimate the degree of physiological function of a mutant enzyme. This question also arises in discussions of the possible physiological advantages which might lead to evolution of iso-zymes and to polymorphism for seemingly neutral enzyme variants. What-ever the answer may be to these questions, the observation remains that failure to distinguish between two enzymes catalyzing the same reaction can cause the basic defect to be missed during research into an inborn error of metabolism. It can also cause the disorder to be missed during subsequent diagnostic assays.

When two enzymes catalyze the same reaction within a cell, misleading results can be generated if one of the two enzymes represents only a minor component of the total activity. This error is one of interpretation of mo-lecular mechanisms rather than one of diagnosis. Consider a deficiency in enzymic activity of the type which is accompanied by a small amount of residual activity (Fig. 2). This residual activity is regarded by some inves-tigators as holding a clue to whether the deficiency results from regulation or from structural mutation. If the deficiency arises from regulation, one might expect the residual enzyme to be qualitatively identical to the nor-

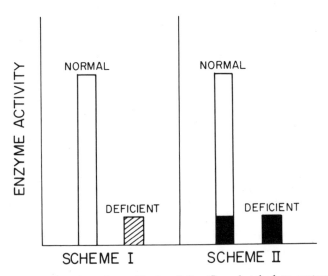

FIG. 2.—Two explanations for residual activity. Cross-hatched = mutant enzyme, allelic to normal. Solid = enzyme determined by a structural locus other than that for normal enzyme.

mal enzyme. If the deficiency arises from an alteration in the structural gene of the enzyme, the residual enzyme might have abnormal qualitative characteristics. Those investigators who wish to use this approach, however, should realize that the residual enzyme could have qualitatively abnormal characteristics for another reason: it might represent a minor component that is determined at an unaffected structural locus (Fig. 2). This minor component could pass unnoticed in the presence of large amounts of the predominating enzyme in normal cells. Under these circumstances, the discovery of a new "variant" would have no validity.

For a time, a minor component was suspected of accounting for several types of apparent "variants" of human G-6-PD which were accompanied by partial deficiencies of G-6-PD. A small fraction of the total G-6-PD activity in mammaliam liver arises from hexose-6-phosphate dehydrogenase, a microsomal enzyme which seems to be structurally and genetically distinct from G-6-PD (Ohno et al., 1966; Shaw, 1966, Shaw and Barto, 1965; Srivastava and Beutler, 1969). This minor component utilizes the substrate analog galactose-6-phosphate more readily than does G-6-PD. Since many variants of human G-6-PD were being reported as doing the same, this raised the possibility that these were not variants at all, but simply the expression of hexose-6-phosphate dehydrogenase, which was predominating in the face of G-6-PD deficiency. Two developments rendered this possibility unlikely: this hexose-6-phosphate dehydrogenase activity was shown not to be present in red cells (the tissue from which G-6-PD was extracted for characterization), and variants which utilized galactose-6-phosphate readily were diverse among themselves. Some were electrophoretically abnormal; others were electrophoretically normal. Indeed, when the residual activity of different enzyme-deficient people exhibits different characteristics, the mechanism represented by scheme II in Fig. 2 would seem to be unlikely.

Although the same enzymic reaction can be catalyzed by two genetically distinct enzymes, it is also true that two apparently distinct isozymes can be determined by the same structural gene, either because they share a common subunit or because they are secondary modifications of the same protein. The latter mechanisms seems to account for the different electrophoretically distinct bands of alkaline phosphatase seen in certain strains of *Escherichia coli*. This enzyme is a dimer determined at a single structural locus, yet several electrophoretic components are observed. The various components are concomitantly affected by genetic influences on the enzyme. Recent studies of the structure of the enzyme suggest that this molecular heterogeneity results from some secondary modifications of the structure of the enzyme after it is synthesized (Natori and Garen, 1970). An example of secondary modification which holds current interest is the synthesis of proinsulin and the subsequent cleavage of proinsulin into the two different polypeptide chains of insulin (Rubenstein and Steiner, 1970). Seemingly distinct electrophoretic bands of an enzyme may be interconvertible. Blume and co-workers (1971) found that one electrophoretic component of pyruvate kinase could be converted to another by the addition of fructose diphosphate or by aging of the enzyme. Kirkman and Hanna (1968) demonstrated that some electrophoretic components of red cell G-6-PD are interconvertible and may simply be different states of the same enzyme protein. These also are concomitantly affected whenever a deficiency or electrophoretic abnormality of the G-6-PD occurs.

Residual Activity of the Affected Enzyme

The residual activity in cells with a partial enzymic deficiency can represent the contribution of an unaffected enzyme, which is controlled at another genetic locus, but it can also represent activity remaining from the enzyme which is primarily affected in some quantitative or qualitative way by the mutation. The great diversity of enzymic phenotypes, including electrophoretic abnormalities, and the familial patterns indicate that this is true for the many variants of G-6-PD which are accompanied by deficiency in activity of G-6-PD (Kirkman, 1971). Studies of this enzyme are simplified by the fact that it is an aggregate of a single type of polypeptide chain, and that it is determined by a single structural locus on the X chromosome. Accordingly, the human male can make only one type of red cell G-6-PD. For reasons that will become clearer later, the white cells of G-6-PD-deficient subjects are often far less deficient in activity than are red cells. In each subject in which white cell G-6-PD has been examined, however, it exhibits the same abnormalities of electrophoretic migration and other characteristics as red cell G-6-PD. These various observations would be difficult, if not impossible, to reconcile with the possibility that the abnormal characteristics arise from an independent, minor component.

Most obvious of the examples of residual activity in an affected enzyme are those variant enzymes which *appear to have normal activity, yet have very little function in vivo.* They pose one of the most serious of current problems in research and diagnosis of human enzymic defects. Many of these are variants with abnormally high Michaelis constants (K_m's). It may be recalled that each enzyme molecule, like any other catalytic molecule, can work with only a limited amount of substrate at any given moment. As the concentration of substrate is increased, the rate of the reaction approaches a maximal rate which is determined by the number of enzyme molecules present (Fig. 3). It is in the presence of such high concentrations of substrate that activity of many enzymes can be measured

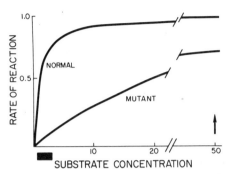

Fig. 3.—Plot of activity of a hypothetical enzyme at various concentrations of substrate. Bar = range of concentration of substrate in vivo. Arrow = concentration of substrate in assay. Mutant has high K_m.

with greatest simplicity and accuracy. Most enzymic assays, therefore, call for the addition of substrate in relatively large amounts. In vivo, however, the enzyme may be required to work with much lower concentrations of substrate. The efficiency with which an enzyme can work at low concentrations of substrate is determined by the K_m, which is simply defined as the concentration of substrate which allows an enzyme to function at half of its maximum capability. The higher the K_m, the higher the substrate concentration must be if the enzyme is to function effectively. Since genetic influences can change the K_m and maximal velocity independently, some mutant enzymes can give the impression of functioning normally at high substrate concentration, but they function very poorly at substrate concentrations in the physiological range (Fig. 3). This deceptive property is encountered in the most prevalent type of deficiency of pseudocholinesterase, a condition which causes profound over responsiveness to the muscle relaxant succinylcholine (Davies et al., 1960; Goedde et al., 1968). It is encountered also in type VIa (phosphorylase kinase-defective) glycogen storage disease (Huijing, 1970) and in chronic hemolytic anemia resulting from certain types of pyruvate kinase defects (Sachs et al., 1967; Miwa et al., 1968). In each instance, the standard enzymic assays might indicate falsely that the enzymic activity is normal; in each instance, the enzyme is almost functionless under physiological conditions. Variant enzymes with elevated K_m's are relatively common among enzyme defects of man. Another example is found in pentosuria (Wang and van Eys, 1970), one of the inborn errors discussed by Sir Archibald Garrod earlier in the century. High K_m's are seen in defects of hexokinase (hemolytic anemia), α-galactosidase (Fabry's disease), methemoglobin reductase (methemoglobinemia), G-6-PD (Oklahoma variant with hemolytic anemia), and argininosuccinate synthetase (citrullinemia) (Necheles et al., 1970; Romeo and Migeon, 1971; Schwartz et al., 1970; Kirkman et al., 1960; Tedesco and Mellman, 1967). Certain variants of pyruvate kinase (Oski and Bowman, 1969) and G-6-PD (Kirkman, 1971; Yoshida et al., 1971) have K_m's that are lower than normal, but this change is not so likely to lead to a misdiagnosis as is an elevated K_m.

The recent studies of pyruvate kinase serve to emphasize another way in which enzyme variants can appear to have greater function in a standard assay than in vivo. The activities of some enzymes do not vary with substrate concentration in the manner shown in Fig. 3. The plot of activity versus substrate concentration may more nearly follow a sigmoid curve. Such enzymes may undergo unfolding or dissociation under certain conditions, and activity of the enzyme may be affected by physiological substances which interact with the enzyme molecule at some point other than the catalytic site. Few enzymic assays are carried out in a manner that would allow the enzyme to be exposed to the types and concentrations of such allosteric effectors as occur in vivo. Accordingly, the activity which a variant enzyme exhibits in an assay may be considerably greater or less than the activity it has in the cell. This phenomenon may explain why red cells of certain patients with chronic hemolytic disease accumulate intermediates of the Embden-Meyerhoff pathway in a manner suggesting deficiency of pyruvate kinase, yet they have nearly normal activity of pyruvate kinase by standard assay. Munro and Miller (1970) found that fructose-1,6-diphosphate, a potent allosteric effector for normal pyruvate kinase, lowers the K_m for phosphoenolpyruvate of normal pyruvate kinase, but it raises the K_m of a mutant form of pyruvate kinase. Blume and co-workers (1971) demonstrated that normal pyruvate kinase is brought to half maximal activation by 0.1 μM fructose diphosphate, but one variant of the enzyme required 100 times this concentration for half maximal activation. Presumably, the activity of this variant in the presence of fructose-1,6-diphosphate in vivo is much lower than that of normal pyruvate kinase. Similarly, Afolayan and Luzzatto (1971) suggest that normal G-6-PD B) and the enzyme of G-6-PD-deficient Negroes (G-6-PD A−) differ in allosteric responsiveness to reduced nicotinamide adenine dinucleotide phosphate (NADPH). They describe how this might account for certain discrepancies between the two enzymes in their activity in vivo and in vitro.

In a subsequent section, we will consider a third mechanism by which activity of a defective enzyme may appear falsely to be normal, but the examples already cited should allow the worker in medical genetics to be warned: *normal activity of an enzyme in a cellfree assay does not mean that the enzyme has normal activity within the cell.* When studies of whole-cell or whole body metabolism point to deficiency of an enzyme, that enzyme may need to be examined in a number of different ways before its defective function becomes apparent.

MECHANISMS OF ENZYMIC DEFICIENCIES

Studies of microbial mutants have revealed two important mechanisms by which enzymic activity may be lacking: (a) the enzyme (protein) is synthesized but lacks the ability to function or (b) the enzyme (protein) is not synthesized. Examples of the first type are certain mutants of tryptophan synthetase in *Neurospora* and *E. Coli* (Suskind, 1955; Lerner and Yanofsky, 1957). By preparing antibodies against highly purified normal enzyme, an investigator can test for the presence of material which cross-reacts with the antibody. Such cross-reacting material (CRM) is assumed to be mutant enzyme protein which has lost its catalytic function but has retained its antigenic similarity to normal enzyme. Tedesco and Mellman (1971) have recently presented evidence that cells from subjects with galactosemia have a substance which is CRM for normal galactose-1-phosphate uridyl transferase. Immunological studies by Stites et al., (1971) and by Zimmerman et al. (1971) indicate that hemophilia A is also a CRM-positive mutation. Similar evidence exists for some forms of hemophilia B (Brown et al., 1970). In a way, the previously discussed enzyme variants with high K_m's must also be placed in this category. The nearly normal activity they exhibit at high concentrations of substrate is evidence of the presence of enzyme protein, yet this protein does not function well at physiological concentrations of substrate.

Apart from these examples, however, most studies thus far reveal that a significant deficiency in enzyme protein underlies deficiencies in activity. Hodgkin et al., (1965) found no CRM in the complete type of pseudocholinesterase deficiency. Robbins (1960) found none in the muscles of a subject with muscle phosphorylase deficiency. The leukocytes of patients with myeloperoxidase deficiency also seem to lack CRM for the affected enzyme (Salmon et al., 1970). In contrast to deficiency of red cell catalase in mice (Feinstein et al., 1967, 1968), catalase deficiency in man seems to be CRM negative (Nishimura, 1961; Hosoi, 1968; Hosoi et al., 1969), although a small amount of CRM with $\frac{1}{6}$ the molecular weight of active catalase is detectable in red cells of affected, heterozygous, and normal subjects (Shibata et al., 1967). In addition, von Willebrand's disease seems to be a CRM-negative defect of factor VIII (Zimmerman et al., 1971; Stites et al., 1971). Since deficiencies in activity of red cell G-6-PD are not complete, it is not surprising that a small amount of CRM for G-6-PD is present in these conditions, yet Yoshida et al. (1967) found the amount of CRM to be greatly reduced in red cells of subjects with A−,

Seattle, and Mediterranean types of G-6-PD deficiency, and Rosa et al. (1970), found a twofold difference, or less, in ratio of CRM to G-6-PD activity when they compared normal G-6-PD with that of males with the Mediterranean and Canton types of G-6-PD deficiency. Since these variants have less than $\frac{1}{6}$ normal G-6-PD activity, these findings indicate that the deficiency in activity results largely from a deficiency in amount of enzymic protein.

It should be kept in mind that failure to find CRM material does not necessarily mean that the enzyme protein is missing: the mutation may have caused the protein to lose its immunological identity to a normal enzyme, and the antibody against the normal enzyme may not be sufficiently potent to allow detection of the modified protein. Yoshida points out that immunoprecipitation could depend upon the presence of the enzyme in a normal, multimeric state. Subunits or dissociated forms of the enzyme might be underestimated or missed (Gelehrter et al., 1970). Nevertheless, the frequency with which enzyme deficiencies in man are being found to be CRM negative is noteworthy. For deficiencies in activity of G-6-PD, an independent approach also indicates that the deficiency cannot be attributed to enzyme protein with greatly reduced function. Although the amount of enzyme in G-6-PD-deficient red cells is too small to allow complete purification by present methods, a system of partial purification and electrophoresis allows a minimum estimate for the specific activity of the pure enzyme protein (Kirkman, 1966). These indicate that G-6-PD A−, Seattle, Mediterranean, several types of variants accompanied by chronic hemolytic disease, and possibly Canton, all have a specific activity at least $\frac{1}{3}$ as great as that of normal G-6-PD. Since activity is greatly reduced in red cells of many of these variants, the deficiency must be attributed to a deficiency of enzyme protein rather than to reduced catalytic deficiency.

A surprising development in the study of G-6-PD deficiency is the frequency with which residual activity exhibits one or more abnormal qualitative characteristics. The justification for believing that this does not represent activity of a genetically independent, minor component has already been given. Thus, the deficiencies in activity of G-6-PD cannot be attributed simply to a decreased rate of synthesis of normal enzyme. In some way, the mutation has resulted in derangement of both structure and amount of the enzyme protein. The finding of reduced amount of enzyme protein raises the question of whether the reduced amount results from decreased synthesis or inhanced destruction. This question can be answered conveniently in the human red cell. The human red cell loses DNA and RNA very early. During much of the remaining three months of its lifespan, the red cell is without capability for protein synthesis. It must meet metabolic needs with whatever proteins were present at the reticulocyte stage. Human red cells undergo change in resistance to osmotic shock and change in density as they age. These two properties allow a sample of red cells to be fractionated roughly according to the age of the red cells. Using the technique of differential osmotic shock, Marks and Gross (1959) offered evidence that the deficiency of G-6-PD A− cells results from increased loss of the G-6-PD activity in vivo. More recently, Yoshida et al. (1967), Powell et al. (1966), Kirkman et al. (1968), and Piomelli et al. (1968) have found a similar explanation for tse decreased activity in red cells of subjects with G-6-PD Mediterranean and G-6-PD Seattle. Some evidence has been obtained to suggest similarly enhanced liability in vivo of the enzyme which is defective in congenital methemoglobinemia (Feig et al., 1971) and Swiss-type acatalasia (Aebi et al., 1968).

So nearly normal is the G-6-PD activity in reticulocytes of G-6-PD A− subjects that a clinical problem arises in the diagnosis of this deficiency during severe reticulocytosis. This phenomemon represents a third mechanism by which activity of an enzyme, at least in the human red cell, can be greatly overestimated. If activity is decaying rapidly in vivo, measurements on the whole red cell population simply reflect the average enzymic activity. The average does not necessarily indicate the extent to which the red cells become deficient in activity as they age. This effect has also complicated the search for other types of enzyme defects in red cells of patients with chronic hemolytic disease. These patients often have reticulocytosis. Unless the level of activity of the suspected enzyme is known to be less than that in normal reticulocytes or unless activity is estimated in older, affected red cells, the enzymic defect can be missed. Very little is known about the mechanisms by which these mutant G-6-PD's undergo rapid destruction in vivo. The Mediterranean variant of G-6-PD exhibits moderate thermolability after partial purification. Many of the G-6-PD variants from people with chronic hemolytic disease have profound thermolability and instability on storage in the laboratory.

Thermolability was one of the first abnormal properties to be noted among mutant enzymes (Maas and Davis, 1952; Horowitz and Fling, 1956). Such instability has been reported for the defective hypoxanthine guanine phosphoribosyl transferase of children with Lesch-Nyhan syndrome (Kelly and Wyngaarden, 1970). The opposite characteristic, unusual thermostability, has been found with the α-galactosidase of Fabry's disease (Romeo and Migeon, 1971). Students of biochemical genetics, however, should be warned that thermostability of an enzyme is a property which is very easily influenced by the environment in which the enzyme exists both in vivo and in vitro. Many enzymes are sensitive to traces of heavy metals. Ionic environment, pH, and the presence of cofactors, substrates, and products may influence the stability of an enzyme.

Upon lysis of the cell, many enzymes begin to undergo destruction from intrinsic proteinases of the cell. The studies of Greene et al. (1970) and Kelly (1971) indicate that the unusually high activity of adenine phosphoribosyl transferase (APRT) in red cells of patients with hypoxanthine guanine phosphoribosyl transferase deficiency results from the accumulation of phosphoribosylpyrophosphate in these red cells. This substance seems, in turn, to stabilize the APRT and decrease the rate at which the APRT is inactivated by normal mechanisms within the red cell. Bellanti et al. (1970) suggest that the X-linked recessive form of chronic granulomatous disease results from an unstable white cell G-6-PD. The addition of electrophoretically abnormal G-6-PD to the white cell lyzates of these patients, however, allows one to test whether the increased rate of destruction of the G-6-PD represents an intrinsic defect of the G-6-PD or an effect of the environment of the white cell lyzate, such as proteinases. Such studies reveal that the white cell lyzates of some children with this disease do indeed destroy G-6-PD rapidly, but they destroy added G-6-PD just as readily as their own G-6-PD (Kirkman, unpublished). Conclusions as to whether differences in stability in vitro represent an intrinsic defect of an enzyme usually require carefully performed mixing experiments (W.H.O. Scientific Group, 1967).

Instability of a mutant enzyme helps to explain certain differences in degree of deficiency among various tissues. As mentioned, the human red cell must survive for several months without ability to synthesize protein. The white cell, on the other hand, has a continuing capacity for protein synthesis. Moreover, the life-span of the white cell is measured in hours and days rather than months. One would expect the degree of deficiency in white cells and in many other tissues to be less than in the red cell when the deficiency results from instability of the enzyme molecule in vivo. Such is the case for deficiencies of G-6-PD. The human red cell is the extreme example of a cell with prolonged life-span and limited ability for protein synthesis. In contrast, bacterial cells divide rapidly and have a very high capacity for protein synthesis. It is possible that intrinsic instability will be found to be the cause for human enzymic deficiencies, especially in red cells, far more often than would be expected from studies of microorganisms. The important role which molecular instability plays in mutant human proteins has become apparent also from studies of unstable hemoglobins (Perutz and Lehmann, 1968; Huehns, 1970).

These considerations emphasize that a qualitative and structural abnormality of an enzyme can lead secondarily to an abnormality in quantity of the enzyme protein. Other enzymic abnormalities are beginning to emerge that illustrate how the amount of enzyme protein can be secondarily affected by structural mutation. These findings tend to detract from any simplistic view that abnormalities in quantity of enzyme protein result from regulatory mutations whereas abnormalities in qualitative characteristics of the enzyme represent structural mutations. An unusual variant of human red cell G-6-PD is the Hektoen variant, which causes the red cell to have four times the normal amount of G-6-PD activity. Yoshida (1970) has recently demonstrated that this variant has a substitution of tyrosine for histidine at a single residue. One might assume, therefore, that this protein is a "super" enzyme, having several times the normal catalytic efficiency. In fact, the specific activity of the pure protein is approximately the same as that of normal G-6-PD. Immunological studies of Dern et al. (1969) indicate that the overactivity results from an excessive amount of the enzyme protein within the red cell. Their studies of fractionated red cells of the Hektoen variant indicate that the increased amount of protein cannot be attributed to decreased rate of destruction in vivo. Therefore, an increased rate of synthesis must be assumed. Similarly, Yoshida and Motulsky (1969) have studied a variant of pseudocholinesterase in a subject with resistance to succinylcholine. The level of activity of this enzyme was several times normal. Diisopropylfluorophosphate binding and immunological studies indicated that the amount of enzymic protein was actually increased. They suggest that this variant also represents an abnormality in primary structure, with secondary effects on the amount of enzyme protein.

Rather unexpected is the infrequency with the residual activity is found to represent an enzyme with characteristics identical to that of the normal enzyme, even when allowance is made for the possibility that the residual activity comes from a minor component controlled by another structural locus. Gaffney and Lehman (1969) find some residual activity even in the serum of subjects homozygous for the silent pseudocholinesterase gene. Altland and Goedde (1970) find that many of these exhibit unusual disc electrophoretic patterns. Of 25 such subjects studied by Rubenstein et al. (1970), 16 had neither enzyme activity nor CRM for serum pseudocholinesterase activity, but 8 patients had a small amount of both. A small amount of acetylcholinesterase activity was present in the serum of both normal and affected subjects.

Treatment of Enzyme Defects in Man

Just as the incomplete nature of many enzymic defects has diagnostic significance, the infrequency of functionless mutant enzymes as a cause for human enzymic deficiency has therapeutic significance. Whereas earlier attention was given to the use of special diets or to the avoidance of certain drugs to protect an affected individual from an overaccumulation of substrate, more recent interest is centered on efforts to increase or restore enzymic activity. The observation that a number of enzymic defects result from an elevated K_m raises the possibility that the environment can be modified sufficiently in vivo to allow the mutant enzyme to function with greater efficiency. The administration of a large amount of substrate might not be desirable, for many of these patients suffer from toxic levels of substrate or by-products of substrates. When the elevated K_m is for a vitamin coenzyme, however, a possibility exists that the disorder could be treated by the administration of large amounts of the vitamin. The administration of large amounts of a vitamin might serve to help an enzyme with a high K_m for the vitamin coenzyme to function better. This possible mechanism has been suggested to explain the beneficial results when large amounts of pyridoxine are administered to certain patients with xanthurenic aciduria (Tada et al., 1967) and cystathioninuria (Frimpter et al., 1969).

The effect of vitamins has been more clearly defined in B_{12}-responsive methylmalonic aciduria and in a disorder with combined homocystinuria and methylmalonic aciduria. Infants with methylmalonic aciduria excrete large amounts of this organic acid in their urine, suffer from acidosis, growth failure, and mental retardation, and often die in infancy. The defect has been identified as an impairment in the function of methylmalonyl CoA mutase (Rosenberg et al., 1968; Morrow et al., 1969). This enzyme requires 5'-deoxyadenosylcobalamin, a coenzyme form of vitamin B_{12}. Linblad et al. (1969) and Rosenberg et al. (1968) discovered that some patients with this disorder excrete much less methylmalonic acid after the administration of B_{12} in large amounts. Coupled with a reduced intake of protein, this has proved to be an effective way of managing the disorder in these children (Hsia et al., 1970). Rosenberg and co-workers (1969) find that the fibroblasts of patients with B_{12}-responsive methylmalonic aciduria accumulate less than 10% of the normal amount of 5'-deoxyadenosylcobalamin. The defect in methylmalonate metabolism is overcome by allowing the fibroblasts to grow in the presence of large amounts of B_{12}. Their findings suggest that the primary defect in this variety of methylmalonic aciduria is an impaired ability to convert B_{12} to the coenzyme. Other subjects with methylmalonic aciduria do not respond to the administration of vitamin B_{12}. The latter type is presumed to be a defect in the apoenzyme.

Another form of B_{12}, methylcobalamin, is used by the enzyme N^5-methyltetrahydrofolate homocysteine methyltransferase. Mudd et al. (1969, 1970b) found decreased levels of this enzyme and of 5'-deoxyadenosylcobalamin in the liver of a boy with combined homocystinuria and methylmalonic aciduria. Activity of methylmalonyl CoA mutase was reduced. Fibroblasts from an affected patient had partial restoration of methyltransferase activity and full restoration of methylmalonic acid metabolism when B_{12} was added to culture medium. Presumably, the cells of these subjects are deficient in both the methyl and deoxyadenosyl form of B_{12}, and the defect is one of transport or metabolism of B_{12} before the conversion of B_{12} to these two forms.

Hines (1971) has observed decreased levels of pyridoxal phosphokinase in red cells and livers of patients with pyridoxine-dependent refractory sideroblastic anemia and in the red cells and fibroblasts of a patient with cystathioninuria. McLaren and Zekian (1971) report a child who exhibited signs of vitamin A deficiency, despite normal diet and absence of malabsorption. Large doses of β-carotene failed to correct the disorder, whereas the administration of vitamin A did so. They presumed that this disorder represents a failure of enzymic cleavage of β-carotene. Rosenberg et al. (1969) have summarized the various defects which might underlie vitamin-responsive inborn errors of metabolism. These include: (1) defective transport of the vitamin into the cell, (2) defective conversion of the vitamin to the corresponding coenzyme, and (3) defective formation of the holoenzyme. A beneficial effect would be expected if the administration of a large amount of vitamin served to overcome any of these defects. It might also be expected if a vitamin coenzyme stabilizes a labile, mutant enzyme or induces the synthesis of the apoenzyme. Mudd et al. (1970a) have discussed these last two possibilities and have cited, as an example, the evidence that pyridoxine induces the synthesis of transaminase. Conversely, a deficiency of the appropriate intracellular form of B_{12} seems to have led to a secondary deficiency of methyltransferase in a subject with combined homocystinuria and methylmalonic aciduria. The methyltransferase activity could not be restored to normal levels by the addition of methylcobalamin to cell lyzates (Mudd et al., 1970b). Regardless of the mechanism, these recent observations point to the availability of a new approach to the treatment of certain inborn errors of metabolism.

Another, relatively untried, approach to the treatment of inborn errors of metabolism is the use of hormones or other agents to raise the level of activity of a deficient enzyme. The effects of these agents call to mind the process of enzyme induction in bacteria, but the mechanism need not be the same. Phenobarbital is of current interest to pediatricians as a drug which may facilitate the glucuronidation of bilirubin in newborn infants. The conversion of bilirubin to the diglucuronide of bilirubin (conjugated or direct-reacting bilirubin) occurs much more slowly in normal newborns than in children and adults. Some method of enhancing this process in the newborn would be of considerable value in the prevention and management of hyperbilirubinemia. Excessive levels of unconjugated bilirubin occur in premature and term infants from a variety of causes. These excessive levels can lead to a form of brain damage (kernicterus) in the infant. The effect of phenobarbital has been studied in infants with Crigler-Najjar syndrome and in Gunn rats. Both conditions represent severe deficiencies in activity of glucuronyl transferase. Gartner and Arias (1968) could see no effect of phenobarbital on the serum bilirubin of an infant with Crigler-Najjar syndrome or on the serum bilirubin and hepatic glucuronyl transferase activity of Gunn rats. Yaffee et al. (1966) and Crigler and Gold (1966), however, observed a considerable decline of serum bilirubin concentration when infants with Crigler-Najjar syndrome received phenobarbital. Gartner and Arias attributed the difference in results to the possibility that the responsive infants had a milder form of Crigler-Najjar syndrome. Their initial bilirubin levels were lower than those of infants with the typical disease. Arias et al., (1969) have offered evidence that the disorder is genetically heterogeneous.

One of the many contributions made by the study of mutant human cells in cell culture may be the ease with which such cells can be tested for responsiveness to certain agents. Nadler (1971a), for example, has found evidence for genetic heterogeneity of acid phosphatase deficiency. One form of this disease represents a deficiency of lysosomal acid phosphatase; the other form represents a deficiency of total acid phosphatase activity. Activity of the enzyme is increased when prednisolone is added to cells cultured from a patient with the lysosomal acid phosphatase deficiency. This finding raises the possibility that prednisolone would be of benefit to infants with this serious disorder. Only clinical trials, of course, can confirm this, but cell cultures would seem to provide a safe and useful means for exploring ways of altering metabolism in a manner that might benefit patients.

A major advance in medical genetics has been the development of techniques for antenatal diagnosis of enzyme defects. A list of the inborn errors of metabolism which have been diagnosed by this approach appears in the Table 1. New disorders are being added to the list, as enzymic assays and other biochemical determinations are adapted to amniotic fluid and amniotic cells. Pitfalls in enzyme diagnosis by this approach have been discussed earlier. For couples at risk for having an infant with an inborn error of metabolism, this procedure represents a valuable option which would allow them to be assured of the birth of an infant free of the disorder in question. Couples who wish to take this approach may elect to have the pregnancy terminated if the fetus is shown to be affected. Such couples could attempt to have a normal child with a subsequent pregnancy. This procedure also provides a benefit even when the diagnosis reveals that the fetus does have the suspected defect: the pregnant woman is sometimes lifted from a state of despair by being reassured as to the outcome of the pregnancy. In a certain sense, this represents an approach to

TABLE 1.—*Inborn Errors of Metabolism
That Have Been Diagnosed Antenatally**

Acid phosphatase deficiency (lysosomal)
Adrenogenital syndrome
Fabry's disease
Galactosemia
Lesch-Nyhan syndrome
Maple syrup urine disease
Metachromatic leukodystrophy
Methylmalonicaciduria
Mucopolysaccharidosis (Hurler's syndrome)
Niemann-Pick disease
Pompe's disease (type II glycogen storage disease)
Tay-Sachs disease

* From Milunsky et al. (1970) and Nadler (1971b).

the management of inborn errors of metabolism which is an important as the methods of treatment just described. It is applicable to disorders for which no treatment exists at present. Indeed, it would seem to be particularly appropriate for disorders without other means of treatment.

DETECTION OF HETEROZYGOUS SUBJECTS

Earlier interest in the detection of subjects heterozygous for inborn errors of metabolism stemmed from the requirement for genetic counseling, particularly of X-linked recessive disorders, and from the value of heterozygote recognition in determining more clearly the mode of inheritance of biochemical disorders. Occasionally, the worker involved in genetic counseling of an autosomal recessive disorder is asked if a sibling, aunt, or uncle of an affected person is likely to have a similarly affected child. The risk can be defined with greater accuracy if the worker can determine whether or not this relative is heterozygous for the same disorder. The value of detecting heterozygotes for this purpose, however, is limited. Even if heterozygous, the relative would not be at appreciable risk for having an affected child unless his mate were also heterozygous. In the absence of consanguinity, the chance that the mate would also be heterozygous is small. The large majority of births of affected children would not be anticipated by this approach. Except for sibs, infants born with an autosomal recessive enzymic defect are seldom relatives of similarly affected children.

Just as the development of dietary treatment for phenylketonuria made important the diagnosis of this disorder in early infancy, so has the development of antenatal diagnosis made important methods for detecting couples who are at risk for having a child with an enzyme defect even before the birth of an affected child in the family. It should be admitted that antenatal diagnosis for inborn errors of metabolism is at present used largely for couples who have already had at least one affected child. This method of ascertainment of couples at risk, however, is a very inefficient one. It is particularly inefficient in a society in which emphasis is being placed on limiting the number of children of each couple to possibly 2 or 3. Table 2 illustrates the inefficiency of "waiting for lightning to strike once" before taking action for autosomal recessive diseases. In a hypothetical society in which all couples have only one child, this approach would have zero efficiency; for the couples with an affected child would not be planning to have another child anyway. Nor would this approach be efficient for dealing with couples who have had several normal children and who plan to have no further children after the birth of an affected child. In a hypothetical population in which all couples would have only 2 children, this approach would allow the detection of only 12.5% of the total number of affected children born; for hypothetical couples having 3 children, 23%; 4 children, 32%, and so forth. A far more efficient method of anticipating either autosomal recessive or sex-linked recessive disease would be one in which young couples could be tested for heterozygosity before the first pregnancy.

The detection of persons who are heterozygous for enzymic deficiencies usually rests upon a demonstration that their levels of enzymic activity lie between those of normal and fully affected subjects. Ideally, one might hope that there would be no overlapping of values, that is, that levels for heterozygotes would fall outside the range for either normal or fully affected people. Usually, however, at least a small percentage of heterozygous subjects have values that fall into the range for normal people. Overlapping of this magnitude is not enough to interfere seriously with efforts to identify heterozygotes among relatives of subjects with enzymic deficiencies. Almost as many close relatives will be heterozygous as will be normal (Fig. 4a). Under these conditions, nearly all of the people with

TABLE 2.—*Efficiency of Detection of Fetuses or Newborns with an Autosomal Recessive Disease If the Parents at Risk Are Ascertained Only by the Previous Birth of an Affected Infant*

Final size of sibship	Efficiency, %
1	0
2	12.5
3	23
4	32
5	39

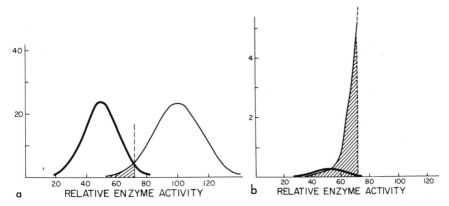

FIG. 4.—(*a*) Distribution curves of enzyme levels for hypothetical population of heterozygous subjects (*left*) and homozygous normal subjects (*right*). Populations are of equal size. (*b*) Same populations as in (*a*) except normals outnumber heterozygotes 100 to 1.

levels in the heterozygous range will actually be heterozygous. Most heterozygotes for an autosomal recessive disease, however, are not close relatives of affected subjects. The efficient anticipation of such disease requires the identification of heterozygotes in the population at large or, at least, in relatively large ethnic or geographic groups at special risk for the disorder.

It is not generally recognized that a test which is satisfactory for family studies can be grossly inaccurate for detecting heterozygotes in the general population, where the ratio of homozygous normal subjects to heterozygous subjects may be many times greater than 1. As the ratio of homozygous normal to heterozygous subjects gets larger and larger, the distribution curve for normals beings to overrun the distribution curve for heterozygous people (Fig. 4*b*). Soon a point is reached at which most people who are labeled as heterozygous are actually homozygous normal. The same test that is correct 97% of the time in the detection of heterozygotes in family studies, could be correct only 20% of the time in detection of heterozygotes in the population at large. Worse still, if the test is correct only 20% of the time in defining individuals as heterozygotes, it will be correct only 4% of the time ($\frac{1}{5} \times \frac{1}{5}$) in defining couples in which both partners are heterozygous. An argument can be made that studies of the parents of the partners should help to confirm whether or not each partner is heterozygous; for heterozygote should have a parent who is either heterozygote or, rarely, a homozygous affected person. This effort is helpful, but it does not offer a full solution to the problem.

These remarks should not be taken to mean that mass screening for heterozygotes by quantitative enzymic assay are futile. On the contrary, laboratory improvements that decrease the standard deviations only slightly could improve the efficiency of heterozygote detection drastically. Moreover, screening for heterozygotes is most likely to be attempted for autosomal recessive diseases with a relatively high incidence (1:10,000 to 1:1000), such as cystic fibrosis in Caucasians, sickle cell disease in Negroes, and Tay-Sachs disease in people of European Jewish ancestry. One may estimate by Hardy-Weinberg ratios that between 2% and 6% of the population should be heterozygous for a disease of that order of prevalence. Under these conditions the homozygous normal to heterozygote ratio is between 50 to 1 and 16 to 1. The frequency of mistaking normal homozygotes for heterozygotes would be less than for rarer diseases. Nevertheless, those who attempt mass screening for heterozygotes should realize that the degree of overlapping is determined not only by the standard deviations but by the ratio of homozygous normals to heterozygotes.

Occasionally, also, values for heterozygotes overlap those of homozygous affected subjects. This represents less of a problem than the one previously discussed, for usually the presence of the homozygous state is apparent from the symptoms of the affected individual. A distinction between the heterozygote and the fully affected individual becomes extremely important, however, in the studies of fetal cells for antenatal diagnosis (Kaback, personal communications). This is a problem at present in the use of metachromasia for the diagnosis of cystic fibrosis. The cells of heterozygotes for cystic fibrosis also exhibit metachromatic staining (Bearn et al., 1970). Unless the heterozygote can be distinguished from the homozygous affected fetus, women at risk for having fully affected infants might have to have an inordinate number of theraputic abortions before conceiving a homozygous normal infant. Such couples have only a 25% chance of having a homozygous normal fetus with each pregnancy. The problem in this instance, however, is analogous to that of detecting heterozygotes among relatives of homozygous affected subjects: the number of heterozygous fetuses will not be greatly different from the number of homozygous affected fetuses. In fact, the ratio should be 2 to 1. The fact that this ratio is not 100 to 1 serves to minimize the frequency of misdiagnosis resulting from overlapping values.

The inconvenience caused by a high proportion of false positives has been noticeable in programs of screening for phenylketonuria among newborn infants. For several types of assays, the borderline in serum phenylalanine values between normal infants and infants suspected of having phenylketonuria is set so as to minimize the chance that the phenylketonuric infant would be missed. This is appropriate, for early diagnosis and dietary management of these infants is believed by many workers to increase the likelihood that the infant will develop with normal intelligence, but the efficiency in detecting affected infancy is achieved at the expense of including many nonphenylketonuric infants in the suspect group. The ratio of false positives to true positives may be 10 to 1 or higher. At some considerable cost in time and laboratory effort, further studies must be undertaken to confirm the presence of phenylketonuria in the suspected infant. Ahlvin (1970) has pointed out that the effort and expense of resolving false positive diagnoses are often not taken into consideration in estimating the cost of a screening program. Perhaps of even greater importance is the cost in mental anguish which can occur when an unusually high percentage of false positive diagnoses exist or when the normal subject becomes unnecessarily alarmed.

Since only a slight broadening of the standard deviation of enzyme values for normals and heterozygotes serves to increase the zone of uncertainty between the two genotypes, it is not surprising that factors which tend to modify the enzyme level also tend to impede the correct designation of homozygous normals and heterozygotes. O'Brien et al. (1970) demonstrated that heterozygotes for Tay-Sachs disease had values for serum hexosaminadase A values that fell below the range for presumably homozygous normal control subjects when this value was expressed as a percentage of the total hexosaminadase level. Values on patients with diabetes mellitus, or on patients who had been hospitalized for other disorders, tended to overlap the values for both heterozygotes and controls. These findings suggest that homozygous normal subjects who have diabetes or other illnesses might be falsely classified as heterozygous by this method. Modification of the opposite sort occurs in a most unfortunate way in Duchenne muscular dystrophy, which is sex-linked recessive. Levels of serum creatine phosphokinase are often slightly to moderately elevated in women who are heterozygous for this disorder. Blyth and Hughes (1971) have recently reported that some women who are heterozygous for this disorder have lower serum enzyme levels during pregnancy. Thus, a considerable danger exists that the sister of an affected male might be falsely classified as homozygous normal during the pregnancy.

Detection of heterozygotes by quantity of enzymic activity is possible during screening of large populations if normal variation and laboratory error are small enough, but the difficulties of this approach serve to emphasis the desirability of having a marker which is more nearly a qualitative one. A familiar example is the use of electrophoresis for the detection of subjects heterozygous for sickle cell disease. The enzymic counterpart of this example is the use of the inhibitor dibucaine for detection of people who are heterozygous for the "atypical" type of pseudocholinesterase. Homozygous affected subjects have a functional deficiency of pseudocholinesterase, which causes them to be susceptible to prolonged paralysis after receiving normally appropriate doses of the muscle relaxant succinylcholine. The mutant enzyme is more resistant to inhibition by dibucaine than normal pseudocholinesterase. Calculation of the percentage inhibition allows a clear delineation of homozygous normal, heterozygotes, and homozygous affected subjects (Kalow and Staron, 1957; Harris et al., 1960). Figure 5 provides another example of the use of a qualitative marker for the detection of heterozygotes. Blood was received in the laboratory of this reviewer from a woman who was suspected of being heterozygous for G-6-PD A−. This variant moves 6 % to 10% faster than normal G-6-PD on electrophoresis. As mentioned, it has lability in vivo, which results in

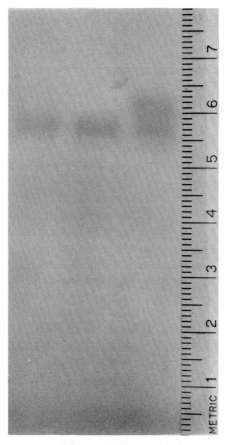

FIG. 5.—Starch gel electrophoretic patterns of G-6-PD. From left to right: hemolyzate from mother, hemolyzate from normal subject, white cell lyzate from mother.

deficiency of activity of this enzyme in red cells, but only slight deficiency in white cells. Owing to the effects of shipment and storage, significance could not be attached to the fact that red cell G-6-PD activity of the sample was slightly lower than average. Electrophoresis of the hemolyzate revealed a band of normal G-6-PD. White cell lyzates exhibited both bands. This pattern clearly indicated that the woman was heterozygous for G-6-PD A−.

An interesting technique has been employed recently for bringing out an expression of heterozygosity in lymphocytes. The lymphocytes of heterozygotes for some inborn errors of metabolism often do not exhibit intermediate levels of activity. Hirschhorn et al. (1969) found that lymphocytes obtained from subjects heterozygous for type II glycogen storage disease failed to show an increase in levels of α-1,4-glucosidase after incubation in the presence of phytohemagglutinin, which stimulates lymphocytes to synthesize protein more rapidly and to undergo mitosis. In contrast, lymphocytes of normal subjects had higher levels of this enzyme after the incubation. Nadler and Egan (1970) found that the addition of this substance to lymphocytes also permitted the detection of subjects heterozygous for lysosomal acid phosphatase deficiency.

Enzymic Assays

An appreciable risk of misdiagnosis accompanies use of enzymic assays for detection of inborn errors of metabolism. The diversity and rarity of these disorders make it difficult for the staff of the average hospital laboratory to acquire either the experience or the appropriate reagents for these assays. Those who are inexperienced in enzymology are sometimes unaware of the lability of enzymes. Moreover, enzymic assays differ from other biochemical procedures in being essentially measurements of rate. Concepts of enzyme kinetics enter strongly into the design and interpretation of these assays. A detailed consideration of enzymic techniques would be inappropriate for this review, but the following are generalizations that might help to prevent some of the mistakes that occur most frequently with enzymic diagnosis.

1. The sample being tested should actually come from the person for whom the test is intended. This obvious statement is not meant to refer to mislabeling of samples. More subtle errors of this type arise. An assay for red cell galactose-1-phosphate uridyl transferase in red cells provides a highly definitive test for galactosemia. Infants with this disorder often develop severe growth failure, jaundice, hepatic damage, cataracts, and mental retardation. Some die. Early diagnosis and placement of the infant on a galactose-free diet tend to spare the infant from these developments. The

jaundice of severe galactosemia in early infancy, however, may prompt the physician to do an exchange transfusion before the diagnosis is suspected. Those experienced in performing this assay on the red cells of newborn infants have been made aware of the necessity of enquiring as to whether or not the infant has been given an exchange transfusion. If so, the blood sample from the infant may represent red cells largely from a doner in the blood bank.

Antenatal diagnosis provides another circumstance in which cells being studied may not come from the subject for whom the test is intended. During amniocentesis, maternal cells occasionally contaminate the sample of amniotic fluid. With subsequent cell culture, these may grow and may even overgrow the culture. If so, the biochemical or cytogenetic diagnosis would be on the mother, not on the fetus. The likelihood of this occurring is diminished if the amniotic fluid is placed in several vials. Often only one maternal cell, if any, is present; therefore, only one vial may be overgrown with maternal cells. Early growth of the cells also suggests that they are of maternal origin. Nevertheless, this represents another circumstance in which the cells studied may not be from the subject for whom the test was intended. The diagnosis in a fetus could be missed if attention were not given to this possibility. Whether for cytogenetic or biochemical diagnosis, brief characterization or assay of certain enzymes in the cultured cells may someday prove useful for distinguishing between maternal and fetal cells and for providing a safeguard against maternal cell contamination. As exemplified by isozyme patterns of lactate dehydrogenase, qualitative and quantitative differences exist between certain enzymes of fetal cells and those of adult cells. One wonders if these enzymes might not prove to be useful markers that would allow a distinction between maternal and fetal cells.

2. Attention should be directed to the possibility that the sample has deteriorated as a consequence of faulty collection, shipment, or storage. The same reservation applies to the use of uncultured amniotic cells, many of which may represent "old" cells that have deteriorated while floating in amniotic fluid in utero. Enzymes differ in susceptibility to destruction. Some are stable under conditions of collection and storage that lead to the rapid destruction of others. Instructions for collection and shipment of samples should be followed closely.

3. The conditions of the enzymic assay should be such that the rate of the reaction observed is proportional to the amount of enzyme present. These conditions include the availibility of adequate amounts of substrate, the avoidance of excessive amounts of enzyme, and the avoidance of accumulation of product of the types and amounts that might inhibit the enzyme. These conditions are not those necessary for determining the func-

tion of the enzyme at low substrate concentration, as previously discussed. Consequently, explorations for previously undiscovered enzyme defects may require simultaneous assays under two conditions: those optimal for detecting K_m and allosteric mutants, and those necessary for detecting simple deficiencies in activity.

4. If the assay is based upon a measurement of the consumption of substrate, the substrate should not be generated during the reaction, nor should it be consumed by any reaction other than the one intended for measurement.

5. If the assay is based upon the generation of product, the product should not be generated by any mechanism other than the one intended for measurement, nor should the product be consumed. The product of the reaction catalyzed by G-6-PD, for example, is NADPH and 6-phosphogluconate (6-PG), but 6-PG is utilized for the generation of another molecule of NADPH by the next enzyme in the metabolic sequence. Consequently, when the rate of G-6-PD is followed in cell lyzates by measurements of the amount of NADPH, the reaction rate of the enzyme is overestimated. Conversely, one of the products of the reaction catalyzed by glutamine phosphoribosyl pyrophosphate transamidase is pyrophosphate. The progress of the reaction is followed by means of determinations of this product. Many cell lyzates, however, are rich in pyrophosphatase. Sodium fluoride, added as an inhibitor of this pyrophosphatase, prevents loss of this product.

The product of many enzyme reactions may more readily be detected by the addition of a reagent enzyme that converts the product into another substance that is easily measured. Sometimes, however, the reagent enzyme itself is contaminated with the very enzyme which is being measured. This is true for some preparations of lactate dehydrogenase, used in the assay for pyruvate kinase, and ornithine transcarbamylase, used in the assay of carbamyl phosphate synthetase.

These complexities emphasize the desirability of centralizing the performance of enzymic assays for rare disorders in national or regional reference laboratories, where the frequency of assays would allow them to be carried out with greater accuracy and economy. Such efforts, however, increase the need for attention to the methods by which samples are collected and transported.

ENZYME DEFECTS AT HIGHER LEVELS OF CELLULAR ORGANIZATION

Nearly all enzymic defects presently known to exist in man are those which affect intermediary metabolism, often resulting in overaccumulation of some metabolite. Representatives of these disorders are the various storage diseases, aminoacidurias, and organic acidemias. With advances in understanding of molecular biology, however, has come an appreciation of biochemical mechanisms operating at higher levels of cellular organizations. Among these are the many enzymic steps involved in replication, repair, and transcription of DNA, and translation. Enzymic mechanisms seem to be involved in acetylation (Allfrey et al., 1964; Pogo et al, 1966) and phosphorylation (Ord and Stocken, 1966) of histones, which some workers believe may influence gene activity. Cyclic AMP seems to be involved not only in the phosphorylation of histones (Langan,- 1968) but also in the mechanism of action of various hormones. Adenyl cyclase of adipose tissue is activated by ACTH, glucagon, catecholamines, prolactin, and thyroid-stimulating hormone, while that of cardiac tissue is activated by catecholamine, thyroid hormone, and glucagon (Drummond and Duncan, 1970). Although defects in metabolic pathways are well known to have secondary effects, a deficiency in enzymic activity at one of these higher levels of cellular organization might be especially likely to exert an effect in many different ways.

Conversely, physicians are aware of conditions which seem difficult to characterize by conventional methods of biochemical analysis. Many of these, of course, may also prove to be enzymic defects of recognized pathways of intermediary metabolism, but one wonders if others might not be defects at the higher levels described. These thoughts come to mind when one considers progeria and severe forms of unexplained dwarfism.

Examples of enzyme defects at these levels are beginning to emerge. Among the disorders of skin is xeroderma pigmentosum, an autosomal recessive disease characterized by development of lesions of the skin, especially when the patient is exposed to sunlight. These patients also develop carcinomas of the skin. Setlow and co-workers (1969) have offered evidence that the basic defect in this disorder is one involving the first step in the repair of DNA which has been damaged by ultraviolet light. An interesting study by Aarskog and Fagerhol (1970) was directed at the possibility that proteolytic enzymes may be involved in the normal mechanisms of meiosis, spindle apparatus formation, and cell division. Among the components of human serum are the inhibitors of proteases, a familiar example being α_1-antitrypsin. These workers determined the electrophoretic phenotype of patients with sex chromosomal mosaicism and of their parents. In 5 of the 7 families, the electrophoretic type was one other than the usual (MM) type seen in healthy Norwegians. Another example is suggested by the studies of Wiesmann et al. (1971) who found evidence to support the possibility that "I-cell" disease is a defect expressed by leakage of lysosomal enzymes from the patient's cells. Cultured fibroblast exhibited low levels of four lysosomal enzymes within the cell and high levels of these enzymes in the culture medium. Their observation raises the possibility that the defect is not primarily a deficiency of these four enzymes but a defect expressed at a higher level of organization.

Emmer and co-workers (1970) studied strains of *E. coli* that were unable to synthesize various inducible enzymes. Cyclic AMP is required for the synthesis of β-galactosidase and other inducible catabolic enzymes in *E. coli*. One strain was deficient in adenyl cyclase activity and had undetectable levels of cyclic AMP. The addition of cyclic AMP allowed enzyme synthesis. A second class of mutant had a defective receptor protein for cyclic AMP. Enzyme synthesis in this second mutant could not be restored by the addition of cyclic AMP, but it could be restored by the addition of normal receptor protein.

EMERGING PROBLEMS

The Molecular Mechanism of Genetically Dominant Diseases

As laboratory tests for detection of heterozygous subjects began to emerge, uncertainty arose over the meaning of the terms dominant and recessive. These developments, however, merely served to emphasize the necessity for defining the phenotype before using these terms. Thus, sickle cell *disease* is recessive, the sickling phenomenon is dominant, and the appearances of sickle hemoglobin and normal hemoglobin on electrophoresis are codominant. Perhaps most genetic disorders have some degree of intermediate dominance, affecting heterozygotes less severely than homozygotes. Nevertheless, when one considers disorders sufficiently severe to shorten life: impair function, or require medical attention, many diseases can be classified as either recessive or dominant. Among the hereditary disorders of man in which the basic defect has been recognized, most are recessive in clinical expression, and many of these represent impairments in enzyme function. At the present time, deficiencies of specific proteins and enzymic activity are conspicuously rare among dominant disorders. A notable exception is the deficiency of inhibitor of C′1 esterase in angioneurotic edema, which is genetically dominant (Donaldson and Rosen, 1964; Alper et al., 1970).

Although approximately half-normal activities are characteristically seen among people who are heterozygous for enzymic deficiencies, this degree of impairment does not seem to be sufficient to result in disease. Possibly this stems from the fact that few enzymes are so rate-limiting as to cause a serious reduction in rate of a metabolic pathway when the enzyme has 40-60% normal activity. Uroporphyrinogen synthetase, however, may be such a rate-limiting enzyme; for Strand and co-workers (1970, 1971) have offered evidence that acute intermittent porphyria may result from a partial deficiency in activity of this enzyme.

The basic defect has been identified in far more recessive than dominant disorders, but the number of dominant diseases of man exceeds the number of recognized recessive diseases (McKusick, 1968). It would appear, therefore, that dominant disorders have been relatively refractory to elucidation by present methods of study. It is possible to hypothesize a mechanism with dominant expression arising from the familiar mechanism of a mutation in the structural locus for a protein. The resultant abnormal protein might have a deleterious effect on the cell, out of proportion to the amount of mutant protein present. Such a protein would do more harm than would occur if it were absent. A number of dominant hemolytic disorders result from the presence in the red cell of an abnormal and unstable hemoglobin (Perutz and Lehmann, 1968; Huehns, 1970). The presence of one of these abnormal hemoglobins seems to shorten the survival of the red cell, despite the presence of normal hemoglobin within the cell. Another example of this type is provided by certain abnormal fibrinogens, which disrupt the formation of normal clots. Mammen and co-workers (1969) have described such a protein (fibrinogen Detroit), which seems to be molecularly abnormal. Hampton and co-workers (1971) have studied families with defective fibrin formation resulting either from a deficiency of an enzyme which cross-links monomers of fibrin (autosomal recessive) or from an abnormal fibrinogen (autosomal dominant).

One class of structural mutants possibly capable of causing dominant disease is the group of enzymes with altered substrate specificity. Extreme examples of these have been found among the variants of G-6-PD (Kirkman et al., 1968; Yoshida et al., 1971). Their existence prompts one to wonder if an enzyme variant might not generate abnormal products either by using a substrate which it is not suppose to use or by acting on its natural substrate in the wrong way. No examples of this are known in man, although certain suppressor mutants of *E. coli* have a genetically dominant trait resulting from altered specificity of soluble RNA. Kobata and Ginsburg (1970) have isolated from human milk an enzyme which is responsible for the attachment of *N*-acetyl-D-galactosamine to terminal galactosyl residues of certain L-focuse-containing oligosaccharides. The product is the substance which determines the familiar blood type A. The enzyme is also present in AB subjects, but missing in subjects of blood type O or B.

Two classes of dominant traits in microorganisms express themselves not by deficiency in enzyme activity but by excessive enzymic activity. Mutations of the structural locus of an enzyme may reduce the ability of the enzyme to be inhibited by the end product of the metabolic pathway in which the enzyme participates. Operator constitutive mutations cause the organism to produce an excessive amount of messenger RNA. Both defects led to an overproduction of metabolites. Acute intermittent porphyria seems to be an autosomal dominant disorder. Tschudy et al. (1965) and Nakao et al. (1966) report that the level of enzyme leading into the pathway of synthesis of porphyrin is abnormally high in the liver of subjects with acute intermittent porphyria. Strand and co-workers (1970, 1971), however, find that patients with acute intermittent porphyria have partial deficiency of uroporphyrinogen synthetase, an enzyme in the middle of the pathway of heme synthesis. They present evidence that the increase in activity of the enzyme earlier in the pathway is due to derepression resulting from decreased amounts of heme.

Similarly, the hyperuricaciduria of Lesch-Nyhan syndrome has been shown by Seegmiller and co-workers (1967) to represent a deficiency of hypoxanthine-guanine phosphoribosyl transferase (HGPRT). This enzyme is active in the retrieval of purine nucleotide from purine bases, and a deficiency of the enzyme leads secondarily to increased rate of synthesis of purines. A partial defect of the same enzyme is responsible for some clinically milder types of hyperuricaciduria (Kogut et al., 1970), including types with renal calculi and gout (Kelly et al., 1969). Thus, while mutants with loss of feedback inhibitability and mutants with overproduction due primarily to disordered regulation may well exist in man, studies to date have not revealed them.

Regulation

Earlier discussions have referred to the scarcity of evidence for a human genetic defect that could be classed primarily as a defect of regulation. A recent review has disclosed a comparable situation among mutants in *Drosophila* (E. Glassman, personal communication). This state of affairs cannot be attributed entirely to lack of opportunity for the detection of such mutants. For example, a certain proportion of regulatory mutants should give rise to reduced amounts of enzyme without changes in the qualitative characteristics of the enzyme. As mentioned, among the previously cited deficiencies of G-6-PD, most are not fully deficient, yet the residual enzyme in each instance tends to exhibit one of several dozen sets of abnormal characteristics. The most likely candidate for a regulatory abnormality of G-6-PD was G-6-PD Hektoen, whose synthesis at an excessive rate causes the affected red cell to have abnormally high amounts of G-6-PD activity, yet this variant has an amino acid substitution (Yoshida, 1970). Oroticaciduria has also served as a possible candidate for being a regulatory mutant. It is unusual among inborn errors of metabolism in that it is a deficiency of two enzymes, orotidylic pyrophosphorylase and orotidylic decarboxylase, which catalyze consecutive steps in the synthesis of pyrimidines. These two activities may arise from the same protein or protein complex, however, for Appel (1968) found that the ratio of the two activities remained constant throughout extensive purification from bovine brain. The activities remained constant also throughout heat-inactivation studies. This conclusion is complicated by the recent finding of a case of deficiency of orotidylic decarboxylase, without deficiency of orotidylic pyrophosphorylase (Fox et al., 1969), but this can be explained on the basis that a mutation could affect one activity of the complex without affecting the other activity. Examples of this phenomenon are known in microbial systems (Jones, 1971).

Littlefield (1969) has reviewed the studies on regulation in animal cells and has pointed out that strong evidence for bacterial-type regulation in these cells does not exist. He also described reservations that should be kept in mind when one attempts to study regulation in cultured mammalian cells. These points should not be taken as arguments that regulatory mechanisms do not exist in man, only that studies of genetic disorders have not revealed convincing examples of defects which seem to be primarily those of a regulatory system. Evidence of mechanisms of regulation emerges, however, from the secondary effects just discussed, from studies of cultures of rat hepatoma cells (Tomkins et al., 1969), and from recent studies of cell hybrids. Illustrative of the last approach is the work of Klebe et al. (1970), which was directed at determining which chromosome exerts negative control on a kidney-associated esterase, ES-2. This esterase is present in mouse renal adenocarcinoma cells. Somatic cell hybridization of the renal cells with either mouse or human fibroblasts leads to a decided reduction in ES-2 esterase activity. Since mouse-human hybrids gradually lose human chromosomes, these workers were able to associate the negative control with human chromosome C_{10}.

Other Problems

Among the hereditary disorders in man, typified by Huntington's chorea and adult-onset muscular dystrophies, are those in which the affected individual seems to live a normal life for years before exhibiting manifestations of the disease. The nearly normal life enjoyed briefly by infants with sickle cell disease and β-thalassemia is explained by the preponderance of fetal hemoglobin in the red cells of normal newborn infants. Each is a defect involving the structure or rate of synthesis of the β chain. The gene for the β chain does not become active until later in fetal development, and the affected infants begin to suffer from the disease only when they reach that age when adult hemoglobin ($\alpha_2\beta_2$) comprises a major portion of the hemoglobin of the red cell. Such switching from one gene to the other seems to occur as a developmental process in man, however, only during fetal life and early infancy. As yet, there is no evidence of a developmental switching from one gene to another during childhood or adulthood. Some metabolic diseases seem to owe their more gradual onset to the fact that the enzyme is not as deficient in activity as it is in infantile forms of the same disease. This seems to be the explanation for adult form of Gaucher's disease (Brady, 1970) and juvenile GM_2 gangliosidosis (Okada et al., 1970, 1971). The same substance accumulates in these individuals as in the more severely affected infants; presumably, the rate of accumulation is slower. One wonders if even milder enzymic defects might not lead to accumulation of substances, or alterations of intercellular environment, that would hasten the senescence of cells in certain tissues. These are intriguing problems and problems for which an explanation might have considerable practical application. The distressing feature of Huntington's chorea, for example, is the fact that the affected individual may beget children before realizing that he carries this abnormal gene. Early diagnosis of this disease, in the absence of treatment, would be a depressing accomplishment for affected individuals, but it might lead to control of the disease. The diseases of late onset, however, remain to be explained at a molecular level.

Methods of cell culture and hybridization now allow tests for complementation between different cells with a metabolic abnormality. This approach has been a powerful technique for the elucidation of genetic control of bacterial enzymes. It is already proving to be useful for studies of human enzyme defects. The procedure is a functional and cellular test of allelism, analogous to the *trans* test in microbial genetics. An examination for restoration of function is made on hybrid cells formed by the fusion of cells from 2 subjects. If the abnormality of the 2 subjects resides in the same gene—for example, in the structural gene for the same polypeptide chain—then little or no restoration of function would be expected. If the abnormality resides in different genes, function would be observed. The procedure is capable of revealing that two or more structural genes determine a single enzyme, or that two or more enzymes participate in a metabolic pathway. Nadler and co-workers (1970) observed such complementation in hybrid cells from certain patients with deficiency in galactrose-1-phosphate uridyl transferase, the enzyme which is deficient in activity in galactosemia. Hybrids from other patients did not exhibit complementation.

An interesting outcome from tests for complementation has been the observation that human cells may exhibit complementation even when placed in the same culture flask without cell fusion. The recent studies of Danes and Bearn (1970) illustrate the immense value of this procedure in classifying mucopolysaccharidoses, revealing previously unrecognized subtypes of each disorder, and determining whether or not 2 patients have the same disorder. Such complementations between unfused cells can occur if metabolites or enzymes of the involved pathway are able to get from one cell to the next. The extensive studies of Neufeld and her co-workers (1970) are compatible with the possibility that the exchanged substance is the enzyme. Wiesmann et al. (1971) found that cellular levels of arylsulfatase A in fibroblasts from patients with metachromatic leukodystrophy could be raised to one-third normal by incubation of the cells with partially purified arylsulfatase A. Kyriakides and co-workers (1971) noted that fibroblasts from subjects with Wolman's disease (acid lipase deficiency) lost their excessive accumulation of lipid when exposed to medium preincubated with normal cells. The possibility that certain enzymes can leave and enter cells is an exciting one. One might have assumed that the relatively large size of most enzymes would have prevented their passage across cell membranes. This may not be true. The observation that cells cultured from patients with enzyme defects can be "treated" raises the possibility of treatment of the patient himself with enzyme. Whether or not adequate levels of administered enzymes can be achieved in the patient, in the face of possible destruction by immune and other mechanisms, remains to be seen, but the possibility is exciting.

SUMMARY

Recent studies of the rapidly expanding number of recognized enzymic defects of man have brought both confirmation and major changes of various concepts about the nature of these defects. Many additional examples of genetic heterogeneity have been uncovered, and additional examples of intermediate expression in the heterozygote have been found. On the other hand, sufficient information is available to suggest that the mechanisms of enzymic deficiency in man differ significantly from those which receive emphasis in studies of microorganisms. Many human enzymic deficiencies are incomplete. The nature and properties of the residual activity have diagnostic and therapeutic significance. Genetic modification of an enzyme can affect kinetic characteristics and stability so that seriously impaired function of the enzyme in vivo would be missed during a routine assay. Enzymic diagnosis can be complicated also by the presence of two genetically independent enzymes catalyzing the same reaction. Although large and genetically determined variations in amounts of enzyme protein exist, present evidence indicates that these are not primarily regulatory defects. They seem to be secondary to structural changes in the enzyme. Lability in vivo seems to play an important role in causing enzymic deficiency in human red cells. Cell culture and hybridization provide new opportunities for unraveling the mechanisms and nature of enzymic deficiencies in mammalian cells. Recent developments of methods of antenatal diagnosis of biochemical defects emphasize both the opportunities and serious responsibilities accompanying studies of hereditary enzymic defects in man.

REFERENCES

Aarskog, D., and M. K. Fagerhol. 1970. Protease inhibitor (Pi) phenotypes in chromosome aberrations. J. Med. Genet. 7:367-370.

Aebi, H., E. Bossi, M. Cantz, S. Matsubara, and H. Suter. 1968. Acatalas(em)ia in Switzerland. In Beutler, E. (Ed.), Hereditary Disorders of Erythrocyte Metabolism, pp. 41-61. New York, Grune & Stratton.

Afolayan, A., and L. Luzzatto. 1971. Genetic variants of human erythrocyte glucose-6-phosphate dehydrogenase. Biochemistry 10:420.

Ahlvin, R. C. 1970. Biochemical screening—a critique. New Eng. J. Med. 283:1084-1086.

Allfrey, V. G., R. Faulkner, and A. E. Mirsky. 1964. Acetylation and methylation of histones and their possible role in the regulation of RNA synthesis. Proc. Natl. Acad. Sci. U.S.A. 51:786-794.

Alper, C. A., F. S. Rosen, J. Pensky, M. A. Klemperer, and V. H. Donaldson. 1970. Heterogeneity of genetic variants in hereditary angioneurotic edema. J. Clin. Invest. 49:3a.

Altay, C., C. A. Alper, and D. C. Nathan. 1970. Normal and variant isoenzymes of human blood cell hexokinase and the isoenzyme patterns in hemolytic disease. Blood 36:219-227.

Altland, K., and H. W. Goedde. 1970. Heterogeneity in the silent gene phenotype of pseudocholinesterase of human serum. Biochem. Genet. 4:321-338.

Appel, S. H. 1968. Purification and kinetic properties of brain orotidine 5-phosphate decarboxylase. J. Biol. Chem. 243:3924-3929.

Arias, I. M., L. M. Gartner, M. Cohen, J. B. Ezzer, and A. J. Levi. 1969. Chronic nonhemolytic unconjugated hyperbilirubinemia with glucuronyl transferase deficiency. Clinical biochemical, pharmacologic and genetic evidence for heterogeneity. Amer. J. Med. 47:395-409.

Austin, J., D. Armstrong, and L. Shearer. 1965. Metachromatic form of diffuse cerebral sclerosis. V. The nature and significance of low sulfatase activity. Arch. Neurol. 13:593-614.

Bearn, A. G., B. S. Danes, and V. A. McKusick. 1970. Metachromasia elaborated. New Eng. J. Med. 282:102-103.

Bellanti, J. A., B. E. Cantz, and R. J. Schlegel. 1970. Accelerated decay of glucose-6-phosphate dehydrogenase activity in chronic granulomatous disease. Pediat. Res. 4:405-411.

Beutler, E., M. C. Baluda, P. Sturgeon, and R. Day. 1966. The genetics of galactose-1-phosphate uridyl transferase deficiency. J. Lab. Clin. Med. 68:646-658.

Blume, K. G., R. W. Hoffbauer, D. Busch, H. Arnold, and G. W. Löhr. 1971. Purification and properties of pyruvate kinase in normal and in pyruvate kinase deficient human red blood cells. Biochim. Biophys. Acta 227:364-372.

Blyth, H., and B. P. Hughes. 1971. Pregnancy and serum CPK levels in potential carriers of "severe" X-linked muscular dystrophy. Lancet 1:855-856.

Brady, R. O. 1970. Cerebral lipidoses. Ann. Rev. Med. 21:317-334.

Brown, P. E., C. Hougie, and H. R. Roberts. 1970. The genetic heterogeneity of hemophilia B. New Eng. J. Med. 283:61-64.

Cori, G. T., and C. F. Cori. 1952. Glucose-6-phosphatase of the liver in glycogen storage disease. J. Biol. Chem. 199:661-667.

Crigler, J. F., Jr., and N. I. Gold. 1966. Sodium phenobarbital induced decrease in serum bilirubin in an infant with congenital nonhemolytic jaundice and kernicterus. J. Clin. Invest. 45:998-999.

Danes, B. S., and A. G. Bearn. 1970. Correction of cellular metachromasia in cultured fibroblasts in several inherited mucopolysaccharidoses. Proc. Natl. Acad. Sci. U.S.A. 67:357-364.

Davies, R. O., A. V. Marton, and W. Kalow. 1960. The action of normal and atypical cholinesterase of human serum upon a series of esters of choline. Canad. J. Biochem. Physiol. 38:545-551.

Dawson, G., and A. O. Stein. 1970. Lactosyl ceramidosis: catabolic enzyme defect of glycosphingolipid metabolism. Science 170:556-558.

Dern, R. J., P. R. McCurdy, and A. Yoshida. 1969. A new structural variant of glucose-6-phosphate dehydrogenase with a high production rate (G6PD Hektoen). J. Lab. Clin. Med. 73:283-290.

Donaldson, V. H., and F. S. Rosen. 1964. The action of complement in hereditary angioneurotic edema: the role of C'1 esterase. J. Clin. Invest. 43:2204-2213.

Drummond, G. I., and L. Duncan. 1970. Adenyl cyclase in cardiac tissue. J. Biol. Chem. 245:976-983.

Emmer, M., B. deCrombrugghe, I. Pastan, and R. Perlman. 1970. Cyclic AMP rector protein of E. coli: its role in the synthesis of inducible enzymes. Proc. Nat. Acad. Sci. U.S.A. 66:480-487.

Feig, S. A., D. G. Nathan, and H. A. Zarkowsky. 1971. Age liability of normal and variant methemoglobin reductase. Pediat. Res. 5:409-410.

Feinstein, R. N., J. T. Braun, and J. B. Howard. 1967. Acatalasemia and hypocatalasemic mouse mutants. II. Mutational variations in blood and solid tissue catalases. Arch. Biochem. Biophys. 120:165-169.

———, H. Suter, and B. N. Jaroslow. 1968. Blood catalase polymorphism: some immunological aspects. Science 159:638-640.

Fox, R. M., W. J. O'Sullivan, and B. G. Firkin. 1969. Orotic aciduria. Differing enzyme patterns. Amer. J. Med. 47:332-336.

Frimpter, G. W., R. J. Andelman, and W. F. George. 1969. Vitamin B₆-dependency syndromes. Amer. J. Clin. Nutr. 22:794-805.

Gaffney, P. J., and H. Lehman. 1969. Residual enzyme activity in the serum of a homozygote for the silent pseudocholinesterase gene. Hum. Hered. 19:234-238.

Gartner, L. M., and I. M. Arias. 1968. Pharmacologic and genetic determinants of disordered bilirubin transport and metabolism in the liver. Ann N. Y. Acad. Sci. 151:833-841.

Gelehrter, T., A. G. Motulsky, and G. S. Omenn. 1970. Genetic control mechanisms in man and other mammals. Science 169:791-792.

Glassman, E. 1971. Personal communication.

Goedde, H. W., K. Altland, and W. Schloot. 1968. Therapy of prolonged apnea after suxamethonium with purified pseudocholinesterase. Science 151:742-751.

Greene, M. L., J. A. Boyle, and J. E. Seegmiller. 1970. Substrate stabilization: genetically controlled reciprocal relationship of two human enzymes. Science 167:887-889.

Hampton, J. W., R. O. Morton, D. Bannerjec, and E. Kalmal. 1971. Defective fibrin cross-linkages: a genetic and biochemical study of these families. J. Clin. Invest. 50:42a.

Harris, H., M. Whittaker, H. Lehmann, and E. Silk. 1960. The pseudocholinesterase variants. Esterase levels and dibucaine numbers in families selected through sexamethonium sensitive individuals. Acta Genet. Statist. Med. 10:1-16.

Hines, J. D. 1971. Quantitative assessment of blood and tissue pyridoxal phosphokinase concentration in patients with vitamin B_6-dependent states. J. Clin. Invest. 50:45a.

Hirschhorn, K., H. L. Nadler, W. I. Waithe, B. I. Brown, and R. Hirschhorn. 1969. Pompe's disease. Detection of heterozygotes by lymphocyte stimulation. Science 166:1632-1633.

Hodgkin, W. E., Giblett, H. Levine, W. Bauer, and A. G. Motulsky. 1965. Complete pseudocholinesterase deficiency: genetic and immunologic characterization. J. Clin. Invest. 44:486-493.

Horowitz, N. H., and M. Fling. 1956. Studies of tyrosinase production by a heterocaryon of Neurospora. Proc. Nat. Acad. Sci. U.S.A. 43:498-501.

Hosoi, T. 1968. Fluorescent antibody technique utilized for studies on cellular distribution of erythrocytic antigens. Acta Haemat. Jap. 31:138-150.

———, S. Yahara, H. B. Hamilton, N. Fujiki, T. Sasaki, and Y. Ishihara. 1969. Studies of human erythrocyte catalase by fluorescent antibody technique. The distribution of catalase in acatalasia and hypocatalasia. Blood 34:25-31.

Hsia, Y. E., A. C. Lilljeqvist, and L. E. Rosenberg. 1970. Vitamin B_{12}-dependent methylmalonic-aciduria: amino acid toxicity, long chain ketonuria, and protective effect of vitamin B_{12}. Pediatrics 46:497-507.

Huehns, E. R. 1970. Diseases due to abnormalities of hemoglobin structure. Ann. Rev. Med. 21:157-178.

Huijing, F. 1970. Glycogen-storage disease type VIa: low phosphorylase kinase activity caused by a low enzyme substrate affinity. Biochim. Biophys. Acta 206:199-201.

Jones, M. E. 1970. Regulation of pyrimidine and arginine biosynthesis in mammals. Adv. Enzym. Regulat. 9:19-50.

Kaback, M. M. 1971. Personal communication.

———, and R. R. Howell. 1970. Infantile metachromatic leukodystrophy. New Eng. J. Med. 282:1336-1340.

Kalow, W., and N. Staron. 1957. On the distribution and inheritance of atypical forms of human serum cholinesterase as indicated by dibucaine numbers. Canad. J. Biochem. Physiol. 35:1305-1320.

Kelly, W. N. 1971. Studies on the adenine phosphoribosyltransferase enzyme in human fibroblasts lacking hypoxanthine-guanine phosphoribosyltransferase. J. Lab. Clin. Med. 77:33-38.

———, M. L. Greene, F. M. Rosenbloom, J. F. Henderson, and J. E. Seegmiller. 1969. Hypoxanthine-guanine phosphoribosyl transferase deficiency in gout. Ann. Intern. Med. 70:155-206.

———, and J. B. Wyngaarden. 1970. Studies on the purine phosphoribosyltransferase enzymes in fibroblasts from patients with the Lesch-Nyhan syndrome. Clin. Res. 18:394.

Kirkman, H. N. 1966. Deficiency of the mutant protein in persons with glucose-6-phosphage dehydrogenase defects. Fed. Proc. 25:337.

———. 1971. Glucose-6-phosphate dehydrogenase. Adv. Hum. Genet. 2:1-60.

———, and J. E. Hanna. 1968. Isozymes of human red cell glucose-6-phosphate dehydrogenase. Ann. N. Y. Acad. Sci. 151:133-148.

———, C. Kidson, and M. Kennedy. 1968. Variants of human glucose-6-phosphate dehydrogenase. Studies of sample from New Guinea. In Beutler, E. (Ed.), Hereditary Disorders of Erythrocyte Metabolism, pp. 126-145. New York, Grune & Stratton.

———, N. D. Riley, and B. B. Crowell. 1960. Different enzymic expressions of mutants of human glucose-6-phosphate dehydrogenase. Proc. Nat. Acad. Sci. U.S.A. 46:938-944.

Klebe, R. J., T. R. Chen, and F. H. Ruddle. 1970. Mapping of a human genetic regulator element by somatic cell genetic analysis. Proc. Nat. Acad. Sci. U.S.A. 66:1220-1227.

Kobata, A., and V. Ginsburg. 1970. Uridine disphosphate N-acetyl D-galactosamine: D-galactose α-3-N-acetyl-D-galactosaminyltransferase, a product of the gene that determines blood type A in man. J. Biol. Chem. 245:1484-1490.

Kogut, M. D., G. N. Donnell, W. L. Nyhan, and L. Sweetman. 1970. Disorder of purine metabolism due to partial deficiency of hypoxanthine-guanine phosphoribosyltransferase. Amer. J. Med. 48:148-161.

Koler, R. D., R. H. Bigley, and P. Stenzel. 1968. Biochemical properties of human erythrocyte and leukocyte pyruvate kinase. In Beutler, E. (Ed.), Hereditary Disorders of Erythrocyte Metabolism, pp. 249-259. New York, Grune & Stratton.

Kyriakides, E. C., B. Paul, and J. A. Balint. 1971. Wolman's disease: demonstration of lipid accumulation and acid lipase deficiency and their apparent correction in vitro in cultured fibroblasts. Clin Res. 19:478.

Langan, T. A. 1968. Action of adenosine 3',5'-monophosphate-dependent histone kinase in vivo. J. Biol. Chem. 244:5763-5765.

Lerner, P., and C. Yanofsky. 1957. An immunological study of mutants of Escherichia coli lacking the enzyme tryptophan synthetase. J. Bact. 74:494-501.

Lindblad, B., K. Lindstrand, S. Svanberg, and R. Zotterstorm. 1969. The effect of a cobamide coenzyme in methylmalonic acidemia. Acta Pediat. Scand. 58:178-180.

Littlefield, J. W. 1969. Weak evidence for bacterial-type regulation in animal cells. In Genetic Concepts and Neoplasis, Baltimore, Williams & Wilkins.

Maas, W. K., and B. D. Davis. 1952. Production of an altered pantothenate-synthesizing enzyme by a temperature-sensitive mutant of Escherichia coli. Proc. Nat. Acad. Sci. U.S.A. 38:785-797.

Mammen, E. F., A. S. Prasad, M. I. Barnhart, and C. C. Au. 1969. Congenital dysfibrinogenemia: fibrinogen Detroit. J. Clin. Invest. 48:235-249.

Marks, P. A., and R. T. Gross. 1959. Erythrocytic glucose-6-phosphate dehydrogenase deficiency: evidence of differences between Negroes and Caucasians with respect to this genetically determined trait. J. Clin. Invest. 38:2253-2262.

McKusick, V. A. 1968. Mendelian Inheritance in Man: Catalogs of Autosomal Dominant, Autosomal Recessive, and X-linked Phenotypes. Baltimore, Johns Hopkins.

McLaren, D. S., and B. Zekian. 1971. Failure of enzymic cleavage of B carotene. The cause of vitamin A deficiency in a child. Amer. J. Dis. Child. 121:278-280.

Mehl, E., and H. Jatzkewitz. 1968. Cerebroside 3-sulfate as a physiological substrate of arylsulfutase. A. Biochim. Biophys. Acta 151:619-627.

Milunsky, A., J. W. Littlefield, J. N. Kanfer, E. H. Kolodny, V. E. Shih, and L. Atkins. 1970. Prenatal genetic diagnosis. New Eng. J. Med. 283:1370-1381.

Miwa, S., T. Nishina, H. Ohyama, and I. Kumatori. 1968. Congenital hemolytic anemia due to functionally abnormal pyruvate kinase. Trans. 12th Int. Congr. Hemat. p. 117.

Morrow, G., L. A. Barnes, and G. J. Cardinale. 1969. Congenital methymalonic acidemia: enzymatic evidence for two forms of the disease. Proc. Nat. Acad. Sci. U.S.A. 63:191-197.

Mudd, S. H., W. A. Edwards, P. M. Loeb, M. S. Brown, and L. Laster. 1970a. Homocystinuria due to cystathionine synthetase deficiency: the effect of pyridoxine. J. Clin. Invest. 49:1762-1773.

―――, H. L. Levy, and R. H. Abeles. 1969. A derangement in B_{12} metabolism leading to homocystinemia, cystathioninemia, and methylmalonic aciduria. Biochem. Biophys. Res. Comm. 35:121-126.

―――, ―――, and B. G. Morrow. 1970b. Deranged B_{12} metabolism: effects on sulfur amino acid metabolism. Biochem. Med. 4:193-214.

Munro, G. F., and D. R. Miller. 1970. Mechanism of fructose diphosphate (FDP) activation of a mutant pyruvate kinase (PK) from human RBC. Clin. Res. 18:395.

Nadler, H. L. 1971a. Genetic heterogeneity in acid phosphatase deficiency. Pediat. Res. 5:421.

―――. 1971b. Indications for amniocentesis in the early prenatal detection of genetic disorders. Birth Defects 7:5-9.

―――, C. M. Chacko, and M. Rachmeler. 1970. Interallelic complementation in hybrid cells derived from human diploid strains deficient in galactose-1-phosphate uridyl transferase activity. Proc. Nat. Acad. Sci. U.S.A. 67:976-982.

―――, and T. J. Egan. 1970. Deficiency of lysosomal acid phosphatase, a new familial metabolic disorder. New Eng. J. Med. 282:302-307.

Nakao, K., O. Wada, T. Kitamura, K. Uono, and G. Urata. 1966. Activity of amino-laevulinic acid synthetase in normal and prophyric human livers. Nature (London) 210:838-839.

Natori, S., and A. Garen. 1970. Molecular heterogeneity in the amino-terminal region of alkaline phosphatase. J. Molec. Biol. 49:577-588.

Necheles, T. F., U. S. Rai, and D. Cameron. 1970. Congenital nonspherocytic hemolytic anemia associated with an unusual erythrocyte hexokinase abnormality. J. Lab. Clin. Med. 76:593-602.

Neufeld, E. F., and J. C. Fratantoni. 1970. Inborn errors of mucopolysaccharide metabolism. Science 169:141-146.

Nishimura, E. T., T. V. Kobana, S. Takahara, H. B. Hamilton, and S. C. Madden. 1961. Immunologic evidence of catalase deficiency in human hereditary acatalasemia. Lab. Invest. 10:333-340.

O'Brien, J. S., S. Odada, A. Chen, and D. L. Fillerup. 1970. Tay-Sachs disease. Detection of heterozygotes and homozygotes by serum hexosaminidase assay. New Eng. J. Med. 283:15-20.

Ohnno, S., H. W. Payne, M. Morrison, and E. Beutler. 1966. Hexose-6-phosphate dehydrogenase found in human liver. Science 153:1015-1016.

Okada, S., and J. S. O'Brien. 1969. Tay-Sachs disease: generalized absence of beta-D-N-acetylhexosaminidase component. Science 165:698-700.

————, M. L. Veath, J. Leroy, and J. S. O'Brien. 1971. Ganglioside GM₂ storage disease: hexosaminidase deficiency in cultured fibroblasts. Amer. J. Hum. Genet. 23:55-61.

————, M. L. Veath, and J. S. O'Brien. 1970. Juvenile GM₂ gangliosidosis: partial deficiency of hexosaminidase. Amer. J. Pediat. 77:1063-1065.

Ord, M. G., and L. A. Stocken. 1966. Metabolic properties of histones from rat liver and thymus gland. Biochem. J. 98:888-897.

Oski, F. A., and H. Bowman. 1969. A low K_m phosphoenolpyruvate mutant in the Amish with red cell pyruvate kinase deficiency. Brit. J. Haemat. 17:289-297.

Patrick, A. D., and B. D. Lake. 1969. Wolman's disease. Caused by a deficiency of acid lipase. Nature 222:1067-1068.

Perutz, M. F., and H. Lehmann. 1968. Molecular pathology of human haemoglobin. Nature 19:902-909.

Piomelli, S., L. M. Corash, D. D. Davenport, J. Miroglia, and E. L. Amorosi. 1968. In vivo lability of glucose-6-phosphate dehydrogenase in Gd^{A-} and Gd Mediterranean deficiency. J. Clin. Invest. 47:940-948.

Pogo, B. G. T., V. G. Allfrey, and A. E. Mirsky. 1966. RNA synthesis and histone acetylation during the course of gene activation in lymphocytes. Proc. Nat. Acad. Sci. U.S.A. 55:805-812.

Powell, R. D., G. J. Brewer, R. L. DeGowin, and P. E. Carson. 1966. Effects of glucose-6-phosphate dehydrogenase deficiency upon the host and upon host-drug-malaria parasite interactions. Milit. Med. 131:1039-1056.

Robbins, P. W. 1960. Immunological study of human muscle lacking phosphorylase. Fed. Proc. 19:193.

Romeo, G., and B. R. Migeon. 1971. Fabry's disease: evidence for structural mutation of α-galactosidase. Pediat. Res. 5:420-421.

Rosa, R., Y. Alexandre, J. Kaplan, and J. Dreyfus. 1970. Comportement immunologique de la glucose-6-phosphate-déhydrogénase érythrocytaire chez des mutants déficients. Clin. Chim. Acta 29:209-214.

Rosenberg, L. E., A. C. Lilljeqvist, and Y. E. Hsia. 1968. Methylmalonic aciduria: metabolic block localization and vitamin B₁₂ deficiency. Science 162:805-807.

————, A. Lilljevest, Y. E. Hsia, and F. M. Rosenbloom. 1969. Vitamin B₁₂ dependent methylmalonic-aciduria: defective B₁₂ metabolism in cultured fibroblasts. Biochem. Biophys. Res. Comm. 37:607-614.

Rubenstein, A. H., and D. F. Steiner. 1970. Proinsulin: the single chain precursor of insulin. Med. Clin. N. Amer. 54:191-199.

Rubinstein, H. M., A. A. Dietz, L. K. Hodges, T. Lubrano, and V. Czebotar. 1970. Silent cholinesterase gene: variations in the properties of serum enzyme in apparent homozygotes. J. Clin. Invest. 49:479-486.

Sachs, J. R., D. J. Wicker, R. D. Gilcher, M. E. Conrad, and R. J. Cohen. 1967. P. K. deficient hemolytic anemia inherited as an autosomal dominant. Blood 30:881.

Salafsky, I. S., and H. L. Nadler. 1971. α1,4 glucosidase activity in Pompe's disease. Pediat. Res. 5:422.

Salmon, S. E., M. J. Cline, J. Schultz, and R. I. Lehrer. 1970. Myeloperoxidase deficiency. Immunologic study of a genetic leukocyte defect. New Eng. J. Med. 282:250-253.

Sawin, P. B., and D. Glick. 1943. Atropinesterase, a genetically determined enzyme in the rabbit. Proc. Nat. Acad. Sci. U.S.A. 29:55-59.

Schwartz, J. M. P. Paress, J. M. Ross, K. Fagelman, F. W. DiPillo, and R. Rizek. 1970. A Puerto Rican variant of NADH methemoglobin reductase in hereditary methemoglobinemia. Clin. Res. 18:396.

Seegmiller, J. E., F. M. Rosenbloom, and W. N. Kelley. 1967. Enzyme defect associated with a sex-linked human neurological disorder and excessive purine synthesis. Science 155:1682-1684.

Segal, S., S. Rogers, and P. G. Holtzapple. 1971. Liver galactose-1-phosphate uridyl transferase: activity in normal and galactosemic subjects. J. Clin. Invest. 50:500-506.

Setlow, R. B., D. Regan, J. German, and W. L. Carrier. 1969. Evidence that xerodermia pigmentosum cells do not perform the first step in the repair of ultraviolet damage to their DNA. Proc. Nat. Acad. Sci. U.S.A. 64:1035-1041.

Shaw, C. R. 1966. Glucose-6-phosphate dehydrogenase: homologous molecules in deer mouse and man. Science 153:1013-1015.

————, and E. Barto. 1965. Autosomally determined polymorphism of glucose-6-phosphate dehydrogenase in *Peromyscus.* Science 148:1099-1101.

Shibata, Y., T. Higashi, H. Hirai, and H. B. Hamilton. 1967. Immunochemical studies on catalase II. An anticatalase reacting component in normal, hypocatalasic, and acatalasic human erythrocytes. Arch. Biochem. Biophys. 118:200-209.

Srivastava, S. K., and E. Beutler. 1969. Auxillary pathways of galactose metabolism. J. Biol. Chem. 244:6377-6382.

Stites, D. P., E. J. Hershgold, J. D. Perlman, and H. H. Fudenberg. 1971. Factor VIII detection by hemagglutination inhibition: hemophilia A and von Willebrand's disease. Science 171:196-197.

Strand, L. J., B. F. Felsher, A. G. Redeker, and H. S. Marver. 1970. Heme biosynthesis in intermittent acute porphyria: decreased hepatic conversion of porphobilinogen to porphyrins and increased delta aminolevulinic acid synthetase activity. Proc. Nat. Acad. Sci. U.S.A. 67:1315-1320.

————, ————, ————, and ————. 1971. Intermittent acute porphyria (IAP): new evidence for a basic defect in uroporphyrinogen synthetase (URO-S). J. Clin. Invest. 50:89a-90a.

Suskind, S. R., C. Yanofsky, and D. M. Bonner. 1955. Allelic strains of *Neurospora* lacking tryptophan synthetase: a preliminary immunochemical characterization. Proc. Nat. Acad. Sci. U.S.A. 41:577-582.

Suzuki, Y., and K. Suzuki. 1971. Krabbe's globoid cell leukodystrophy: deficiency of galactocerbrosidase in serum, leukocytes, and fibroblasts. Science 171:73-75.

Tada, K., Y. Yokayama, H. Nakagawa, T. Yoshida, and T. Akakawa. 1967. Vitamin B_6 dependent xanthurenic aciduria. Tohoku J. Exp. Med. 93:115-124.

Taylor, A. T., M. A. Stafford, and O. W. Jones. 1971. Phenotype expression of thymidine kinase during human fetal development. J. Clin. Invest. 50:91a.

Tedesco, T. A., and M. J. Mellman. 1971. Normal, Duarte variant, and galactosemic alleles code for immunologically identical Gal-1-P uridyl transferase enzyme protein. Pediat. Res. 5:421.

————, and W. J. Mellman. 1967. Argininosuccinate synthetase activity and citrulline metabolism in cells cultured from a citrullinemic subject. Proc. Nat. Acad. Sci. U.S.A. 57:829-834.

Tomkins, G. M., T. D. Gelehrter, D. Granner, D. Martin, Jr., H. H. Samuels, and E. B. Thompson. 1969. Control of specific gene expression in higher organisms. Science 166:1474-1480.

Tschudy, D. P., M. G. Perlroth, H. S. Marver, A. Collins, G. Hunter, Jr., and M. Rechcigl, Jr. 1965. Acute intermittent porphyria: the first "overproduction disease" localized to a specific enzyme. Proc. Nat. Acad. Sci. U.S.A. 53:841-847.

Wang, Y. M., and J. van Eys. 1970. The enzymatic defect in essential pentosuria. New Eng. J. Med. 282:892-896.

W.H.O. Scientific Group. 1967. Standardization of procedures for the study of glucose-6-phosphate dehydrogenase. W.H.O. Techn. Rep. Ser. 366:1-53.

Wiesmann, U. N., J. Lightbody, F. Vassella, and N. N. Herschkowitz. 1971. Multiple lysosomal enzyme deficiency due to enzyme leakage. New Eng. J. Med. 284:109-110.

———, E. E. Rossi, and N. N. Herschkowitz. 1971. Treatment of metachromatic leukodystrophy in fibroblasts by enzyme replacement. New Eng. J. Med. 284:672-673.

Williams, H. E., and J. B. Field. 1961. Low leukocyte phosphorylase in hepatic phosphorylase-deficient glycogen storage disease. J. Clin. Invest. 40:1841-1845.

Yaffe, S. J., G. Levy, T. Matsuzawa, and T. Baliah. 1966. Enhancement of glucuronide-conjugating capacity in a hyperbilirubinemia infant due to apparent enzyme induction by phenobarbital. New Eng. J. Med. 275:1461-1465.

Yoshida, A. 1970. Amino acid substitution (histidine to tyrosine) in a glucose-6-phosphate dehydrogenase variant (G6PD Hektoen) associated with overproduction. J. Molec. Biol. 52:483-490.

———, E. Beutler, and A. G. Motulsky. 1971. Table of variants of human glucose-6-phosphate dehydrogenase. Personal communication.

———, and A. G. Motulsky. 1969. A pseudocholinesterase variant (E Cynthiana) associated with elevated plasma enzyme activity. Amer. J. Hum. Genet. 21:486-498.

———, G. Stamatoyannopoulos, and A. G. Motulsky. 1967. Negro variant of glucose-6-phosphate dehydrogenase deficiency (A−) in man. Science 155:97-99.

Zimmerman, T. S., O. D. Ratnoff, and A. E. Powell. 1971. Immunologic differentiation of classic hemophilia (factor VIII deficiency) and von Willebrand's disease. J. Clin. Invest. 50:244-254.

CHAPTER 5

Prevention of Rh Isoimmunization

C. A. Clarke

Professor of Medicine and Director, Nuffield Unit of Medical Genetics, Department of Medicine, University of Liverpool, Liverpool, England.

THE STORY OF THE RESEARCH leading up to the successful prophylaxis of Rh hemolytic disease has been told many times before (Clarke, 1966; McConnell, 1966; Clarke, 1967; Clarke, 1968a; Clarke, 1968b; Clarke, 1969; Friedman, 1969; Robertson, 1969; Robertson and Dambrosio, 1969); Woodrow, 1970), and there are only two justifications for writing about it again. The first is that there was a W.H.O. meeting in Geneva in October, 1970, at which most interesting discussions took place between representatives of many countries and many of these are incorporated here (see W.H.O. report, 1971). (I am most grateful to Dr. H. C. Goodman, Chief of the Immunology Division, and to Dr. Zdenek Trnka, Secretary of the Scientific Group on the Prevention of Rh Sensitisation, for permission to use this new material.) The second is that by being included in this series the work is formally recognized as being "genetics," a source of satisfaction to the writer, who has it constantly held against him that it is not.

BACKGROUND TO THE RESEARCH

In mimicry, certain butterflies, particularly tropical ones, resemble others, the models (often belonging to quite different families), which are distasteful to predators, particularly birds. Models and mimics usually fly together, and birds which have sampled the distasteful models tend to leave the mimics alone even though these are highly palatable. Breeding data superficially appear to demonstrate that there is a single gene difference between the various morphs within a mimetic species. However, we have been able to show that the matter is not as simple as this, for crossing over sometimes occurs and there is good evidence that the single gene is in fact a supergene composed of several closely linked loci (Clarke and Sheppard, 1959; Clarke and Sheppard, 1960; Clarke et al., 1968). It was this type of finding (first in *Papilio dardanus* Brown and then in *Papilio memnon* L.) and the many examples of genic interaction in the *Papilio* species which directed our attention to the rhesus blood group system. Here, if multiple loci are involved, crossovers could account for the rarer genotypes and there is a marked interaction between the Rh and ABO systems.

<h2 style="text-align:center">IDEAS LEADING TO THE PROPHYLAXIS</h2>

Because of the natural protective mechanisms against Rh immunization afforded by ABO incompatibility between mother and fetus (Levine, 1943), the Liverpool research group felt that this protection might be copied by injecting Rh-negative mothers having Rh-positive ABO-compatible babies (a much more common situation than ABO incompatibility) with passive Rh antibody after delivery. Levine's original observation has been confirmed by many workers, one of the most relevant papers being that in which Nevanlinna and Vainio (1956) drew attention to the importance of the ABO group of the immunizing fetus, usually the normal baby preceding the first affected one. We obtained contributory evidence when we investigated 91 families, in all of which Rh hemolytic disease had occurred (Clarke, et al., 1958). As many as 23 of these were from ABO-incompatible matings between mother and father, and in 14 of the families we were able to determine the immunizing fetus with certainty. We found that this fetus was always compatible on the ABO system with its mother, the probability of finding this by chance being in 1 in 500. Incompatibility between mother and father does not, of course, necessarily imply incompatibility between mother and fetus since, for example, a group O mother may marry a man, who, though typing as group A, is in fact heterozygous AO. It is generally agreed that ABO incompatibility between mother and fetus gives a good measure of natural protection and the contrary view expressed by Ascari et al. (1969) need not be taken too seriously because these authors have to some extent equated ABO incompatibility between mother and father with that between mother and baby.

The mechanism of protection by ABO incompatibility is discussed later, and for the present all that need be said is that it seemed logical to try to imitate the natural protection by giving anti-D antibody to the mother after delivery in the 80% of cases where the mother and fetus were ABO-compatible. The hypothesis was that the anti-D would destroy any Rh (D)-positive cells which had entered the maternal circulation, and that therefore the effect of the immunizing fetus would be obviated, the woman starting her subsequent Rh positive pregnancy as if it were her first. The idea was first put forward by Finn (1960), and in a series of papers over the next few years we reported our initial work in Rh-negative male volunteers (Finn et al., 1961; Clarke et al., 1963; Woodrow et al., 1965; and Clarke et al., 1966). Briefly, we found that when we gave anti-D plasma containing predominantly IgM (19S) antibody, we seemed to enhance immune antibody formation but if the injection was mainly of IgG (7S) the men were usually protected.

Workers in the United States approached the matter differently (Freda and Gorman, 1962; Freda et al., 1964). Instead of trying to prevent immunization by destroying the fetal cells, they hoped to inhibit it by injecting an excess of Rh antibody, the attempt being based on the idea of Theobald Smith (1909) who showed that mixtures of diphtheria toxin and antitoxin, with antibody in excess, did not immunize when injected. From the point of view of the results of the treatment, it does not matter which of the two theories is correct, but the great contribution of the United States group was that they used anti-D gamma globulin, this having the advantages of being given intramuscularly and of being free from the risk of transmitting virus hepatitis. In our original experiments we used intravenous plasma, but we changed over entirely to gamma globulin after hearing about their work. However, the final word on the choice of treatment may not yet have been said, since the discovery of the Australia antigen (Blumberg et al., 1965) may now make it possible to select "risk-free" plasma. This would certainly be cheaper than gamma globulin and could even be more effective, although it would still have the disadvantage that it needs to be given intravenously (see pp. 195-197).

EXPERIMENTAL PROTECTION IN VOLUNTEERS: PRELIMINARY
EXPERIMENTS

Before considering giving anti-D to recently delivered women it was clearly necessary, for ethical reasons, to try it out first in Rh-negative male volunteers. Those who took part in the original Liverpool experiment were 26 Rh-negative blood donors; each was injected with 5 ml of Rh-positive ABO-compatible adult blood tagged with radioactive chromium. Approximately half of the men were kept as controls, while the others were injected shortly afterwards with 10 ml of anti-D serum, this having a titer of 1:64 in saline. The reason we gave saline or complete antibody was because we knew that the naturally occurring anti-A and anti-B concerned with the protection conferred by ABO incompatibility was mainly of this type. The results of this experiment were unexpected and a setback, since 8 out of 15 of those treated formed immune antibody whereas only one of the 11 controls did so. In other words, we thought we had enhanced rather than suppressed immunization (Finn et al., 1961), though with hindsight it seems more likely that we had done neither (see below).

After the failures, we reconsidered the whole matter and decided to give *incomplete* (7S) instead of complete (19S) anti-D. This was partly because Stern et al. had shown in 1961 that when Rh-positive red cells, coated in vitro with incomplete anti-D, were given to Rh-negative men they did not make antibody, probably because the D antigen sites were blocked.

In our next experiment (Clarke et al., 1963), therefore, we gave intravenously 35-40 ml of plasma containing predominantly incomplete anti-D. We then found that only 3 out of 21 "treated" men developed immune antibodies, one after one and 2 after four injections of Rh-positive blood given intramuscularly, whereas 11 out of 21 controls did so after between one and four stimuli, the difference being statistically significant ($p = 0.02$).

The relevance of clearance of the injected red cells to protection is uncertain, and while it is likely that the greater the speed with which cells are taken from the circulation, the less the likelihood of immunization, the clearance rate had been not inconsiderable in our first experiment and there we thought we had enhanced antibody formation. Recently, Mollison (personal communication, 1970) has repeated our earlier work with Rh-negative men using a purified IgM given intravenously. With his first injections he has obtained clearance curves much the same as we had in our first experiments (see Fig. 1), but the interesting thing is that, as far as the experiments have gone, the IgM has neither enhanced nor suppressed immunization—there has been simply no effect. It is possible, therefore, that our rather alarming initial results were just fortuitous.

The next major contribution to the field of protection came from Freda

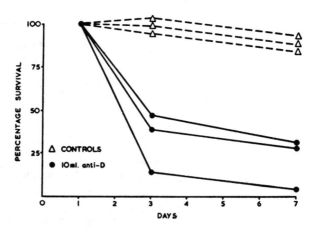

FIG. 1.—Remaining percentage radioactivity at various times after injection of 5 ml of Rh-positive blood tagged with ⁵¹Cr into 6 Rh-negative male volunteers. The treated men were given 10 ml of anti-D serum with a titer of 1:64 both in saline and in albumin. (Reprinted by permission from Finn et al., 1961.)

and Gorman (1962) and Freda et al. (1964) in the United States. As already mentioned, they used anti-D gamma globulin instead of whole serum and their protection experiments were similar to our own, 9 Rh-negative group O male volunteers being challenged once a month with 2 ml of Rh-positive whole blood on five successive occasions. Five of the men acted as controls, while the other 4 received 5 ml of gamma globulin (with an indirect antiglobulin titer of 1:64,000) *before* each injection of blood. The rationale for this was that, if a specific antibody is administered passively to an individual, subsequent injections of the corresponding antigen may fail to immunize. None of the 4 treated men produced antibodies, whereas 4 out of 5 of the controls did so. In the same paper, the authors reported that in a second experiment 27 further volunteers were given one intravenous injection of 10 ml of Rh-positive blood and, 3 days later, 4 ml of gamma globulin were given to 14 of them, the remainder acting as controls. In this series, none of the treated men made immune antibody while 6 of the 13 controls did so.

In Germany, Schneider (1963) also carried out experiments on much the same lines as those in Liverpool. He used only 0.5 ml of Rh-positive fetal blood as his antigenic stimulus because he thought that transplacental hemorrhages as large as 5 ml were rare. He used a correspondingly small amount (at first only 1 ml) of anti-D *serum,* and 5 of his 20 treated subjects developed immune antibodies. Later, 10 to 26 ml of anti-D serum were used; then more rapid clearance of the fetal cells was obtained, and none of the 13 treated subjects developed an immune antibody (Preisler and Schneider, 1964).

In England the anti-D gamma globulin was prepared for us by Dr. W. d'A. Maycock, Mr. L. Vallet, and their staff at the Lister Institute of Preventive Medicine, London, and it was derived from the pooled sera of 11 of our hyperimmunized male volunteers. The anti-D titer of this gamma globulin was extremely high, reaching 1 in 262,000 by the indirect Coombs test.

Using this preparation, we next carried out an experiment to see whether fetal blood injected into female volunteers could be cleared as rapidly as adult blood from males, and whether the women could be protected. Ten Rh-negative postmenopausal female volunteers were each given 5 ml of Rh-positive, ABO-compatible fetal blood intravenously, and in 5 of them this was followed by an intramuscular injection of 5 ml of the gamma globulin. The procedure was repeated 3 and again 6 months later. Clearance of the fetal cells was rapid, and none of the treated women developed immune anti-D, though one of the controls did so. The result, though it does not demonstrate that protection was achieved, makes it very improbable that we were enhancing antibody production.

At the present time our batches of gamma globulin are assessed by radioassay for anti-D content in micrograms per milliliter by Dr. Hughes-Jones (see Hughes-Jones, 1967, and "Methods of Assay of Anti-D" below), but this was not so when we began the research.

After these experiments on Rh-negative volunteers, we decided that it was justifiable to start clinical trials in primiparae who had just been delivered of ABO-compatible babies and in whom we judged the risk of immunization to be high. However, before discussing these it is necessary to consider the general question of fetal red cells in the maternal circulation and their relationship to immunization during or following a pregnancy or after an abortion.

Recognition and Counting of Fetal Cells in the Maternal Circulation

The presence of fetal red cells in a sample of adult blood may be detected by the "acid elution" method (Kleihauer et al., 1957). In films prepared by this method fetal red cells stain darkly whereas normal adult red cells appear colorless (see Fig. 2). However, most films of cord blood stained by the acid elution method contain less than 100% of the darkly staining cells; thus the acid elution method usually gives an underestimate

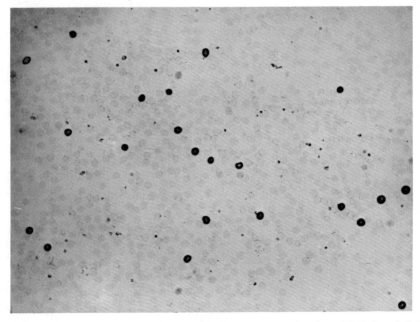

FIG. 2.—Fetal cells in the maternal circulation, detected by the acid elution (Kleihauer) technique.

of the number of fetal cells present. Other methods of recognizing fetal red cells have been developed, but they have been used by only a few laboratories, mainly for research purposes (Szelényi and Hollán, 1967).

One difficulty in interpreting blood films prepared by the acid elution (Kleihauer) method is that some samples of normal adult blood contain a few staining cells; these do not stain as darkly as most fetal cells, however, and are sometimes referred to as intermediately stained cells. Such cells are more commonly encountered in the blood of pregnant than of nonpregnant women, and where they occur it may be impossible, therefore, to decide whether or not fetal red cells are present. Virtually all observers have shown that, in the case of an ABO-incompatible baby, fetal red cells are found less frequently and in much smaller amounts (see Table 1).

Quantitation

The acid elution method cannot be applied to red cells in solution but only to fixed films of blood. Accordingly, results have to be expressed as a proportion of fetal to adult cells, this being much more accurate than counting the number of cells seen in 50 low-power fields.

In about 85% of blood samples from recently delivered women the proportion of fetal to adult cells is less than about 1 in 20,000 and at these levels accurate quantitation cannot be achieved by this method.

TABLE 1.—*Comparison of Fetal Cell Counts in Fetomaternal ABO Compatibility and Incompatibility*

Fetal blood	Significant fetomaternal bleeding*	Insignificant fetomaternal bleeding*	No bleeding	Total
ABO-compatible, D-positive	85 (18.6%)	184 (40.2%)	189 (41.2%)	458 (100%)
ABO-compatible, D-negative	70 (20.2%)	147 (42.2%)	131 (37.6%)	348 (100%)
ABO-incompatible, D-positive	5 (4.2%)	28 (23.5%)	86 (72.3%)	119 (100%)
ABO-incompatible, D-negative	3 (4.0%)	20 (26.7%)	52 (69.3%)	75 (100%)
Total	163	379	458	1000

*Fetomaternal bleeding which gives fetal cell counts of 5 or more per 50 low-power fields is called significant, while bleeding giving counts of from 1 to 4 inclusive is called insignificant. It will be seen that, when the fetal blood is ABO-incompatible with the mother, there is a marked decrease in the proportion of both significant and insignificant fetomaternal bleeding (Bowley, personal communication, 1968). (Reprinted by permission from Clarke, 1968a.)

Practical Value of the Quantitation of Fetal Cells in the Prevention of Rh Immunization (W.H.O., 1971)

The dose of anti-D which suppresses Rh immunization appears to be directly related to the number of Rh-positive red cells which enter the circulation (Woodrow and Donohoe, 1968; see also "Relationship Between Dose of Anti-D and Size of Stimulus," below). The current standard injection (about 200 μg) prevents immunization by amounts of D-positive red cells up to about 100 ml, so that it is desirable to apply a test which will detect those cases in which more than 10 ml of fetal red cells are present in the circulation. When relatively large amounts of Rh-positive red cells (e.g., 50 ml) are present in the circulation of an Rh-negative woman, they can be readily detected by incubating the sample with anti-D serum and then doing an antiglobulin test. Unfortunately, it is difficult to recognize D-positive cells in this way unless they constitute at least 2% of the total number of red cells present. In a woman with a normal red cell volume, 10 ml of fetal red cells constitute less than 1% of the total. Such a proportion can, however, be readily detected by the acid elution (Kleihauer) method. Assuming that only about 80% of fetal red cells are recognized by this technique and that the average mother's red cell volume at term is 1500 ml, the presence of 10 ml of fetal red cells in the maternal circulation corresponds to a proportion of approximately one fetal red cell to 200 adult cells. If an area of the film containing 10,000 cells is examined and not more than two or three darkly staining cells are observed, one may assume that the proportion of fetal to adult red cells is well below 1:200.

When the number of cells encountered in a preliminary scan suggests the possibility that the proportion could be as high as 1 in 200, an estimate of the actual proportion present should be made. The amount of anti-D to be given when it reaches or exceeds 1 in 200 is discussed on pp. 192-195.

A point to bear in mind when assessing the extent of transplacental hemorrhage is the fact that following abortion or Caesarean section fetal red cells may be slowly absorbed from the uterine or the peritoneal cavity (Haering, 1967). In such cases it may be advisable, therefore, to have a second blood film examined after 3 to 5 days.

Some estimate can be made of the number of women who will become immunized to Rh following a large but undetected transplacental hemorrhage. The incidence of a TPH of 10 ml or more is of the order of 2 to 3 per thousand. However, the incidence of Rh immunization when a dose of 200-300 μg of anti-D is given will not be as high as this: first, not all D-negative subjects will respond; second, this dose of anti-D will probably not fail to suppress immunization in all subjects. It is, therefore, unlikely that in these circumstances more than 1 in 1000 women will become immunized because of undertreatment.

In view of the very considerable labor of examining blood smears from all Rh-negative women recently delivered of an Rh-positive infant, it may be questioned whether the procedure is worthwhile when a dose of 200-300 μg is being given routinely.

On the other hand, there are a few circumstances in which there is a good case for making a test to discover whether an unusually large transplacental hemorrhage has occurred; these are (1) observation of anemia in a newborn infant; (2) unexplained intrauterine death; (3) manual removal of a placenta; and (4) amniocentesis.

Rh Immunization During a First Pregnancy

Evidence is now accumulating that occasionally some Rh-negative primigravidae form Rh antibodies either during their first Rh-positive pregnancy or very soon after delivery. A relatively high incidence of such immunization (2-3%) has been reported from Canada (Godel et al., 1968; Chown et al., 1969; and Aickin, 1970), and this may be due to the extreme sensitivity of the enzyme tests which they use, for an indirect antiglobulin technique alone would have detected less than 50% of the Rh antibodies they found.

It is possible that the use of less sensitive screening techniques may explain why some centers have reported a very low incidence of Rh immunization of primigravidae during pregnancy or very soon after delivery, and a corresponding higher incidence of apparent failure of Rh immunoglobulin to prevent Rh antibody formation by 6 months after delivery or during a second Rh-positive pregnancy. (See Tables 11 and 12 for some Canadian results.)

There is evidence that Rh antibody detectable only by an enzyme or "automated" technique probably represents active Rh immunization which usually cannot be reversed by administration of Rh immunoglobin at that time. Thus in one series (Chown et al., 1969) of 20 women given 300 μg of Rh immunoglobulin immediately after the first demonstration of such an antibody, only 6 showed no demonstrable Rh antibody 6 to 9 months after delivery. One of the 6 developed Rh antibodies in her second pregnancy and delivered an erythroblastotic baby. Since none of the remaining 5 have become pregnant again, there is no proof that they are not still immunized. On the other hand, Nossal (1967) writes that "when the anti-Rh is given the process of division and differentiation of the potential antibody-forming cells rapidly comes to a halt, there being a com-

plete block of the recruitment of new cells—though there is no effect on a
mature antibody-forming cell." If the Canadian view of the number becoming immunized by their first pregnancy, and of the inability of routine
anti-D to protect in this situation is correct, then 10 to 15% of the 17%
of Rh-negative women destined to develop Rh antibodies may not be
protected by postdelivery anti-D. Prevention of Rh antibody formation in
at least some of these susceptible women will require other types of treatment, possibly injection of anti-D during pregnancy (see pp. 191-192).
Failure of protection in every case following injection of Rh immunoglobulin in the presence of very weakly demonstrable Rh antibody has,
however, not yet been proved (some cases may be false positives), and
for this reason its continued use when this situation arises is still advisable.

Rh Immunization Following the First Full-Term Delivery

A first pregnancy with an Rh-positive, ABO-compatible infant causes
primary Rh immunization in about 17% of Rh-negative women who have
a subsequent Rh-positive baby. In about one-half of these cases, and particularly where the TPH is 1 ml or more, anti-D is usually detectable
within 6 months of the delivery of the first infant; in the remaining cases,
where the initial TPH is 0 or very few cells, it is detectable only during
the second Rh-positive pregnancy (whether ABO-compatible or not).

Table 2 shows the relationship of immunization to the size of TPH.
Factors which are thought to increase the change of TPH are amniocentesis,
external version, and antepartum hemorrhage—and possibly repeated abdominal examinations.

TABLE 2.—*Relationship of Fetomaternal Hemorrhage After Delivery to Rh Immunization 6 months Later (First delivery, Rh-positive ABO-Compatible Baby)* *

| | \multicolumn{8}{c}{Fetal cell score} |
	0	1	2	3–4	5–10	11–39	40+	Total
Anti-D present	13 (4)†	6 (2)	8 (2)	10 (3)	11 (2)	9 (1)	4	61 (14)
Anti-D absent	346	141	73	50	42	33	14	699
Total	359	147	81	60	53	42	18	760
Percent with anti-D	3.6	4.1	9.9	16.7	20.8	21.4	22.2	8.0

†Figures in parentheses denote anti-D detected by papain technique only.
*Reprinted by permission from Woodrow and Donohoe (1968).

Primary immunization is known to be dependent on a number of other factors:

1. As already stated, when the infant's red cells are incompatible with the mother's plasma, i.e., when there is ABO incompatibility, the chance of primary Rh immunization is reduced, the effect being greater with A than with B incompatibility.

2. The Rh phenotype of the baby is of some slight influence, R^2r cells providing a better antigenic stimulus than R^1r cells (Murray, 1957).

3. An important factor is the ability of the mother to respond to the D antigen, as it is known that there exists a considerable biological variation between individuals in this respect (see "Production of Anti-D Immunoglobulin," below).

Rh Immunization Following Abortion

There is a theoretical risk of isoimmunization during pregnancy as soon as the Rh antigens concerned appear on fetal red cells, and these have been found before 6 weeks' gestation (Bergström et al., 1967). To make this risk actual, red cells must pass from the fetal to the maternal circulation; this can also occur at less than 6 weeks' gestation (Woodrow et al., 1965; Clarke and Sheppard, 1969). Fetomaternal hemorrhage has been found in 4% of normal pregnancies of up to 6 months' gestation (Edwards, personal communication, 1970) and in 10% during the last trimester (Davey, personal communication, 1970). The early TPHs are usually very small, less than 0.1 ml of fetal blood, but this does not necessarily mean that they represent an inadequate immunizing stimulus. Several large series have shown that, in untreated subjects, about 6% of cases of Rh isoimmunization following delivery occur in women who had no, or few, fetal cells in the circulation at that time (though the reason for this may, in some cases, be due to earlier "priming" (see page 184). Theoretically, therefore, abortion may cause immunization, but the problem is how often in fact it does so.

The experience of most obstetricians is that immunization during a first pregnancy is extremely rare, and yet abortion is not a very unusual prior event. Some people (*Brit. Med. J.,* 1969) have argued that because, in their view, 0.5 ml of blood is necessary to immunize, a small fetus is unlikely to spill this amount and therefore immunization due to an abortion is a rare event. However, Woodrow et al. (1965) have estimated the regression of the probability of immunization on the size of transplacental hemorrhage. Using this estimation (see Fig. 3), the sizes of the transplacental hemorrhages in therapeutic abortion reported by Katz (1969) (Table 3), and the information contained in Table 2, it would appear that

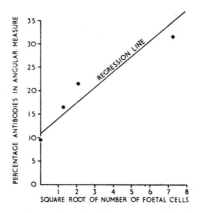

FIG. 3.—Weighted regression of the incidence of antibody formation on fetal cell score. Regression coefficient *b* equals 3.24 and is highly significant ($P < 0.001$). The *y* axis intercept *a* equals 10.83. It will be seen that the *y* axis (percentage producing antibodies) has been transformed to angles and the *x* axis (fetal cell score) to the square root of the cell score. This is because the direct relation between the two parameters was nonlinear. (For the purposes of the regression calculation, the data were grouped into four categories, each containing as nearly as possible the same number of individuals developing an antibody. This was because of the small antibody specificity—the Fab and the $F(ab')_2$ fragments. The black dots are where the chains are linked to each other. (Reprinted by permission from Nossal, 1969.)

TABLE 3.—*Estimation of Fetal Cell Scores**

	Number of cases	Fetal cells				Incidence, %
		0	1	2–5	>5	
In normal pregnancy						
Period of gestation:						
<16 weeks	41	35	3	3	0	14.6
16 to 40 weeks	50	38	6	5	1	24.0
In abortion before surgery						
Type of abortion:						
Threatened	34	26	4	4	0	23.5
Incomplete	36	27	5	3	1	25.0
After curettage and the effect of oxytocic drugs						
Drugs:						
No drugs	55	30	6	16	3	45.5
Oxytocic drug and minimal blood loss	26	13	5	7	1	50.0

*Reprinted by permission from Katz (1969).

the risk of immunization may be higher than many people think, possibly at least 1.0% of the "at risk" women who have had abortions therapeutically. Furthermore, Matthews' (1968) failure to find any cases of immunization in 97 Rh-negative women is inconclusive because the expected numbers in full-term deliveries would only be about 4 (having excluded the expected number of Rh-negative babies and the ABO-incompatible ones).

Retrospective information from Freda et al. (1970) appears to show that the average risk of immunization after abortion is between 3 and 4%, but this varies considerably with the age of the fetus: "virtually negligible at one month, definitely appreciable at two months (2 per cent) and very substantial at three months and beyond ($\pm$ 9 per cent)." In Scotland, Wallace (personal communication, 1970) quotes McDougall as attributing immunization to a first pregnancy abortion in 4 out of 774 immunized women, the total number of first pregnancy abortions in the series being 69. Bowman (1970) describes one case with antibodies in a second pregnancy where the sensitizing stimulus had been an earlier abortion at 16 weeks, and Murray et al. (1970) report Rh antibodies 6 months after abortion in 3 out of 23 cases tested where no antibodies had been present before operation. All these women were multiparae; one had had an abdominal hysterotomy, and 2 had had suction curettage.

However, it may well be that the risk of immunization by therapeutic abortion is lower than has been calculated (see Clarke, 1969), either because the fetal cells at this stage are less antigenic, or for some other reason, such as immunological inertia in the mother during pregnancy (see McConnell, 1969), but there is no definite proof of this in man and in rabbits it does not occur (Woodrow et al., 1971). In guinea pigs, on the other hand, trophoblast cells survive longer as allografts in pregnant than in virgin recipients, and interestingly the effect is more marked in cells deriving from a female conceptus (Borland et al., 1970).

Information is available on the size of the TPH in both spontaneous and induced abortions. The view of most people (see Matthews and Matthews, 1969, for example) is that artificial termination is much more likely to be associated with the leakage of fetal cells into the maternal circulation than is spontaneous abortion, in which some abnormality of placentation may have been present to cause the abortion. In support of this, Hollán (personal communication, 1970) in Hungary, comparing TPH after therapeutic abortion with that after normal delivery, found a similar incidence in both. Thus 18 cases out of 112 observed after curettage had fetal cells (2 a "moderate" and 16 a "small" number) compared with 13 out of 77 normal deliveries (1 a "large," 2 a "moderate," and 10 a "small number. Kogoj-Bakis and Vujaklija-Stipanovic (personal communication, 1970) found that in 500 curettage cases who had had no cells before operation (278 carried out at 6 to 8 weeks, and 222 at from 8 to 12 weeks) 19 had cells afterwards, and of these 3 had a substantial number. From Australia, Davey (personal communication, 1970) quoted Edwards as having shown a twofold increase in the fetal cell score in women who had had a curettage. Barron (1969), however, considers that with suction curettage there is no more risk of TPH than there is following a spontaneous abortion. The Newcastle workers (Murray et al., 1970) report on the frequency and size of the TPH in 483 patients admitted to hospital for abortion, 392 being therapeutic and 91 spontaneous. The blood was tested before, immediately before, and some time after evacuation of the uterus, and, in the opinion of the authors, there was very little risk of immunization by any type of abortion since where TPH occurred in nearly all cases the volume of blood was small (<0.1 ml). Bowman (1970), however, found 1 ml and 1.2 ml of fetal blood respectively in the circulation of 2 girls who had a therapeutic abortion, one at 15 weeks and the second at 18 weeks (he treated both).

In spite of all the conflicting opinions, one thing stands out—immunization does sometimes follow abortion, and therefore to be on the safe side it is recommended (see W.H.O., 1971) that any Rh negative woman without antibodies who has an abortion at any stage of pregnancy should be given anti-D, whether there is evidence of TPH or not. This is especially so if it is true that hemolytic disease of the newborn is more likely to be severe following immunization by abortion than by a normal full-term pregnancy (Bowman, personal communication, 1970).

CLINICAL TRIALS

When it became clear from experiments in the Rh-negative volunteers that prevention of Rh immunization was usually possible, clinical trials, initially with controls, were begun in many centers, the anti-D gamma globulin being given up to 72 hours after delivery in those previously nonimmunized Rh-negative mothers where the baby was Rh-positive. Some series consisted of primiparae only, whereas others included multiparae, and in some only ABO-compatible babies were included. The first step in each trial was to assess the immune Rh antibody status of the mother 6 months after delivery, but the crucial test lay in the presence or absence of Rh antibody at the end of the subsequent Rh-positive pregnancy.

Tables 4-15 give the most recent information that we know of; the results in the various centers are next commented on.

The First Liverpool Group Trial (Combined Study, 1966, 1971)

This trial began in 1964 and ended in 1968 except for the follow-up of the subsequent pregnancies; the figures are given in Tables 4 and 5. The trial was designed to give the greatest amount of information on the efficacy of the treatment while injecting as few women as possible, and each center adopted the same protocol. Since the likelihood of immunization was found to be related to the size of the transplacental hemorrhage (TPH) at delivery (Woodrow and Donohoe, 1968; also see Table 2), only previously untransfused primiparae who had had a TPH with a Kleihauer score of five fetal cells or over per 50 low-power fields, and who had had an Rh-positive, ABO-compatible baby were included. These were thought to be high-risk cases, and alternate ones were kept as controls. The dose was 5 ml of anti-D gamma globulin, containing about 1000 μg of anti-D, given intramuscularly within 48 hours of delivery. The gamma globulin was prepared by Dr. W. d'A. Maycock and his staff at the Lister Institute, London. It will be seen from Tables 4 and 5 that the results were successful, there being only 2 failures in the series. The trial demonstrated that we had in fact picked a high-risk group (immunization rate in the controls, 22%) and that in this group the subsequent pregnancies were protected—one of the 2 failures recorded in Table 5 being the same as that in Table 4.

TABLE 4.—*Liverpool Group 5 Ml High-Risk Trial:*
Rh Antibodies 6 months Postdelivery

Center	Number	Not immunized	Immunized
	Controls		
Liverpool	92 (40)*	72 (30)	20 (10)
Baltimore	31 (14)	23 (10)	8 (4)
Sheffield	41 (15)	31 (10)	10 (5)
Leeds and Bradford	12 (9)	12 (9)	0 (0)
Total	176 (78)	138 (59)	38 (19)
	Treated		
Liverpool	94 (40)	93 (40)	1 (0)
Baltimore	26 (13)	26 (13)	0 (0)
Sheffield	39 (14)	39 (12)	0 (0)
Leeds and Bradford	14 (11)	14 (10)	0 (0)
Total	173 (78)	172 (75)	1 (0)

*The figures in parentheses are those when the trial was published (Combined study, 1966). They are *included* in the larger figures.

TABLE 5.—*Liverpool Group 5 Ml Trial:*
Rh Antibodies at End of Second Rh-Positive Pregnancy

Center	Number	Not immunized	Immunized
		Controls	
Liverpool	38	30	8 (7)*
Baltimore	4	3	1
Sheffield	19	10	9 (5)
Leeds and Bradford	4	2	2
Total	65	45	20 (12)
		Treated	
Liverpool	59	57	2 (1)
Baltimore	12	12	0
Sheffield	10	10	0
Leeds and Bradford	7	7	0
Total	88	86	2 (1)

*Numbers in parentheses are mothers who had developed antibodies after the first pregnancy. They are *included* in the larger number.

The Second Liverpool Trial (Woodrow et al., 1971)

Here the dose of anti-D gamma globulin was 1 ml (about 200 μg), other centers were not involved, and the injection was given to those primiparae with a fetal cell score of from 0 to 4 in 50 low-power fields. Table 6 shows that the 6 month figures are again very satisfactory, but in the second pregnancies (Table 7) there are 3 failures in the treated as against 7 new immunizations in the controls. This appears paradoxical compared with the first trial, but it seems very likely that these failures are women who had been "primed"* by a TPH early in the first pregnancy, and that though they had no demonstrable antibody (NDA) their hidden antibody had removed the fetal cells. If this is the case, then the anti-D gamma globulin would have been given too late. That this situation can occur has been shown by a study of Woodrow et al. (1969) and also by an experience of our own with an Rh-negative blood donor volunteer (Clarke, 1968b; see also p. 190). It is further borne out by the finding of Woodrow and Donohoe (1968), already mentioned, that women with larger bleeds at delivery tend to make antibody at 6 months, or not at all, whereas those with small or no bleeds make antibodies more frequently

* By "primed" is meant that the woman is immunized, but no antibodies can be demonstrated by routine methods, though shortened red cell survival can often be demonstrated.

TABLE 6.—*Liverpool 1 Ml Trial: Rh Antibodies 6 Months Postdelivery*

	Number	Not immunized	Immunized
Controls	362	349	13
Treated	353	353	0
Total	715	702	13

TABLE 7.—*Liverpool 1 Ml Trial:*
Rh Antibodies at End of Second Rh-Positive Pregnancy

	Number	Not immunized	Immunized
Controls	127	114	13 (4)*
Treated	128	125	3
Total	255	239	16 (4)

*The numbers in parentheses refer to mothers who had developed antibodies after the first pregnancy. They are *included* in the larger number.

after the stimulus of a second Rh-positive pregnancy. This has also been the experience of Spensieri et al. (1968).

Some National Health Service (U.K.) Results

England and Wales. Prophylactic treatment of primiparae under the National Health Service started in January, 1968. Dosage has varied between 140 μg and 200 μg and the follow-up at 6 months has revealed 26 failures out of 5693 treated (0.46%). Table 8 gives the details (Maycock, personal communication, 1970).

Scotland. Wallace (personal communication, 1970) in Glasgow had 14 women with antibodies at 6 months out of 1005 treated, but in 10 of them there was evidence of probable previous immunization (Table 9). In Edinburgh, Robertson (1968; personal communication, 1969) independently of the N.H.S., had no failures at 6 months in 100 treated compared with 15 in 112 controls. The numbers in the second pregnancies are not big enough to give an adequate assessment of the efficiency of the prophylaxis—12 controls with 2 more immunized compared with 9 injected and none immunized.

United States of America

Here multiparae as well as primiparae are included, and the Kleihauer test is not carried out as a routine. It will be seen (Table 10) that the results are slightly better than those in Liverpool, a fact which is remarkable

TABLE 8.—*National Health Service:*
*England and Wales, Results to December, 1969**

Total primigravidae injected: 5693
  Dose: 140 μg or 200 μg
Of 5666 followed up at 6 months, 5635 had no antibodies
  26 definite failures (0.46%)
  In addition:
    4 failures possibly due to previous abortions
    1 failure probably due to a previous transfusion
  In 7 of the 26 cases the antibody might still be the remains of the injected passive antibody

Results where Kleihauer score is known

Total primigravidae injected: 4581
  Dose: 140 μg or 200 μg
Analysis of 20 failures:

Kleihauer score	0		1–20	21–100	101–500	>501
Treated primiparae	703 (1)†		3346 (8)	409 (1)	92 (3)	31 (7)

  10 failures in 4458 with Kleihauer of <100
  10 failures in 123 with Kleihauer of >101
  I.e., 140–200 μg give good protection up to 5 ml TPHs

---

*Maycock, personal communication (1970).
†The numbers in parentheses indicate the number of failures.

since multiparae were excluded there. The explanation is uncertain, but it may be that the American commercial anti-D (RhoGAM) has greater affinity—and it is also true that in the earlier United States cases a large dose was given—though for some time now about 300 μg has been given with equally good results.

In St. Louis, Mo., Hamilton (1970; personal communication, 1970) appreciated the importance of the second pregnancy on reading our 1961 paper (Finn et al., 1961), and he never troubled to test at 6 months at

TABLE 9.—*National Health Service: Scotland**

Total primigravidae injected: 1005
Analysis of 14 failures:
  Dose: 200 μg National Health Service gamma globulin
  14 immunized out of 991
  Of the 14:
    3 had had previous abortions
    4 were already immunized
    3 got anti-D very quickly
    ———
    10
  This leaves four true failures, or 0.4%: 2 had no cells and 2 had from 0–4 cells.

---

*Wallace, personal communication (1970).

TABLE 10.—*United States: Ortho Trials (RhoGAM)**

	Total	Immunized	Not immunized	% immunized
Tested 6 months postdelivery				
Treated	3389	6	3383	0.2
Controls	1476	102	1374	6.9
Subsequent pregnancies				
Treated	390	5	385	1.3
Controls	155	23	132	12.9

*Pollack, personal communication (1970). RhoGAM is commercial gamma globulin made by Ortho Pharmaceuticals, Raritan, N. J., U.S.A.

all. He treated women with plasma, not gamma globulin, and in 219 subsequent Rh-positive pregnancies he has only found evidence of sensitization in 2 cases, using the direct Coombs test on the babies' cord blood. Although this is very satisfactory, yet the W.H.O. Scientific group on the Prevention of Rh Sensitisation think that plasma should not be used because of the risk of transmitting the virus of hepatitis.

Canada

Here Chown's group in Winnipeg and another in Toronto have been very active, and some results using the standard postnatal treatment are given in Tables 11 and 12. Bowman thinks that the excellence of the results is due to the fact that his group use very sensitive techniques to detect antibodies and that those women who are immunized during their first pregnancy (see pp. 177-178) are nearly always excluded from the trial.

West Germany

Workers here were very early in the field (Schneider and Preisler, 1965), and some results are shown in Table 13. It is of interest that the immunization rate in their controls is much lower (4.4%) than it is in the United Kingdom or the United States, and this may be due to excep-

TABLE 11.—*Canada: Some Data on Rh Prevention from Manitoba and Northwestern Ontario, 6–9 Months Results**†

Dose of anti-D IgG within 72 hours of delivery	Primiparae	Multiparae	Total	Rh antibodies
300 μg	544	649	1193	0

*Bowman, personal communication (1970).
†All Rh-negative women, without previous Rh antibodies, delivering Rh-positive babies (ABO-compatible and ABO-incompatible cases included).

TABLE 12.—*Canada: Some Data on Primigravidae from Manitoba Producing D-Positive Babies Followed Through or into Second Pregnancy**

First pregnancy	Un-delivered	D-negative baby	D-positive Baby ABO-incompatible without antibodies	D-positive Baby ABO-compatible without antibodies	Antibody detected in second pregnancy
37 controls † (untreated at end of first pregnancy)	0	6	3	27	1 (Boulet)‡
262 treated, ABO-compatible D-positive first baby	92	24	6	139	1 (Poitras)§
41 treated, ABO-incompatible D-positive first baby	14	6	17	4	0

*Bowman, personal communication (1970).

†There was a second immunization in the controls excluded from table because not tested 6 months postpartum first delivery.

Notes:

‡Boulet: Untreated at first pregnancy; baby ABO-compatible D-positive. No antibody when tested at 17 weeks in second pregnancy. Papain antibody at 22 weeks. Fully developed antibody at 26½ weeks. Baby D-positive ABO-compatible, direct Coombs positive.

§Poitras: Given plasma (not gamma globulin) after first pregnancy; baby ABO-compatible D-positive; 17 ml TPH. No antibody postpartum or up to 39 weeks of second pregnancy. At delivery, antibody, 2 albumin, 4 saline. Baby direct Coombs positive 4.

Summary of results:

‡Boulet: 1 of 28 ABO-compatible D-positive first pregnancy, untreated series.

§Poitras: 1 of 29 ABO-compatible D-positive first pregnancy, treated with plasma (not gamma globulin). May have been a primary sensitization. The other 111 ABO-compatible D-positive cases with IgG were treated, and none developed antibodies in their second pregnancy.

tionally good obstetric care (preventing TPH). Some centers in Germany and elsewhere are giving intravenous gamma globulin in doses adjusted to the amount of transplacental hemorrhage (see pp. 192-195; see also Schneider, 1971).

Australia

The Australians up to 1970 had issued 37,120 doses, the amount given being from 170 μg to 250 μg and the series started in 1967. Table 14 gives the results of those who had been followed up for 6 months or more. In the series restricted to Western Australia (Table 15, 3008 women had been given a dose of 170-250 μg, and in the same table are given possible reasons for the 10 failures. There are no controls, all women being offered treatment.

TABLE 13.—*Current Results in the Combined West German Series*

	Total	Immunized	Not immunized	% immunized
Tested 6 months postdelivery				
Controls	2458 (685) †	96 (26)	2362 (659)	3.9 (3.8)
Treated	3091 (1178)	15 (4) †	3076 (1174)	0.49 (0.34)
Subsequent pregnancies (the next after entering the trial)				
Controls	363 (131)	29 (15)	334 (116)	7.8 (11.5)
Treated	138 (76)	0	138 (76)	0 (0)

*Schneider, personal communication (1970); reprinted by permission of the editor of *Clinical Genetics.*

†Numbers in parentheses are primiparae with ABO-compatible babies and no history of abortion. They are *included* in the larger figures.

‡Dr. Schneider reports that some of these women later lost their antibodies.

Thus by the end of the subsequent pregnancy in the controls 11.7 (15.3) % have become immunized, compared with 0.49 (0.34) in the treated.

TABLE 14.—*Australia: 37,120 Doses (Dose 170–250 μg) Issued;*
*Therapy Started August, 1967**

Follow-Up	Number	Immunized	Not immunized	%
Six months	3307	21	3286	0.64
Next pregnancy	432	3	429	0.66

*Davey, personal communication (1970); reprinted by permission of the editor of *Clinical Genetics.*

18 other failures reported (some doubtful).

TABLE 15.—*Western Australia:*
*Dose 170–250 μg, Results up to December, 1969**

Total injected	Tested at 6 months	Immunized	Not immunized	% immunized
3008	692	10	682	1.4

*Davey, personal communication (1970); reprinted by permission of the editor of *Clinical Genetics.*

Analysis of 10 failures:
9 out of 10 had no fetal cells.
Possible reasons:
Insufficient dose.
Too late for early "bleeds."
Inactive preparation.
Neutralization by anti-gamma globulin.

Holland

A great deal of work has been carried out in Holland; see below under "Increased Dosage in Relation to the Size of Transplacental Hemorrhage."

Sweden

Table 16 gives the results as far as we know them in Sweden (Bartsch et al., 1970).

FAILURES AND METHODS OF PREVENTING THEM

Nothing is 100% in biology or medicine, and though there have been failures of the treatment these have been comparatively few, the general finding in many countries being around 0.5% at 6 months and a total of about 1% by the end of the subsequent pregnancy. This must be compared with an immunization rate of about 8.5% at 6 months and a further 8.5% by the end of the subsequent pregnancy, i.e., 17% in all, if nothing at all is done.

There seem to be two, or possibly three, main reasons for failures. The first is that a woman is sometimes primed by her first baby but has no demonstrable antibodies during or immediately after it, and she may, therefore, be included in the trial. The fact that she is a failure only becomes apparent (usually) during the second Rh-positive pregnancy, a fresh stimulus of Rh-positive cells being necessary to render the occult antibody overt. Such a case occurred in one of our volunteers. An Rh-negative man

TABLE 16.—*Sweden: 6 Months Results or Later,*
*Multigravidae and Primigravidae**

	Total	Immunized	Not immunized	% immunized
All babies Rh-positive ABO-compatible				
Treated with 500–750 μg anti-D (Kabi)	694	8 †	686	1.15 (?)
Treated with 250 μg anti-D (Kabi)	884	3 ‡	881	0.34
Controls	388	17	371	4.3
Subsequent Rh-positive pregnancies				
Treated (both dosage groups)	30	0	30	0

*Adapted from Bartsch et al., personal communication (1970), by permission of the editor of *Clinical Genetics.*

†Weak papain at 6 months and not examined later. Probably remains of passive antibody.

‡All multigravidae. These are true failures.

aged 70, NDA on routine testing, was given 5 ml of Rh-positive fetal blood. Thirty minutes later his fetal cell score was 114, but 48 hours later it was 0 and at that time anti-D began to be detectable. It was then found out that he had had a blood transfusion in the 1914-18 war, and clearly primary immunization had taken place as a result. Had he been a young woman he might have been treated and later regarded as a failure.

A failure may also occur because of a TPH early in a second pregnancy; this may sometimes immunize *during that pregnancy,* but if this happens, clearly the anti-D given after the first delivery cannot be said to have failed.

Third, there is also the possibility that the rate at which the Rh-positive cells are cleared from the circulation is inefficient, though the relationship of this to subsequent immunization is not known.

In considering results and failures generally, it must be remembered that only healthy subsequent Rh-positive babies are a true measure of success because with increasingly sensitive methods of detection of antibodies it is very difficult to be sure, even after 6 months or more, whether anti-D found in the circulation is active or the remains of the passive anti-D, particularly if rather a large dose of anti-D has been given (see p. 197). The best evidence of all of the success of the treatment would be a demonstrable drop in the incidence of Rh hemolytic disease. There is as yet little information on this, but at one busy Liverpool maternity hospital the number of exchange transfusions in 1969 was 12, having been around 30 per year for several years previously (Hibbard, 1970, personal communication).

Mention will now be made of possible methods by which these various types of failure can be dealt with.

Administration of Anti-D During Pregnancy

Because of the risk of priming by a TPH during a first pregnancy, Canadian workers began by treating women during pregnancy (Zipursky et al., 1965; Zipursky and Israels, 1967). The number of cases was not large but their results were good, and it was only because treatment postdelivery turned out to be generally so successful that they did not continue. Now that there is seen to be a small regular failure rate, a new large trial has been set up in Canada, and the background to this is as follows. Bowman (1970) found that in Manitoba 21 of 1061 primigravidae (2.0%) who produced Rh-positive babies had developed Rh antibodies by the third day postdelivery. All 21 developed in women who produced ABO-compatible Rh-positive babies, of which there were a total of 909 (incidence, 2.3%). Thus approximately 2% of women at risk in Manitoba would not be protected by a single postnatal injection of Rh-immune globulin. These women represent 15 to 20% of all women who will be immunized by an initial Rh-positive pregnancy unless they are given Rh-immune globulin after delivery. Five of the 21 women developed their Rh antibody between 29 and 34 weeks' gestation and the remaining 16 did so between 37 weeks' gestation and the third day postdelivery (just prior to injection of Rh-immune globulin).

Bowman believes that if Rh-immune globulin given postpartum is going to leave a failure rate of 2.0%, the logical treatment would be to administer it during pregnancy, well before 34 weeks' gestation, and he and his colleagues set up a trial in Winnipeg in June, 1969. Since the purpose of this is to determine whether the present failure rate of 1 to 2% which occurs with postdelivery injection alone can be reduced, conclusive information will not be available for some time. The dose in the Winnipeg series is 200 to 300 μg at weekly intervals during the last trimester of pregnancy; this is followed by a further dose after delivery if the baby is Rh-positive. So far 188 women treated before delivery have given birth to Rh-positive babies (137 ABO-compatible), and there has been a reduction of fetal red cells in the maternal circulation from 14.1% in the control group (21 of 149) to 5.9% (11 of 188) in the treated. Fears of putting the fetus at risk because of 7S anti-Rh IgG crossing the placenta are, Bowman thinks, groundless. Actively Rh-immunized women having Rh antibody titers of the same degree as that produced by the given dose (never higher than 1:2 in albumin) do not have babies with clinical erythroblastosis, and in Zipursky and Israels' earlier experiments (1967) there was no evidence of clinical disease in any of the Rh-positive babies delivered after the injections. In Bowman's series the treatment has also been shown to be harmless. While Bowman's new series cannot yet be assessed, a single case has been reported (from South Africa) by Grobbelaar and Mostert (1970) in which a TPH of about 10 ml occurred at the twenty-ninth week of the first pregnancy, and 400 μg of anti-D 96 hours later failed to prevent primary immunization.

The matter of treatment with anti-D during pregnancy was fully discussed by the W.H.O. Scientific Group (W.H.O., 1971) and the consensus was that this should at present be restricted to clinical trials and always be followed by postdelivery administration if the baby is Rh-positive. However, ultimately it may prove to be the most effective means of preventing Rh immunization.

Increased Dosage in Relation to the Size of Transplacental Hemorrhage

For practical purposes, a "large" transplacental hemorrhage may be defined as one for which a routine dose of 200-300 μg of anti-D IgG is not enough. This means that the lower level of large bleeds ought to be placed at about 10 ml of fetal red cells. This suggestion was made by Borst-Eilers (personal communication, 1970), the choice being based on the observations of her own group and on results reported by Gorman (1970) (see Table 17). The term massive could be reserved for transplacental hemorrhages involving at least 50 ml of fetal red cells.

The incidence of large and massive transplacental hemorrhages is low (in 0.2 to 0.3% of deliveries), but they carry a relatively high risk of primary immunization. Borst-Eilers (personal communication, 1970) found that in a series of 2803 Dutch women 4 (0.14%) showed a TPH of 25 to 100 ml. of blood, and in only 2 instances (0.07%) a hemorrhage of more than 100 ml of blood had occurred (Table 18).

An incidence of one massive TPH per 1000 deliveries is thought to be reasonably accurate. Borst-Eilers makes the point that in the majority of large and massive TPHs no underlying cause can be found, nor are any means known by which they could be prevented.

TABLE 17.—*Anti-D Immunoprophylaxis in Male Volunteers**

Amount of Rh-positive blood injected, ml	Percentage of individuals forming anti-D	
	Treated, 300 μg RhoGam	Controls
15	0%	45%
20	0%	47%
35	22%	50%
50	31%	58%
100	29%	55%

Gorman, personal communication (1970).

TABLE 18.—*Transplacental Hemorrhage in a Series of 2803 Dutch Women**†

Size of TPH	Number of women
No fetal cells seen	1337 (48%)
0.1 ml	1177 (42%)
0.1–1 ml	223 (8%)
1–10 ml	53 (1.9%)
10–25 ml	7 (0.3%)
25–100 ml	4 (0.14%)
>100 ml	2 (0.07%)
Total	2803

*Borst-Eilers et al., personal communication (1970).
†Postdelivery samples examined by Kleihauer test.

The risk of immunization rises with the size of the TPH (see Table 2, and see Table 19 for data from the Netherlands (Borst-Eilers, personal communication, 1970). Dosage, therefore, becomes extremely important after a large TPH, and all workers are in agreement that the usual 200 μg is inadequate and that large and massive TPHs must be recognized as soon as possible. This is usually easy, since they always give rise to a striking degree of neonatal anaemia, sometimes even to intrauterine death. When a mother is Rh-negative, either of these is an absolute indication to examine the maternal blood for the presence of fetal red cells, and furthermore, in order to calculate the necessary dose of anti-D, at least some rough estimation of the amount of fetal blood involved ought to be made.

On the other hand, TPHs between 25 and 100 ml of blood do not necessarily give rise to clinical symptoms. One can only recognize these by actually looking for them, and this means performing Kleihauer tests on postdelivery blood samples of all Rh-negative women. Where this is not feasible, a certain failure rate (of about 1 to 2 per 1000) is to be expected.

Large-scale clinical trials have shown that failures may also occur because of early TPH, and the hemorrhage may be large here, too. Dudok de Wit and Borst-Eilers describe a case (1968) of a TPH of 180 ml 2 weeks before delivery, while Lunay et al. (1970) found a concentration of 9% fetal red cells 9 days before delivery. Early bleeding is sometimes deduced from the fact that at the time of delivery the mother's circulation contains an amount of fetal red cells which is greater than the total amount present in a normal baby at term (Bowman and Chown, 1968; Dudok de Wit and Borst-Eilers, 1968; Lunay et al., 1970). The appearance of anemia in the newborn, together with signs of enhanced red cell production, also suggest a blood loss over a longer period of time.

In considering 25 cases of massive TPH or mismatched transfusion in which protection with anti-D IgG was attempted, Borst-Eilers (1970) em-

TABLE 19.—*Relation Between Size of TPH and Risk of Rh Immunization*

Size of TPH (Kleihauer test postdelivery)	Number of women examined	Number immunized (anti-D present at 3–6 months)
No fetal cells seen	340	7 (2%)
<0.1 ml	154	11 (7%)
0.1–1 ml	63	10 (16%)
1–10 ml	8	5 (62%)
Total	565	33 (6%)

Borst-Eilers, personal communication (1970).

phasizes that, besides noting the dose in relation to the amount of Rh-positive cells, one must take into account the batch of anti-D used (since these vary), the time interval between TPH and treatment, and the ability of the mother to react to the D antigen. Not every Rh-negative individual is capable of producing Rh antibodies, so an apparent success with a low dose of anti-D might well be due to this factor. Bearing in mind these reservations, she concludes that with anti-D immunoglobulin administered intramuscularly, apparent protection has been achieved with doses ranging from 4 to 50 μg of anti-D per milliliter of fetal red cells with a mean ratio of 25:1, while failures have been reported with doses ranging from 2 to 20 μg of anti-D per milliliter of fetal red cells, the mean ratio being 8:1. With intramuscular injection there seems no harm in giving the entire dose of anti-D at the same time, though when injecting anti-D intravenously divided doses are advisable (see below).

Eklund and Nevanlinna (1971) report 3 cases of mismatched transfusion in which 8000, 5000, and 3900 μg of intravenously administered anti-D protected against 4000, 800, and 400 ml of Rh-positive blood respectively. The first patient received plasma and had a mild transfusion reaction, but the other 2 were treated with gamma globulin and showed no adverse effect. All patients were treated with divided doses of anti-D. Keith et al. (1970) also report a similar case.

Acceleration of Clearance by the Intravenous Administration of Anti-D

Comparison of clearance of fetal red cells gives evidence that an intravenous dose of anti-D clears a TPH twice as fast as the same dose administered intramuscularly. It may also be that the same dose, microgram per microgram, is more effective in protecting against Rh immunization when given by the intravenous route. Thus this method may prove to be of considerable value where large transplacental hemorrhages have been demonstrated, or when for one reason or another administration of anti-D has been delayed. When a TPH of greater than 10 ml of fetal red cells is demonstrated, the suggested dose of intravenous anti-D is 12 μg per ml of fetal red cells. Hoppe (personal communication, 1970) states that the preparation for an intravenous injection should not contain aggregates showing anticomplementary activity, that IgG anti-D preparations with cleavage of the IgG molecule should not be used, and that the anti-D concentration should be high in relation to the total protein (IgG) content (at least 100 μg anti-D/10 mg of total protein). If gamma globulin solutions of the usual concentration (16%) or larger amounts are used, shocklike incidents may occur on intravenous injection (though mainly in cases of immunoglobulin deficiency).

The workers who have carried out the largest intravenous studies are Börner and his colleagues in the Federal Republic of Germany, Huchet in Paris, and Jouvenceaux and his colleagues in Lyons, though many East European countries are also using the method. In South Africa, Shapiro and his colleagues use intravenous plasma (see Clarke, 1970).

Huchet (personal communication, 1970) in Paris carried out a comparison of the intramuscular and intravenous routes and found that in seven TPHs ranging from 10 to 175 ml which were treated by intravenous immunoglobulin there was no latency period, and that the fetal red cell elimination curve was clearly linear as from the time of injection in all cases. For the (usual) 300 μg intravenous injections, the half-life periods ranged from 1¼ hours to 3 hours. In 2 cases with massive TPH treated with a single intravenous injection of 600 μg, the half-lives were 1 hour and 30 minutes and 1 hour and 20 minutes respectively. In these 2 cases, however, the injections were followed, after between 3 and 5 hours, by shivering with hyperthermia (38.5°C in the first case and 39°C in the second) and very transitory malaise. After these incidents (clinically comparable to transfusion shock), the introduction of intravenous doses above 300 μg in a single injection was suspended, no matter what the volume of the fetal bleeding. The injection of large quantities of antibody was spread over several hours. The total time elapsing before obtaining a count below 1 fetal cell per 100,000 adult cells was not greater than 24 hours in any of the cases.

In contrast, where six transplacental hemorrhages ranging from 2 to 85 ml were treated by the intramuscular injection of an immunoglobulin which also contained 300 μg of anti-D, there was a slow elimination period to start with and a second, rapid elimination phase. The greater the volume of transplacental fetal red cells, the longer the latency period. The total time elapsing before obtaining a count below 1/100,000 varied from 36 to 130 hours, according to the volume of fetal red cells to be got rid of.

Comparison of these results indicates that, with equal weights of anti-D antibody injected for a given volume of fetal bleeding, the intravenous route is superior to the intramuscular, both as regards the rapidity of the initial action and the effect on the speed of elimination of fetal red cells. Consequently, a smaller intravenous dose can be used, and this route is particularly indicated in cases of massive TPH.

Börner et al. (1969), using a highly purified anti-D gamma globulin prepared for intravenous injection by Dr. Hoppe of Hamburg, gave adapted doses on a sliding scale according to the size of the TPH. This dose was adjusted so that there was always detectable free anti-D antibody in the maternal serum even after the total elimination of the fetal red blood cells.

Of 50 women thus treated, none became immunized after 6 months; details of 27 of them are shown in Table 20.

Later, Deicher (personal communication, 1970) reported only one failure at 6 months in 3695 cases injected by the intravenous route, and there were no side effects. Jouvenceaux et al. (1968) also report more rapid clearance of cells by the intravenous than by the intramuscular route.

It will be interesting to see how the intravenous results develop. If failures are usually due to priming during an initial pregnancy, then giving anti-D gamma globulin intravenously after delivery would not seem to be the answer. If, on the other hand, failures are more usually due to big TPHs, then the intravenous route might be a very valuable method of therapy.

Failures and the Problem of False Positive Antibody Tests

In assessing the failure rate at 6 months postdelivery, a difficulty which is sometimes encountered is that of deciding whether an antibody detected by a sensitive technique indicates actual immunization or whether it simply represents the tail end of the "passive." There is no certain way of deciding about this except by a "wait and see" attitude—if actively immunized, the antibody is likely to become stronger whereas the "passive" will disappear with time. Wallace (personal communication, 1970) has some interesting data bearing on the matter. He injected approximately 1000 μg of anti-D into each of 12 Rh-negative volunteers to find out how long it could be detected. In 3 cases none was found by the autoanalyzer (which should detect as low a concentration as 0.002 μg/ml) at 6 months, and in one case it had disappeared by 5 months. The remaining 9 all had anti-D after 6 months, and they are being followed until it is no longer detected.

TABLE 20.—*Intravenous Gamma Globulin, Demonstration of Free Anti-D Antibody in the Maternal Serum After Complete Elimination of Rh-Positive Fetal Red Cells**

Approximate Kleihauer score	Intravenous dose of IgG anti-D, μg	Longest time for removal of fetal cells, hours	Anti-D detectable after stated number of hours	Number of cases
0	62	—	6	6
1	62	4	6	6
1–2	148	12	12	5
2–10	148	24	24	7
10–30	186	24	24	3

*Adapted from Börner et al. (1969) by permission of the authors and of the editors of *Geburtshilfe und Frauenheilkunde*.

If human IgG immunoglobulin has a half-life of 25 days, the level of anti-D in the serum 6 months postinjection would be about 0.002 μg/ml. Of the 9 volunteers who still had anti-D after 6 months, 5 had 0.003 μg/ml and 3 others had 0.002, 0.004, and 0.005 μg/ml respectively. This is a most useful yardstick, since some laboratories are claiming to detect anti-D by enzyme techniques 6 months postdelivery when only 22 μg has been injected, though at the time of testing the laboratories were unaware of how much anti-D had been given. Taking into account the half-life of anti-D it would be quite impossible to detect any of it at 6 months if so small a dose had been given, and the results are either false positives or the women have become immunized, and only time will show which is correct.

LATER EXPERIMENTS IN VOLUNTEERS

While the clinical trials were under way, with results suggesting that the prophylaxis was successful, experiments continued to be carried out in male volunteers, particularly to gain experience about the efficacy of protection using a lower dose of anti-D. One study was by American workers (Pollack et al., 1967). Four groups of 10 Rh-negative men were given 10 ml of O Rh-positive whole blood intravenously at monthly intervals for a total of three injections. Twenty-four hours following its administration, three of the four groups were given 1.0 ml, 0.5 ml, and 0.25 ml respectively of a RhoGAM* preparation containing 1200 μg of anti-D antibody per milliliter. Blood samples were tested for anti-D monthly for 9 months, and the final results are summarized in Table 21. It will be seen that 300 μg appeared to be protective against 10 ml of whole blood, but the men were not challenged further.

Experiments with smaller volumes of anti-D were carried out by Mollison and Hughes-Jones (1967). They injected 34 volunteers with 1 ml of

TABLE 21.—*Results of Male Volunteer Experiment**

Group	Dose of anti-D	Number with anti-Rh at 9 months	% with antibody
I	0	6 of 10 men	60
II	1200 μg	0 of 10 men	0
III	600 μg	0 of 10 men	0
IV	300 μg	0 of 10 men	0

*Reprinted by permission from Pollack et al. (1967).

* Commercial gamma globulin made by Ortho Pharmaceuticals, Raritan, N.J.

Rh-positive red cells (some R^1r and some R^2r). Some received no anti-D, some 15 μg, and some 75 μg. Six months later, a proportion of the subjects were challenged with 1 ml of ^{51}Cr-labeled Rh-positive red cells. Only 2 (both of whom had initially been injected with red cells alone, without anti-D) developed immune anti-D antibody, one doing so 6 months after the initial injection and the second a month after the second challenge. Although these results (by serological testing) suggested that the incidence of primary immunization had been very low, the results of the ^{51}Cr red cell survival tests gave a very different picture. They are shown in Table 22, and it will be seen that, among the 13 subjects who initially received red cells alone, 4 had slightly and 3 grossly subnormal cell survival at 7 to 11 days after challenge with labeled red cells; this had revealed that 7 of the 13 were probably immunized, as were 2 of the 8 who had received cells plus 15 μg anti-D. By contrast, of the 13 originally injected with cells plus 75 μg of anti-D none was immunized.

In summary, these experiments suggest that 75 μg is probably an effective dose in suppressing primary immunization by 1 ml of red cells; 15 μg anti-D is probably not fully protective, but there is no evidence that it increases the risk of primary immunization.

It is useful at this stage to consider the relationship between protection and the rate of clearance of Rh-positive cells from the circulation by the giving of passive anti-D. Mollison and Hughes-Jones (1967) gave previously untransfused Rh-negative subjects an intravenous injection of approximately 0.3 ml of Rh-positive red cells, and at about the same time, or 24-28 hours previously, an intramuscular injection of 1-1000 μg of anti-D. Following the injection of the red cells there was a variable period before the onset of red cell destruction. When the antibody had been injected at the same time as the red cells the delay was due partly to the time taken for the antibody to reach the circulation; when it was given at least 24 hours before the cells there was still some delay due to the time

TABLE 22.—*Challenge with 1 Ml of ^{51}Cr-Labeled Red Cells Alone, 6 Months After Initial Injection**

Initial treatment received	^{51}Cr survival at 7–11 days		
	Normal	Slightly subnormal	Grossly subnormal
1 ml cells alone	6	4	3
1 ml cells plus 15 μg anti-D	6	2	0
1 ml cells plus 75 μg anti-D	13	0	0

*Mollison et al., 1969.

required for it to be taken up by the red cells, and in all, the delay before the onset of the maximum rate of red cell destruction varied from about 0.2 hours following the injection of 1000 μg of antibody to approximately 100 hours following the injection of 1 μg.

The maximum rate of red cell destruction was calculated to be approximately proportional to the square root of the amount of antibody on the cells. After the injection of the smallest amount of antibody (1 μg) of high binding capacity the concentration on the red cells was calculated to be about 0.03 μg/ml of Rh-positive cells in the circulation, corresponding to about 10 molecules of antibody per cell. This dose produced clearance with a $T1/2$ (i.e., half-life) of the order of 100 hours as already mentioned.

Assuming that the minimal amount of anti-D on the red cells must be 0.03 μg/ml for destruction to take place, an important point in relation to prevention of Rh isoimmunization was raised by an observation of Hughes-Jones (1967). He found that, when 1 ml of Rh-positive cells was present in the circulation, 21 times as much of a weakly binding antibody (with an equilibrium constant $K = 1 \times 10^7$ liters per mole) were required to give a concentration of anti-D bound to red cells of 0.03 μg/ml red cells, compared with a stronger binding antibody ($K = 1 \times 10^9$ liters per mole). When there were 400 ml of cells in the circulation, however, only three times as much of the weaker antibody was needed. That is, the performance of the antibody is more important when there are only a few cells.

A particularly interesting aspect of clearance in Rh-negative male volunteers is described by Woodrow et al. (1969). They gave 11 Rh-negative male volunteers successive small injections of Rh-positive blood, 4 being given in addition anti-D plasma 30 minutes after the first injection of blood. They found that in 7 cases (one of them treated) rapid clearance of the cells took place after challenge in the absence of detectable antibody, and that 6 of these volunteers eventually made anti-D. It is worth noting that in several instances blood from different Rh-positive donors when injected in turn into the same volunteer showed shortened survival; this provides good circumstantial evidence that an immune state had developed, directed specifically against the D antigen. The question of specificity is discussed again on p. 207.

Relationship Between Dose of Anti-D and Size of Stimulus

Pollack et al. (1971) studied 178 Rh-negative male volunteers in an experiment designed to determine the relation between the dose of IgG anti-D and the size of the stumulus, and the following background information is relevant.

1. Immunization is an all-or-none phenomenon in which the probability of immunization increases as the dose of Rh antigen increases. Thus, if no foreign antigens gain access to the circulation, the probability of immunization is zero, whereas as the dose is infinitely increased, it reaches a limit asymptotically* that will be a value at or less than unity.

2. Since previous data have established that a relationship exists between the dose of antibody and the efficiency of suppression, antibody must combine with the antigen in vivo to exert its effect. This does not make any assumptions as to the exact mechanism involved. However, the fact that antibody can be detected on the Rh-positive cells in the circulation after intramuscular administration of anti-D is supporting evidence that at least the interaction of Rh antibody with antigen occurs within the vascular bed.

3. The binding of antibody to antigen must conform to some adsorption equation (Pollack et al., 1971). While an exact mathematical description of the in vivo equation may be quite different from that in vitro, it will, nevertheless, be empirically related to a calculation based on observation from male volunteer experiments. It follows from what has been said previously that not every antibody preparation will have the same numerically equivalent adsorption equation, nor must it be assumed without evidence that all red cells containing the Rh antigen will bind antibody to exactly the same extent and then be suppressed by equivalent doses of Rh antibody.

The aim of Pollack's experiment, which was started in early 1969, was to determine in a statistically unequivocal way the molar ratio of bound to free antigen that will ensure complete suppression of immunization. It is to be emphasized that the actual molar ratio achieved in vivo is impossible to determine, and what was needed was a molar ratio, obtained by in vitro testing, which gave complete protection, for this can be empirically related to the results of male volunteer experiments. Further, if a sufficient number of donor red cells could be used in the experiment so that the results with extremes of antigen concentration could be obtained, the molar ratio value derived could then be statistically related to the volume of cells which a single dose of an antibody preparation will neutralize. Pollack felt that only by such a study could the dose of antibody be linearly related to the circulating red cell volume.

It was necessary to determine by clinical studies the ratio of bound to

---

* Asymptotic = approaches a maximal level but never finally gets there.

free antigen that gives absolute freedom from immunization and to do this in such a way that many different types of Rh-positive erythrocytes could be studied.

The general design of the study is shown in Table 23; 178 Rh-negative men were divided into six groups consisting of a treated and control series. Each of the volunteers in each group received a single intravenous injection of whole Rh-positive blood starting at 25 ml and increasing to 100 ml of whole blood. Thirty blood donors were used to provide the blood, and within 72 hours each treated man received exactly 1 ml of immune globulin containing 267 µg of anti-D; the control series received a gamma globulin preparation devoid of antibodies to human red cells.

The volunteers were carefully followed serologically for 6 months, and those individuals found to have no detectable Rh antibodies were challenged with 0.2 ml of whole blood. One week later, a serum sample was obtained from all the volunteers and serological analysis was used to determine the outcome of the experiment. The results of the study are shown in Table 24, where it appears that this particular lot of anti-D will protect against 13.0 ml of packed cells or 35 ml of whole blood, though it must be remembered that the probability of immunization rises with an increasing dose of antigen.

Three conclusions may be drawn from these data. The first is that apparently only 65-70% of Rh-negative individuals are susceptible to being immunized to a single injection of Rh-positive red cells, no matter how large, though it is impossible from this to conclude that 30-35% of all Rh-negative individuals are genetically incapable of being immunized. Only subsequent injections of blood given to the nonresponders several months later will resolve this point.

The second is the difference between the slopes of the control and treated series, and the linearity of the transformed data (see Pollack et al.,

TABLE 23.—*Male Volunteer Study to Determine Relationship of Potency to Effectivity of Rh-Immune Globulin Preparations**

1. 25 ml, 35 ml, 45 ml, 55 ml, 75 ml, and 100 ml of whole Rh-positive blood injected intravenously into 6 groups of Rh-negative male volunteers.
2. Three days later, 267 µg of RhoGAM or 1 ml of normal IgG given to treated or control series respectively.
3. Serum samples obtained from each man at monthly intervals for 6 months.
4. Each volunteer then given 0.2 ml of Rh-positive blood intravenously as a booster.
5. Serum sample obtained 1 week later.

*Pollack, personal communication (1970).

TABLE 24.—*Incidence of Immunization in Groups of Volunteers Given Varying Volumes of Rh-Positive Blood Showing 95% Confidence Ranges of Fraction Immunized, 1969–1970**

Volume of packed R.B.C. given	11. 6	13. 4	18. 1	21. 2	30. 1	37. 5
Range	10. 9-12. 4	12. 6-14. 6	16. 6-19. 6	20. 8-21. 3	28. 4-32. 3	35. 9-41. 7
			Untreated group			
Fraction immunized	7/16	6/12	11/19	5/8	7/11	13. 20
	(43. 8%)	(50. 0%)	(57. 9%)	(62. 5%)	(63. 6%)	(65. 0%)
95% confidence range	0. 190-0. 702	0. 211-0. 789	0. 335-0. 798	0. 245 .0-915	0. 308-0. 891	0. 407-0. 846
			Treated group			
Fraction immunized	0/19	0/18	3/18	2/8	4/12	6/17
	(0%)	(0%)	(16. 7%)	(25. 0%)	(33. 3%)	(35. 3%)
95% confidence range	0-0.177	0-0.186	0. 034-0. 414	0. 032-0. 651	0. 099-0. 651	0. 142-0. 617

*Pollack et al, (1971).

1971). If passively administered antibody acted merely to reduce the concentration of antigen reaching immunocompetent cells, the slopes ought to have been the same. One possible explanation for the difference is that antibody acts on some target organ, e.g., the macrophage, to interfere with processing, for the significance of the change in slope is that the antigenicity of the red cells is reduced. Such a mechanism will also explain the differences between the asymptotic values for the control and treated series, if this is confirmed by a larger study.

The third conclusion is that antibody does indeed bind to the antigen surface of the red cells and therefore that the potency assay of the Rh-immune globulin can be safely related to its effectivity. The ratio of bound antigen to free antigen which Pollack was seeking was computed from 13 ml of red cells containing 300 pmoles of antibody adsorbing sites per milliliter. He found that it was possible to calculate a constant which can be used for any IgG anti-Rh preparation which has been assayed according to the methods he describes, and this leads to a very simple method of reporting potency of anti-Rh preparations in terms of the number of milliliters of Rh-positive red cells which can be effectively neutralized by 1 ml of the preparation.

If this suggested method of reporting potency is used, it will allow physicians to prescribe the correct dose of antibody to give for excessively large fetomaternal hemorrhages. It is not suggested that it could be used to reduce the amount of immune globulin for microhemorrhages, since such small volumes of circulating fetal blood cannot be quantitated with the same precision as the larger volumes. The standard dose of immune globulin by these criteria should perhaps be one that prevents immunity to 10 ml of Rh-positive erythrocytes (Pollack et al., 1971).

RISKS OF THE PROPHYLAXIS

The experience of all workers in the field is that the first injection is essentially safe. We have observed very occasionally a sharp local reaction, sometimes associated with fever, lasting about 24 hours, but this is very exceptional and usually (with intramuscular injection) there is no upset of any kind. No anaphylactic reactions have been encountered as far as we know. Furthermore, using gamma globulin (as opposed to plasma), there seems to be no fear of transmitting hepatitis since if the virus was present in the plasma it is eliminated during the preparation of the gamma globulin by the alcohol or ether fractionation procedures (Mollison, 1967).

We know of cases in which anti-D has been given to Rh-positive individuals (both in error to women and experimentally to men) and there were no ill effects (see also Chown et al, 1970), and it has even been given without much harm to Rh-positive babies by those whose only knowledge of the treatment was that it was the baby who was ill—though there is, of course, potential danger if a *large* dose were administered in error to a newborn. Where the gamma globulin has been given to the mother during pregnancy, no harm has been done to the baby, though occasionally the Coombs test on the cord blood has been positive (See "Administration of Anti-D During Pregnancy," above.) (There is even a rumor of it having been given to the husband!)

There has always been the possibility that the mother might become immunized to substances in the gamma globulin itself, particularly to the Gm protein fraction, but we found no significant difference between 65 treated women and 72 controls with respect to the development of an anti-Gm which was not present immediately prepartum—there were 4 in the treated and 1 in the controls ($p > 0.10$). Furthermore, Vos (1965), in an Australian series, found no significant increase in anti-Gm in treated women. One of our 4 treated patients who made anti-Gm (1) which was not present before delivery, was herself Gm (-1) and so was her husband. However, her mother was Gm (1) and it seems likely that this patient may have been originally primed by her mother and that the gamma globulin acted as a booster stimulus.

The question of serious anaphylaxis if gamma globulin needs to be given again in a subsequent pregnancy has always been present and was raised again recently (Barron, personal communication, 1970), but this would seem to be ruled out by the fact that Davey (1970) has treated over 2000 women for a second time with no ill effects. A reaction is really only to be feared in patients who are hypogammaglobulinemic (Grubb et al., 1965).

MECHANISMS OF PROTECTION

When it became evident from the results in many centers that the passive administration of anti-Rh antibody does in fact suppress primary Rh-isoimmunization, much interest was aroused in the mechanisms involved and relevant animal work which had been going on concurrently was looked at to see if any of it could clarify the problem. Some of the theories will now be considered.

The Hypothesis of Central Inhibition

It has been suggested that passive antibody has a direct effect on immunologically competent cells, so that if stimulated by the appropriate antigen they are prevented from synthesizing antibody (Rowley and Fitch, 1967). This theory was based on the finding that if normal rat spleen (i.e., antibody-producing) cells were exposed in vitro to anti-sheep erythrocyte serum and were *then* transferred to irradiated recipients, the cells did not make an early antibody response when challeged with sheep erthrocytes (Rowley and Fitch, 1964). On the other hand, Pierce (1969) and Ryder et al. (1969) have shown in similar experiments on mice that the early hemolysin response to sheep erythrocytes is *not* prevented by the exposure of lymphoid cells to anti-sheep erythrocyte serum, though it is prevented by the exposure of macrophages to such serum.

It is possible, therefore, that in the Rowley and Fitch (1964) work the reason for the prevention of the hemolysin response was because the macrophages, rather than the lymphoid cells, were involved—i.e., there was interference with access of antigen to antigen-reactive cells—or that tolerance was implicated.

In tolerance there is a true central effect on the antibody-forming cells, since lymphoid cells from animals rendered tolerant to an antigen remain unresponsive to that antigen when they are transferred to X-irradiated syngeneic recipients (Friedemann, 1962; Argyris, 1963; Dietrich and Weigle, 1964); lymphoid cells from animals treated to suppress antibody formation do respond when transferred. Both may be concerned in the prevention of the immune response, it now being appreciated that adult animals, as well as embryos, can be rendered tolerant. Figure 4 shows the clear distinction between tolerance and suppression.

Because of the animal work with its emphasis on central inhibition we suggested that in transplantation surgery human anti-donor gamma globulin might "blindfold" the immunological sites on the recipients' lymphocytes and that this might prevent the formation of immune anti-graft antibodies better than heterologous ALS (anti-lymphocyte serum made by injecting human spleen cells into goats or horses). To test this hypothesis, we prepared some gamma globulin made from a patient who 10 years pre-

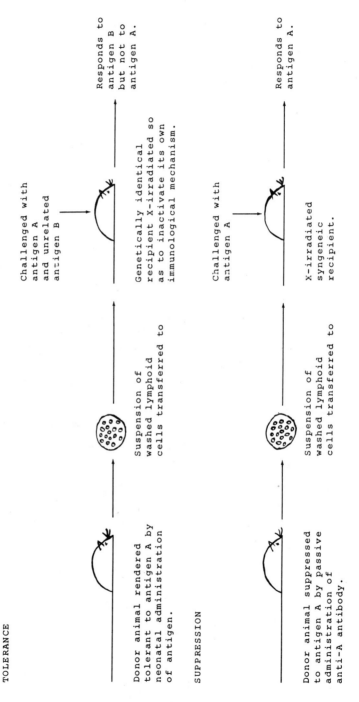

FIG. 4.—Distinction between tolerance and antibody-mediated suppression.

viously had been badly burned and who at that time was treated by temporary skin grafts from his brother-in-law. To hyperimmunize this patient, further brother-in-law skin grafts were carried out and gamma globulin raised which we hoped would increase the survival time of a skin graft from the brother-in-law to a third person, but the necessary volunteer has not so far been forthcoming (see Clarke, 1968b).

More recently, French and Bachelor (1969) procured survival of rat kidney grafts in AS rats for an indefinite period by means of an antiserum. The transplanted kidney was from an August X AS rat, and the antibody was raised by injecting female AS rats with lymphocytes from female August rats. It is believed that the increased survival of the graft occurs because the injected antibody covers a sufficient number of antigen sites on the transplanted kidney to protect it from irreversible damage by immune lymphocytes, but on the other hand sufficient antigen remains not combined with antibody to give some active immunization of the recipient. Therefore, humoral antibody is actively synthesized by the recipient and this continues to protect the graft, competing for antigen sites with the immunologically committed lymphocytes which mediate cellular immunity. The same group (Batchelor et al., 1970) have used the technique with a measure of success in a boy aged 8 who had had a kidney graft. These experiments are much more sophisticated than the one suggested by us, but the same general principle is involved, namely that, as in Rh, passive antibody coats antigenic cells.

Specificity of Suppression

There is evidence that in some systems suppression of antibody formation against one antigenic determinant on a molecule does not suppress antibody formation against a second one. For example, Pollack et al. (1968) prevented anti-Hg antibody production in Hg^AHg^F negative rabbits injected with Hg^AHg^F rabbit erythrocytes by administering passive Hg^A isoantibody but they did not prevent anti-Hg^F antibody formation. Similar findings have been reported by other workers using a variety of antigens (Brody et al., 1967; Dixon et al., 1967). The simplest explanation of this is that passive antibody exerts its effect by covering the corresponding antigenic determinants and hence prevents them from stimulating the appropriate antigen-sensitive cell, with or without the intervention of macrophages. If this theory is correct, then it would be expected that the ability of antibody to suppress would be related to its concentration and affinity (affinity is a measure of the antigen-binding capacity of a population of antibodies). To study this point, Walker and Siskind (1968) assessed the effect of changes in the affinity of anti-hapten-bovine gamma globulin antibody on its ability to suppress the response to hapten-bovine gamma globulin in rabbits. They found that high-affinity antibody can cause suppression at a much lower concentration than can a low-affinity one. This, they argued, is consistent with the theory that antigen binding is involved in suppression, since it follows from the law of mass action that the amount of antigen bound at any given concentration of antibody is a function of the affinity of the antibody. This finding may also resolve the controversy as to whether or not antibody of the IgM type is capable of causing suppression, some workers finding that it can (Rowley and Fitch, 1964; Pearlmann, 1966; Pollack et al., 1968) while others do not (Henry and Jerne, 1968), and the divergences may be explained by the differences in the affinity of the various IgM preparations. Similarly the possibility must now be considered that failure to suppress the anti-D response in the early male volunteer experiment (Clarke et al., 1963) was due to the low affining of the IgM anti-D antibody.

The importance of the interaction between antibody and specific antigenic determinants is also shown by the finding that antibody fragments containing the antigen-binding site are themselves effective in bringing about suppression. Thus Tao and Uhr (1966) and Cerottini et al. (1969) found the $F(ab')_2$ and Fab fragments (see Fig. 5) were able to suppress antibody formation. On the other hand, Sinclair (1969) has found in mice that the ability of anti-sheep erythrocyte serum to inhibit priming to sheep erythrocytes is lost after removal of the Fc piece by pepsin digestion. This suggests that the Fc piece plays some part in increasing the suppressive effect of antibody.

On the other hand, there are studies in which it has been noted that passive antibody acts at the level of the entire antigenic molecule, i.e., in the case of a red cell the total antigenic complex on the surface of the cell. For example, Henney and Ishizaka (1968) found that passive administration of antibody against the Fc portion of human IgG suppressed both anti-Fab and anti-Fc antibody formation in the guinea pig, so that if the operative factor was the covering of the corresponding antigen site only the Fc site would have been covered, and yet the formation of anti-Fab was suppressed. The likely explanation in this case would seem to be that the passive antibody prevented the whole antigenic complex from reaching the antigen-sensitive cells.

More relevant to the situation in man is the apparent lack of specificity of suppression in the interference with Rh isoimmunization due to ABO incompatibility. Pollack et al. (1968) have argued that, since lysed erythrocytes are less immunogenic than unlysed ones, therefore complement-fixing antibodies (such as anti-A and anti-B) against one antigenic determinant on an erythrocyte could lyse the erythrocyte and, as a consequence,

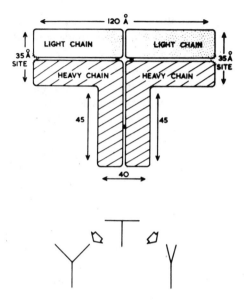

FIG. 5.—Diagram of IgG molecule. There are two combining sites, one at each end of the arms of the T. The two combining sites of an antibody molecule are always the same. The downstroke of the T can be split off, and this portion contains no combining site. It is called the Fc piece. What is left of the molecule can be split at the middle into two fragments, each containing one combining site which retains antibody specificity—the Fab and the F(ab')₂ fragments. The black dots are where the chains are linked to each other. (Reprinted by permision from Nossol, 1969.)

antibody formation against all the antigenic determinants on the erythrocyte would be suppressed. Thus they suggested that the mechanism by which ABO incompatibility interferes with Rh isoimmunization may be due to lysis of Rh-positive erythrocytes by complement-fixing anti-A and anti-B. On the other hand, in rats Elson (personal communication, 1970) found that although lysis of sheep erythrocytes causes diminution in the IgM response there is no reduction in the peak IgG response. In addition, the destruction of the complement-fixing ability of an anti-sheep erythrocyte serum did not reduce its suppressive effect on the IgG response to sheep erythrocytes. Again, Stern et al. (1961) showed that A Rh-negative men injected with A Rh-positive erythrocytes coated in vitro with anti-A *did* develop anti-Rh antibody. Stern (1969) has also investigated an analogous phenomenon in rats, using sheep red cells. These cells possess an antigen which is specific to them alone (isophilic) and also an antigen which they share with many species of animal (heterophilic). When rats were injected with sheep erythrocytes containing *both* these antigens, after having been injected with heterophilic antigen alone, it was found that antibody formation against the isophilic antigen (i.e., the specific sheep red cell antigen) was suppressed. The suppression of anti-isophile antibody was not brought about, however, by the passive administration of small amounts of anti-heterophile antibody 2 hours prior to the injection of the sheep erythrocytes. Stern has taken these results to indicate that the mechanism by which ABO incompatibility interferes with Rh isoimmunization is likely to be because of competition for antigen at a cellular level, and that it is not exclusively humoral (see Bradley and Elson, 1971).

It is clear from the work reviewed above that passive antibody probably does not have a direct "central" effect on antigen-sensitive cells but rather that it affects the "afferent" limb of the immune response by interfering with access of antigen to antigen-sensitive cells. Accepting this, there are two possible mechanisms by which passive antibody exerts a suppressive effect. The first is in situations where suppression is determinant-specific. Here antibody appears to act by covering the corresponding antigenic determinant and rendering it sterically unavailable to antigen-sensitive cells. If this were true of the prevention of Rh isoimmunization in man, then it would mean that in Rh-negative, Kell-negative volunteers challenged with Rh-positive Kell-positive erythrocytes and given passively administered anti-D, only anti-D antibody formation would be prevented whereas anti-Kell would be provoked. On the other hand, if the action were nonspecific, the giving of anti-Kell to these volunteers would prevent them from forming anti-D, and this latter experiment would be much simpler to carry out, because anti-D is more easily provoked than anti-Kell.* In situations where antibody acts at the level of the entire antigenic complex on the red cell, the antibody may act by diverting antigen away from the anatomical area of antigen-sensitive cells or by preventing antigen from reaching antigen-sensitive cells in an immunogenic form, and in the case of the Kell experiment it would mean that neither anti-D nor anti-Kell was formed. We believe that this is the most likely mechanism for two reasons. First, it does not involve making an entirely new hypothesis for the (nonspecific) protection afforded by ABO incompatibility, and second, no anti-Kell antibodies have been produced in a series of 753 women treated by anti-D and tested by us for anti-Kell (and a few would have been expected since the gamma globulin does not contain anti-Kell). No other immune antibodies were produced either (except for Lewis, which is not primarily a blood group antigen), and these findings have to be compared with those of Queenan et al. (1969), who found 299 "irregular" antibodies in 18,378 consecutive obstetric patients. There is also more information from Pollack (personal communication, 1970), who looked at the other anti-

---

* This experiment is at present being carried out in Liverpool.

body status in his 178 Rh volunteers who were being used in protection studies (see "Relationship Between Dose of Anti-D and Size of Stimulus," above). Again, there were none except for an occasional Lewis antibody, and the combined evidence suggests very strongly that what happens in the Rh system is that the partially coated cell is removed from the circulation and opsonized in the macrophages so that no antigen reaches the antibody-forming cells. In other words, the Rh blood groups behave quite differently from animal systems.

ASSAY OF ANTI-D

Three general points are first discussed:

1. *The combining of antibodies* with antigens on human red cells is a reversible process, and is governed by the law of mass action, i.e., rates of formation of the antigen-antibody complex are proportional to the concentrations of antigen and antibody present. There is thus a point at which equilibrium is reached, and the equilibrium constant (K) has a different value for different antibodies—the higher the K, the stronger the binding power of the antibody (see Hughes-Jones, 1967).

2. *The heterogeneity index.* A mixture of antibodies will contain several types of anti-D, and these will behave differently from one another (and the same applies to the other antibodies of the Rh complex). The more heterogeneous the antibody, the lower is its efficiency (a completely homogeneus antibody would be scored as 1).

3. *Titer.* This is a much less accurate measurement. It does not take into account free antibody (and there is always some present), and two antibodies could have the same titer, but if they had different equilibrium constants and heterogeneity indices they would have different binding capacities and therefore their efficiency as antibodies would be different.

It is necessary to compare the titer of anti-D preparations against a standard that has been assayed by one of the two methods discussed below. Even when this is done, a quantitative evaluation of the known preparation will lead to erroneous values if the two differ in their respective equilibrium constants. However, if the anti-D immunoglobulin is prepared from pools of donors, this may not represent a serious problem. Comparison of anti-D concentrations in IgG preparations made from pools of donors using both the autoanalyzer and the radioactive labeling method has shown a close correlation in two series. There is evidence, however, that correlation is poor when assaying an anti-D from a single donor. Comparison between manual agglutination methods and the techniques using radioactivity, with rare exceptions, have shown a poor correlation.

Methods of Assay of Anti-D

The immunosuppressive activity of anti-D immunoglobulin preparations has been related to its antibody concentration (μg/ml), and the most effective assay methods are those using trace labeling with radioactive iodine.

The basic method for the assay of the anti-D content of immunoglobulin preparations involves the iodination of the IgG with ^{125}I and the adsorption of ^{125}I-labeled anti-D onto Rh-positive red cells. The amount of anti-D combined with the red cells can be determined from the radioactive count, but the interpretation of the data is complicated by the fact that the reaction between anti-D and red cells is a reversible reaction and hence, when Rh-positive red cells are added to ^{125}I-labeled anti-D, not all the anti-D is bound, but some remains free in solution. The total anti-D activity can be determined by methods based on the law of mass action (Hughes-Jones, 1967; Hughes-Jones and Stevenson, 1968; Hughes-Jones and Gardner, 1970).

An alternative to the method just described is the use of ^{125}I-labeled anti-gamma globulin, a method which is essentially a quantitative antigamma globulin test. A purified ^{125}I-labeled anti-gamma globulin is made which is calibrated by preparing a series of red cell samples which have absorbed different amounts of ^{131}I-labeled anti-D prepared from a pool of donors. The ^{125}I-labeled anti-gamma globulin is then added to the red cells, and the amount of anti-gamma globulin combined with the ^{131}I-labeled anti-D on the red cells is determined. The calibrated ^{125}I-labeled anti-gamma globulin can then be used to determine the amount of unlabeled anti-D that is bound to red cells. This method has the disadvantage of being less accurate than the direct labeling method since the assumption must be made that the amount of ^{125}I-labeled anti-gamma globulin which combines with the unknown anti-D preparations is the same as that which combined with the ^{131}I-labeled anti-D used for calibration; this may not always be true.

Evidence is accumulating that passively administered anti-D acts by binding the Rh-positive red cells in the circulation, leading to their destruction along with their antigens. Assessment of the biological activity of anti-D should, therefore, include an estimate of both concentration and the value of the equilibrium constant, since both determine the extent to which anti-D is bound to red cells. Up to the present time, however, it has been the practice to assess potency of anti-D immunoglobulin only in terms of concentration. There are two reasons for this. First, assessment of equilibrium constant involves considerably more work than measurement of concentration alone. Second, estimates made on the value of the equilibrium constant on anti-D preparations made from pools of donors have for the most part shown very little variation. Nevertheless the extent to which the equilibrium constant differs must be taken into account in the assessment of the biological activity of anti-D.

PRODUCTION OF ANTI-D IMMUNOGLOBULIN (W.H.O., 1971)

Primary Immunization

If a single injection of Rh-positive red cells is given, the proportion of subjects in whom detectable anti-D is formed within 6 months varies with the dose of red cells, being about 15% when only 1 ml of red cells is injected, 33% when 40 ml of red cells are given, and 65 to 70% following a single transfusion of 500 ml of D-positive blood.

On the other hand, if repeated injections are given, the incidence of antibody formation at 6 months is approximately 50%, even when very small doses of red cells are given. Similar results have been observed over a very wide range of doses and of intervals between injections, from 0.01 ml of red cells given at two weekly intervals to 40 ml given initially, followed by 5 ml at 3 months (Jakobowitz, 1970, personal communication).

It appears that two injections of red cells, each of the order of 1-2 ml, given at an interval of 3 months, will elicit antibody formation within 3 months of the second injection in approximately 50% of subjects, and that no better result is achieved by giving larger amounts of red cells or by more frequent injections (see Mollison et al., 1970).

Only about two out of three D-negative subjects can be immunized to D; those who do not form anti-D after large doses of red cells (20 ml or more) are not immunized by much smaller amounts (0.1 ml), while those who fail to respond to 0.1 ml or less cannot be immunized by subsequent doses of 10 ml. In subjects who produce no detectable anti-D after many injections, survival of D-positive red cells has been shown to be strictly normal, indicating that no immune response has occurred to the D antigen. As no way is yet known to identify such "nonresponders" before immunization, a 30% failure rate must be anticipated in any program of primary immunization.

It would be interesting to see if nonresponse was a genetically determined character, as suggested many years ago by A. S. Wiener. This could be investigated by testing those Rh-negative sisters of Rh-negative propositi immunized to Rh who were married to Rh-positive men.

Secondary Immunization

There is clearly an advantage in choosing as donors of anti-D subjects who are already immunized, as useful levels of anti-D are usually attained within a few weeks of restimulation. In some subjects, the level of anti-body reached within the first 3 weeks is maximal and will not increase after further immunization. In others, antibody levels may continue to rise for more than 12 months when injections of 0.5 to 1 ml of red cells are given at intervals of 5 to 8 weeks. Finally, about 70% of subjects immunized will produce antibody at levels well in excess of 20 μg/ml. Once attained, such levels can be maintained by injections of 0.1 to 0.5 ml of red cells given at intervals of 2 to 9 months, as required. If injections of red cells are discontinued, antibody levels usually fall appreciably within 6 to 12 months.

The equilibrium constant of antibody produced has been shown to in-crease during continuing immunization.

Selection of Red Cells for Immunization

In most attempts at immunization red cells of the phenotype R^2r have been used because it is known that the number of D antigen sites on red cells of this phenotype is relatively large. However, it is now clear that the dose of D antigen required for primary immunization is very small so that it seems probable that any sample of D-positive red cells (other than D^u) will produce similar results. A theoretical advantage of using R^0 red cells is that production of Rh antibodies of specificities other than anti-D is less likely.

When D-positive red cells carrying antigens in addition to D are in-jected into D-negative subjects, a proportion of those who form anti-D form antibodies to these other antigens as well, whereas subjects who do not form anti-D seldom form any other blood group antibodies.

In order to minimize the risk that immunized subjects will form anti-bodies outside the Rh system, the red cell donor should lack such antigens as K and Fy^a which not infrequently stimulate the production of corre-sponding antibodies. This precaution will not, however, always prevent for-mation of antibody reacting with antigens other than D, as anti-CD (G) may be formed, together with anti-D, in as many as one in 3 subjects who are given only R^2r^0 cells.

Washed red cells should be used for immunization, rather than whole blood, as this may reduce the risk of immunization of donors to leukocyte, platelet, and plasma protein antigens, and perhaps also that of transmitting hepatitis. Storage of a large quantity of suitable red cells at low tempera-ture seems a reasonable way to provide safe, washed cells for immuniza-tion over a long period.

Persons selected to provide Rh-positive red cells used for immunization should be healthy blood donors with no history of hepatitis, whose blood has been given to at least 6 (preferably 10) recipients who have been observed for a period of 6 months without developing hepatitis. These donors should be tested for hepatitis-associated antigen (HAA) on each occasion when they give blood by the most sensitive method available. If any of them is found HAA-positive at any time, or develops hepatitis, or comes under suspicion of transmitting hepatitis, his cells should not be used again.

Route of Immunization

To date, immunization has usually been achieved by intravenous injection of red cells. There is no evidence to suggest that better results would be achieved by intramuscular injections.

Safety of Immunization

Accumulating experience of Rh immunization of large numbers of donors suggests no serious risks of the procedure when carried out with adequate precautions: only occasional cases of hepatitis have been reported. However, close supervision of all donors should continue in case any unforeseen complications may eventually develop.

Plasmapheresis

For the production of Rh immunoglobulin, plasma with a high Rh antibody content can be obtained from human volunteers by means of plasmapheresis. This consists of removal of blood and the return of the blood cells to the donor preferably using plastic equipment. The standard procedure is to remove two units (1 unit = approximately 300 ml of plasma) of blood and to return the units of red cells at the same session. Present experience shows that plasmapheresis, when carried out with proper precautions, is essentially a safe procedure.

Antibody Levels in Acceptable Plasmapheresis Donors

1. *Anti-Rh.* Preferably, to be acceptable for plasmapheresis for Rh immunoglobulin, a donor should have a minimal Rh antibody level of 20 to 30 μg/ml. Some centers carrying out plasmapheresis use donors with average levels of 40 to 100 μg/ml.

2. *Other Red Cell Antibodies.* At one time it was feared that appreciable levels of antibodies other than anti-Rh (D), for example anti-C, E, and K, in the plasma of donors would result in antibody levels in Rh immunoglobulin which would be harmful to Rh-negative individuals given Rh immunoglobulin who were positive for these antigens. Since 300 to

600 μg of anti-Rh (D) have been shown to produce no harm to Rh-positive individuals, the lesser amounts of other red cell antibodies in Rh immunoglobulin cannot harm Rh-negative individuals positive for the corresponding antigen. Furthermore, observations from many thousands of cases has shown that it is harmless in practice. For this reason the presence of these antibodies in the plasma of an otherwise acceptable donor should not be a cause for his rejection; nor should the presence of IgM anti-D since plasma fractionation removes most of the IgM from immunoglobulins.

Safeguarding the Plasmapheresis Donor (Speiser and Nevanlinna, 1967; J.A.M.A. 1970)

Acceptance of donors for plasmapheresis should be subject to the same standards as for routine blood donors, although a possible exception could be made for the hemoglobin level. This is because the amount of red cells lost at a double plasmapheresis is only about 2.5 ml, hence the standard for the minimal acceptable hemoglobin level need not be quite so stringent as for normal blood donors. All heptitis-associated antigen-positive donors should be rigorously excluded. However, since there is evidence that hepatitis viruses are removed during the process of immunoglobulin preparation (Cohn method), a donor with a childhood or adolescent history of jaundice consistent with infective hepatitis might be considered acceptable.

A major risk of plasmapheresis is the return of the wrong red cells to the donor. Proper measures should be taken, therefore, to ensure identification of the red cells before they are transfused. The donor should play an active part in this identification.

In order to reduce the risk of minor hazards, such as syncope, the donor should have plasmapheresis carried out in the recumbent position.

Volume of Plasma Removal and Frequency of Plasmapheresis

The Subcommittee of Specialists on Blood Problems of the Council of Europe (1967) has laid down the following recommendations on this point:

1. A single donation should not exceed the amount of plasma from 500 ml of blood.

2. If the first donation is followed by a second, the latter should only be performed after the return to the donor of the red cells from the first donation.

3. Not more than 1000 ml of plasma should be taken from the donor within one 7 day period.

4. Not more than eight single units of plasma should be removed by

plasmapheresis in one month, and not more than 50 single units should be removed in one year.

Since these regulations were promulgated some centers have reported the removal of much larger amounts of plasma, usually 600 to 650 ml per week, for 5 to 7 years without a break. In one instance 1200 ml per week has been taken for 7 years without apparent ill effects.

Plasmapheresis of extremely large volumes has been found to produce falls in serum protein levels. For instance, the withdrawal of 5 liters of plasma in 5 days has been shown to result in an average fall in the total serum protein level of 27% and an average fall in the gamma globulin fraction of 52%. Serum albumin levels returned to normal within 2 weeks, but gamma globulin levels did not reach preplasmapheresis values for 6 to 13 weeks.

Experience in several countries suggests that very intensive plasmapheresis is not required to obtain adequate supplies of plasma for Rh immunoglobulin preparation. If the total serum protein level in the blood falls below 6 g/100 ml the donor should be removed from the program for at least 2 months. The total protein level should exceed 6 g/100 ml again before the donor is allowed to reenter the programme. Any donor who shows a persistent elevation or distortion of his gamma globulin level should be permanently removed from the program.

Possible Long-Term Hazards

Although regular plasmapheresis carried out with proper precautions has minimal short-term risks, it should be stressed that little is known as yet about the possible consequences over a prolonged period of time. Regular careful observation of plasmapheresis donors for possible adverse effects is therefore advised.

Anticipated Requirements for Anti-D Immunoglobulin

If anti-D is to be given to every nonimmunized Rh-negative woman having an Rh-positive child, or an abortion, the number of doses required is arrived at by considering the proportions of Rh-negative women and homozygous and heterozygous Rh-positive men. These are present in the proportions (the Hardy-Weinberg equilibrium) $p^2:2pq:q^2$, where p^2 represents one homozygote, $2pq$ the heterozygote, and q^2 the other homozygote. If q^2 is the homozygous recessive and the frequency of Rh negatives is 16%, $q^2 = 0.16$ and q (which is the frequency of the Rh-negative gene in the population) $= 0.4$. The heterozygotes $2pq$ are, therefore, 48% and the homozygous Rh-positives 36%. Other relevant factors are the birth rate and the number of abortions in the population concerned.

For example, in a population 16% of which is Rh-negative, if the birth rate is 20 per thousand and the abortion rate 2 per thousand per annum, the requirements for anti-D per million of the population will be:

For Rh-negative women with full-term Rh-positive children   1920 doses
For Rh-negative women having abortions (father's Rhesus
    status unknown)   320 doses

                                           Total   2240 doses

To the above requirements, 12.5% should be added to allow for antenatal treatment and experimental use and one arrives at a requirement for this particular community of about 2500 doses per million population per year.

Should antenatal treatment of Rh women in such a community be routinely undertaken, the rate of use of anti-D per million would increase by about 3000 doses per million people per year, if one antenatal dose were given, or by about 6000 if two doses were recommended.

REFERENCES

Aickin, D. R. 1970. Rhesus immunisation before delivery of the first baby. Aust. New Zeal., J. Obstet. Gynaec. 10:95.

Argyris, B. F. 1963. Adoptive tolerance; transfer of the tolerant state. J. Immun. 90:29.

Ascari, W. Q., P. Levine, and W. Pollack. 1969. Incidence of maternal immunization by ABO compatible and incompatible pregnancies. Brit. Med. J. 1:399-401.

Barron, S. L. 1969. Induced abortion and Rh-isoimmunisation. Lancet 1:1159.

Barron, S. L. 1970. Personal communication.

Bartsch, F. K., L. Å. Hanson, L. A. M. Ryttinger, and L. Sandberg. 1970. Personal communication.

Batchelor, J. R., F. Ellis, M. E. French, M. Bewick, J. S. Cameron, and C. S. Ogg. 1970. Immunological enhancement of human kidney graft. Lancet 2:1007-1013.

Bergström, H., L. A. Nilsson, L. Nilsson, and L. Ryttinger. 1967. Demonstration of Rh antigens in a 38-day old foetus. Amer. J. Obstet. Gynec. 99:130-133.

Blumberg, B. S., H. J. Alter, and S. Visnich. 1965. A "new" antigen in leukemia sera. J. A. M. A. 191:541.

Borland, R., Y. W. Loke, and P. J. Oldershaw. 1970. Sex difference in trophoblast behaviour on transplantation. Nature 228:572.

Börner, P., H. Deicher, H. H. Hoppe, H. Hitschhold, S. Holtz, and A. Seifert. 1969. Prophylaxe der Rhesus-Sensibilisierung durch intravenöse Gabe von Immunoglobulin G Anti-D. 1. Klinische Ergebnisse und Untersuchungen zur Anti-D-Dosierung. Geburtsh. Frauenheilk. 29:203-212.

Borst-Eilers, E. 1970. Personal communication.

Bowman, J. M. 1970. Transplacental haemorrhage after abortion. Lancet 1:1108.

Bowman, J. M. 1970. Personal communication.

Bowman, J. M., and B. Chown. 1968. Prevention of Rh immunisation after massive Rh positive transfusion. Canad. Med. Ass. J. 99:385.

Bradley, J., and C. J. Elson. 1971. Suppression of the immune response. J. Med. Genet. 8(3):321-340.

Brit. Med. J. 1969. Leading article: Rhesus sensitization and abortion. 4:61.

Brody, N. I., J. B. Walker, and G. W. Siskind. 1967. Studies on the control of antibody synthesis: interaction of antigenic competition and suppression of antibody formation by passive antibody on the immune response. J. Exp. Med. 126:81.

Cerottini, J., P. J. McConahey, and F. T. Dixon. 1969. The immunosuppressive effect of passively administered antibody IgG fragments. J. Immun. 102:1008.

Chown, B., et al. 1969. Prevention of primary Rh immunisation. 1st report on the western Canadian trial, 1966-1968. Canad. Med. Ass. J. 100:1021-1024.

———, J. M. Bowman, J. Pollack, B. Lowen, and A. Pettett. 1970. The effect of anti-D IgG on D-positive recipients. Canad. Med. Ass. J. 102:1161-1164.

Clarke, C. A. 1966. Prevention of Rh haemolytic disease. Vox. Sang. 11:642.

———. 1967. Prevention of Rh haemolytic disease. Brit. Med. J. 4:7-12.

———. 1968a. Prophylaxis of Rhesus iso-immunisation. Brit. Med. Bull. 24:3.

———. 1968b. Prevention of Rhesus iso-immunisation. Lancet 2:1-7.

———. 1969. Prevention of Rh isoimmunisation. Seminars in Hemat. 6:201-224.

———. 1970. The prevention of Rh iso-immunization. Clin. Genet. 1:183-215.

———, W. T. A. Donohoe, R. B. McConnell, J. C. Woodrow, R. Finn, J. R. Krevans, W. Kulke, D. Lehane, and P. M. Sheppard. 1963. Further experimental studies on the prevention of Rh haemoloytic disease, Brit. Med. J. 1:979.

———, R. Finn, D. Lehane, R. B. McConnell, P. M. Sheppard, and J. C. Woodrow. 1966. Dose of anti-D gammaglobulin in prevention of Rh haemolytic disease of the new-born. Brit. Med. J. 1:213-214.

———, R. Finn, R. B. McConnell, and P. M. Sheppard. 1958. The protection afforded by ABO incompatibility against erythroblastosis due to Rhesus anti-D. Int. Arch. Allerg. 13:380.

———, and P. M. Sheppard. 1959. The genetics of Papilio dardanus, Brown. I. Race cenea from South Africa. Genetics 44:1347-1358.

———, and ———. 1960. The evolution of mimicry in Papilio dardanus. Heredity 14:163-173.

———, and ———. 1969. Rhesus sensitization and abortion. Brit. Med. J. 4:743.

———, ———, and I. W. B. Thornton. 1968. The genetics of the mimetic butterfly, Papilio memnon L. Phil. Trans. Roy. Soc. London, Ser. B 254:37-89.

Combined Study from Centres in England and Baltimore. 1966. Prevention of Rh haemolytic disease: results of the clinical trial. Brit. Med. J. 2:907.

———. 1971. Prevention of Rh haemolytic disease: final results of the "high risk" clinical trial. Brit. Med. J. 2:607-609.

Davey, M. G. 1970. Personal communication.

Deicher, H. 1970. Personal communication.

Dietrich, F. M., and W. O. Weigle. 1964. Immunologic unresponsiveness to heterologous serum proteins induced in adult mice and transfer of the unresponsive state. J. Immun. 92:167.

Dixon, F. J., J. Jacot-Guillarmod, and P. J. McConahey. 1967. The effect of passively administered antibody on antibody synthesis. J. Exp. Med. 125:1119.

Dudok de Wit, C., and E. Borst-Eilers. 1968. Failure of anti-D immunoglobulin injection to protect against Rhesus immunization after massive foeto-maternal haemorrhage. Report of 4 cases. Brit. Med. J. 1:152.

Eklund, J., and H. R. Nevanlinna. 1971. Immunosuppressive therapy in Rh-incompatible transfusion. Brit. Med. J. 3:623-624.

Elson, C. J. 1970. Personal communication.

Finn, R. 1960. Erythroblastosis. Lancet 1:526.

——, C. A. Clarke, W. T. A. Donohoe, R. B. McConnell, P. M. Sheppard, D. Lehane and W. Kulke. 1961. Experimental studies on the prevention of Rh haemolytic disease. Brit. Med. J. 1:1486.

Freda, V. J., and J. G. Gorman. 1962. Ante-partum management of Rh haemolytic disease. Bull. Sloane Hosp. Wom. N.Y. 8:147.

Freda, V. J., J. G. Gorman, and W. Pollack. 1964. Successful prevention of experimental Rh sensitisation in man with anti-Rh gammaglobulin antibody preparation (preliminary report). Transfusion 4:26.

Freda, V. J., J. G. Gorman, R. S. Galen, and N. Treacy. 1970. The threat of Rh immunisation from abortion. Lancet 2:147-148.

French, M. E., and J. R. Batchelor. 1969. Immunological enhancement of rat kidney grafts. Lancet 2:1103-1106.

Friedemann, H. 1962. Transfer of antibody formation by spleen cells from immunologically unresponsive mice. J. Immun. 89:257.

Friedman, E. A. 1969. Prevention of Rh isoimmunisation. In Charles, A. G., and E. A. Friedman (Eds.), Rh Isoimmunisation and Erythroblastosis foetalis, pp. 207-218. London, Butterworth.

Godel, J. G., D. I. Buchanan, J. M. Jarosch, and M. McHugh. 1968. Significance of Rh-sensitization during pregnancy: its relation to a preventive programme. Brit. Med. J. 4:479-482.

Gorman, J. G. 1970. Personal communication.

Grobbelaar, B. G., and G. Mostert. 1970. Ante-natal transplacental haemorrhage. Transfusion 10:76.

Grubb, R., G. Kronvall, and L. Martensson. 1965. Some aspects of the relations between rheumatoid arthritis, antigamma-globulin factors and the polymorphism of human gamma globulin. Ann. N. Y. Acad. Sci. 124:865-872.

Haering, M. von. 1967. Über die Prophylaxie mit Anti-D Globulinen zur Verhinderung der Rhesus-sensibilisierung. Gynaecologia 163:415-424.

Hamilton, E. G. 1970. High-titer anti-D plasma for the prevention of Rh isoimmunisation. Obstet. Gynec. 36:331-340.

Hamilton, E. G. 1970. Personal communication.

Henney, C., and K. Ishizaka. 1968. Studies on the immunogenicity of antigen-antibody precipitates. I. The suppressive effect of anti-L and anti-H chain antibodies on the immunogenicity of human γG globulin. J. Immun. 101:986.

Henry, C., and N. K. Jerne. 1968. Competition of 19S and 7S antigen receptors in the regulation of the primary immune response. J. Exp. Med. 128:133-152.

Hibbard, B. M. 1970. Personal communication.

Hollán, S. R. 1970. Personal communication.

Hoppe, H. H. 1970. Personal communication.

Huchet, J. 1970. Personal communication.

Hughes-Jones, N. C. 1967. The estimation of the concentration and equilibrium constant of anti-D. Immunology 12:565-571.

——, and B. Gardner. 1970. The equilibrium constants of anti-D immunoglobulin preparations made from pools of donor plasma. Immunology 18:347-351.

——, and M. Stevenson. 1968. The anti-D content of IgG preparations for use in the prevention of Rh haemolytic disease. Vox Sang. 14:401-408.

Jakobowitz, R. 1970. Personal communication.

J.A.M.A. 1970. Ad Hoc Committee on Plasmapheresis. Safeguards for plasma donors in plasmapheresis programs. J.A.M.A. 213:747.

Jouvenceaux, A., N. Adenot, F. Berthoux, and L. Révol. 1968. Gamma-globuline anti-D lyophilisée de l'immunisation anti-Rh. In VIIe Congrès National de Transfusion Sanguine (France), pp. 341-347.

Katz, J. 1969. Transplacental passage of fetal red cells in abortion: increased incidence after curettage and effect of oxytoxic drugs. Brit. Med. J. 4:84-86.

Keith, L., A. Cuva, K. Houser, and A. Webster. 1970. Suppression of primary Rh-immunisation by anti-Rh. Transfusion 10(3):142.

Kleihauer, E., H. Braun, and K. Betke. 1957. Demonstration von fetalem Hämoglobin in Erythrozyten eines Blutausstriches. Klin. Wschr. 35:637.

Kogoj-Bakic, V., and K. Vujaklija-Stipanovic. 1970. Personal communication.

Levine, P. 1943. Serological factors as possible causes in spontaneous abortion. J. Hered. 34:71.

Lunay, G. G., R. F. Edwards, and D. B. Thomas. 1970. Chronic transplacental haemorrhage causing acute fetal distress. Brit. Med. J. 2:218.

McConnell, R. B. 1966. The prevention of Rh haemolytic disease. Ann. Rev. Med. 17:291-306.

———. 1969. The immunological relationship between mother and fetus. In Adinolfi, M. (Ed.), Immunology and Development, pp. 159-185. International Medical Publications (Heinemann). London, Spastics.

Matthews, C. D. 1968. Aspects of transplacental haemorrhage. M. D. Thesis, Liverpool.

———, and A. E. B. Matthews. 1969. Transplacental haemorrhage in spontaneous and induced abortion. Lancet 1:694.

Maycock, W. d'A. 1970. Personal communication.

Mollison, P. L. 1967. Blood Transfusion in Clinical Medicine, ed. 4. Oxford, Blackwell.

———, M. Frame, and M. E. Ross. 1970. Differences between Rh(D) negative subjects in response to Rh(D) antigen. Brit. J. Haemat. 19:257.

———, and N. C. Hughes-Jones. 1967. Clearance of Rh-positive red cells by low concentration of Rh antibody. Immunology 12:63-73.

———, ———, M. Lindsay, and J. Wessely. 1969. Suppression of primary Rh-immunisation by passively administered antibody. Experiments in volunteers. Vox Sang. 16:421-439.

Murray, S. 1957. The effect of Rh genotypes on severity in haemolytic disease of the newborn. Brit. J. Haemat. 3:143.

———, S. L. Barron, and R. A. McNay. 1970. Transplacental haemorrhage after abortion. Lancet 1:631-634.

Nevanlinna, H. R., and T. Vainio. 1956. The influence of mother-child ABO incompatibility on Rh immunisation. Vox Sang. 1:26.

Nossal, G. J. V. 1967. Frontiers in Immunology, 5th World Congress in Gynecology and Obstetrics, Sidney. Australia, Butterworth.

———. 1969. Antibodies and Immunity. New York, Basic Books.

Pearlman, D. A. 1966. The influence of antibodies on immunologic responses. I. The effect on the response to particulate antigen in the rabbit. J. Exp. Med. 126:127.

Pierce, C. W. 1969. Immune responses in vitro. II. Suppression of the immune response in vitro by specific antibody. J. Exp. Med. 130:365.

Pollack, W. 1970. Transfusion. In press.

———, W. Q. Ascari, R. J. Kochesky, R. R. O'Connor, T. Y. Ho, and D. Tripodi. Studies on rhesus prophylaxis. 1. The relationship between doses of anti-Rh and the size of the antigenic stimulus. Transfusion, 1971. In press.

———, J. G. Gorman, H. J. Hager, V. J. Freda, and D. Tripodi. 1968. Antibody-mediated immune suppression to Rh-factor. Animal models suggesting mechanism of action. Transfusion 8:134-150.

———, H. O. Singher, J. G. Gorman, and V. J. Freda. 1967. The prevention of isoimmunization to the Rh factor by passive immunization with Rho (D) immune globulin (human). Scientific exhibit, American Association of Blood Banks, Oct. 21-24, New York.

Preisler, O., and J. Schneider. 1964. Versuche, die Sensibilisierung rh-negativen Frauen durch antikörperhaltige Seren zu verhindern. Geburtsh. Frauenheilk. 24:124-131.

Queenan, J. T., D. B. Smith, J. M. Haber, J. Jeffrey, and H. C. Gadow. 1969. Irregular antibodies in the obstetric patient. Obstet. Gynec. 34:767-771.

Robertson, J. G. 1968. Edinburgh (Scotland): Experience with Rh immunoglobulin. Transfusion 8:149-150.

———. 1969. Rhesus isoimmunisation. In Kellar, R. J. (Ed.), Modern Trends in Obstetrics, Vol. 4. London, Butterworth.

———. 1970. Personal communication.

———, and F. Dambrosio. 1969. The Rh problem. In Proceedings of the International Symposium on the Management of the Rh problem, Milan, Italy.

Rowley, D. A., and F. W. Fitch. 1964. Homeostasis of antibody in the adult rat. J. Exp. Med. 120:987.

———, and ———. 1967. Clonal selection and inhibition of the primary antibody response by antibody. In Cinader, B. (Ed.), Regulation of Antibody response, p. 27. Springfield, Ill., Thomas.

Ryder, R. J. W., L. K. Kilham, and R. K. Schwartz. 1969. Immunosuppression by antibody. Transplant. Proc. 1:524.

Schneider, J. 1963. Die quantitative Bestimmung fetaler Erythrozyten im mütterlichen Kreislauf und deren beschleunigter Abbau durch Antikörperseren. Geburtsh. Frauenheilk. 23:562-568.

———. 1971. Arbeitstagung zur Prophylaxe der Rhesus-Sensibilisierung mit Immunoglobulin-anti-D. IV. Geburtsh. Frauenheilk. 6:493-522.

———, and O. Preisler. 1965. Untersuchungen zur serologischen Prophylaxe der Rh-sensibilisierung. Blut 12:4.

Sinclair, N. R. St. C. 1969. Regulation of the immune response. I. Reduction in ability of specific antibody to inhibit long lasting IgG immunological priming after removal of the Fc fragment. J. Exp. Med. 129:1183.

Smith, T. 1909. Active immunity produced by so-called balanced or neutral mixtures of diphtheria toxin and antitoxin. J. Exp. Med. 2:241-256.

Speiser, P., and H. R. Nevanlinna. 1967. Protection of donors undergoing plasmapheresis. Report to Council of Europe Sub-Committee of specialists on blood problems, Strasbourg.

Spensieri, S., A. E. Carnevale, and P. L. Caldana. 1968. Rh isoimmunisation and transplacental transfer of foetal erythrocytes. Monit. Obstet. Ginec. Endocr. Metab. 39(6)(Suppl.):889-906.

Stern, K. 1969. Inhibition of immune response to sheep red cells in rats preimmunised with heterophilic antigen. Clin. Exp. Immun. 4:253.

————, H. S. Goodman and M. Berger. 1961. Experimental isoimmunisation to hemoantigens in man. J. Immun. 87:189.

Szelenyi, J. G., and S. R. Hollán. 1967. A new method for the cytological differentiation of foetal and adult erythrocytes. Vox Sang. 12:234.

Tao, T., and J. W. Uhr. 1966. Capacity of pepsin-digested antibody to inhibit antibody formation. Nature 212:208.

Vos, G. H. 1965. The frequency of ABO-incompatible combinations in relation to maternal Rh antibody values in Rh immunised women. Amer. J. Hum. Genet. 17:202.

Walker, J. G., and G. W. Siskind. 1968. Studies on the control of antibody synthesis. Effect of antibody affinity upon its ability to suppress antibody formation. Immunology 14:21.

Wallace, J. 1970. Personal communication.

W.H.O. 1971. Prevention of Rh Sensitization. Report of a W.H.O. Scientific Group. Technical Report series, 468.

Woodrow, J. C. 1970. Rh Immunisation and Its Prevention. In Jensen, K. G., and S. A. Kilman (Eds.), Series Haematologica 3, No. 3, Munksgaard, Copenhagen.

————, C. A. Clarke, W. T. A. Donohoe, R. Finn, R. B. McConnell, P. M. Sheppard, D. Lehane, H. Russell, W. Kulke, and C. M. Durkin. 1965. Prevention of Rh haemolytic disease: a third report. Brit. Med. J. 1:279.

————, C. A. Clarke, R. B. McConnell, S. H. Towers, and W. T. A. Donohoe. 1971. Prevention of Rh haemolytic disease: results of the Liverpool "low risk" clinical trial. Brit. Med. J. 2:610-612.

————, and W. T. A. Donohoe. 1968. Rh-immunization by pregnancy: results of a survey and their relevance to prophylactic therapy. Brit. Med. J. 2:139-144.

————, C. J. Elson, and W. T. A. Donohoe. 1971. Effect of pregnancy on the isoantibody response in rabbits. Nature 233:62-63.

————, R. Finn, and J. Krevans. 1969. Rapid clearance of Rh positive blood during experimental Rh immunisation. Vox Sang. 17:349-361.

Zipursky, A., and L. G. Israels. 1967. The pathogenesis and prevention of Rh immunization. Canad. Med. Ass. J. 97:1245.

————, J. Pollack, B. Chown, and L. G. Israels. 1965. Transplacental iso-immunisation by foetal red blood cells. Orig. Art. Ser. 1:184.

CHAPTER 6

Disorders of Ganglioside Metabolism

Roscoe O. Brady
Edwin H. Kolodny *

Laboratory of Neurochemistry, National Institute of Neurological Diseases and Stroke, National Institutes of Health, Bethesda, Maryland.

WITHIN THE PAST TWO YEARS, important developments have occurred regarding the fundamental pathophysiology of two disparate aspects of ganglioside metabolism. The first of these is the demonstration of the nature of the metabolic defects in lipid storage diseases in humans in which abnormal quantities of gangliosides accumulate. The second is the discovery of alterations of ganglioside composition and metabolism in cultured cells which have been transformed with the tumorigenic DNA viruses SV40 or polyoma virus. It is the purpose of the present review to acquaint the reader with these developments and to explore the physiological consequences which result from these abnormalities. We shall also attempt to indicate developments which may be anticipated in the future in these areas.

Gangliosides are complex acidic glycolipids whose solubility in water varies with the number and nature of hexose and sialic acid residues which are attached to a lipid moiety common to all of the gangliosides. This lipid portion is called ceramide. It is composed of the long chain amino alcohol sphingosine (Fig. 1a) and a long chain fatty acid linked through an amide bond to the nitrogen atom on carbon 2 of sphingosine (Fig. 1b). Stearic acid is the predominant fatty acid of brain gangliosides. The most common ganglioside in certain peripheral tissues such as liver and the stroma of erythrocytes is a relatively simple substance called hematoside or G_{M3} (Fig. 1c) which consists of one molecule each of glucose, galactose, and either N-acetyl or N-glycolylneuraminic acid attached to the

---

* Present address: Eunice Kennedy Shriver Center for Mental Retardation, Waltham, Massachusetts.

(a) Sphingosine:

$$CH_3-(CH_2)_{12}-CH=CH-CH(OH)-CH(NH_2)-CH_2OH$$

(b) Ceramide:

$$CH_3-(CH_2)_{12}-CH=CH-CH(OH)-CH-C*H_2OH$$

$$\begin{array}{c} | \\ N-H \\ | \\ C=O \\ | \\ (CH_2)_{16} \\ | \\ CH_3 \end{array}$$

Asterisk (*) indicates point of attachments of various substituents

(c) Hematoside (G_{M3}):   Ceramide−glucose−galactose-N-acetylneuraminic acid

(d) Tay-Sachs ganglioside (G_{M2}):
Ceramide−glucose−galactose-N-acetylgalactosamine

$$| \\ N\text{-Acetylneuraminic acid}$$

(e) Monosialoganglioside (G_{M1}):
Ceramide−glucose−galactose-N-acetylgalactosamine−galactose

$$| \\ N\text{-Acetylneuraminic acid}$$

(f) Disialogangliosides (G_{D1a}):
Ceramide−glucose−galactose-N-acetylgalactosamine−galactose

$$| \qquad\qquad\qquad\qquad | \\ N\text{-Acetylneuraminic acid} \qquad N\text{-Acetylneuraminic acid}$$

(g) Disialoganglioside (G_{D1b}):
Ceramide−glucose−galactose-N-acetylgalactosamine−galactose

$$| \\ N\text{-Acetylneuraminic acid} \\ | \\ N\text{-Acetylneuraminic acid}$$

(h) Trisialoganglioside G_{T1}:
Ceramide−glucose−galactose-N-acetylgalactosamine−galactose

$$| \qquad\qquad\qquad\qquad | \\ N\text{-Acetylneuraminic acid} \qquad N\text{-Acetylneuraminic acid} \\ | \\ N\text{-Acetylneuraminic acid}$$

FIG. 1.—Structures of the gangliosides.

ceramide moiety. It is a very minor component of the brain gangliosides; however, as we shall see in the second portion of this review, it is the major ganglioside of the virus-transformed cells. The addition of one molecule of N-acetylgalactosamine to G_{M3} results in the formation of the monosialotrihexosylceramide commonly called Tay-Sachs ganglioside or G_{M2} (Fig. 1d). This substance, too, is normally a minor component of brain gangliosides, but it becomes the predominant ganglioside in the brain of infants with Tay-Sachs disease. Furthermore, this change in ganglioside pattern is not due to a decrease in the quantity of the usually more prevalent higher ganglioside homologs which have a tetrahexosyl oligosaccharide side chain (Figs. 1e-1h), but is the result of an accumulation of a tremendously increased quantity of G_{M2}.

Let us now consider the salient aspects of Tay-Sachs disease in some detail. Actually, this is the first of the lipid storage diseases to be recognized as an inherited abnormality. Siblings with this condition were originally described in the early 1880s by Waren Tay, the English ophthalmologist, who observed the occurrence of a cherry-red spot in the macula of the eye of children with a previously undiagnosed clinical condition. In 1887, the American neurologist Bernard Sachs reported his clinical observations of a child who, in addition to the ocular manifestations, also showed progressive, severe mental retardation. Both of these clinicians recognized this disorder as a hereditary condition, and in time it was named in their honor.

Tay-Sachs disease is probably the most frequently occurring of the lipid storage diseases. It occurs in about 1 in 6000 to 1 in 10,000 births of infants of Ashkenazic Jewish ancestry. The frequency in non-Jews is much less. About 50 patients are born each year with this disease in the United States, approximately ¾ of whom are of Jewish parentage. The children appear nearly normal during the first few postnatal months. Thereafter their acquisition of skills is somewhat slower than that of normal siblings, and by the seventh or eighth month, failure to develop coordinated motor activity is easily noticeable. The children then become progressively less attentive but startle easily, and may have convulsive episodes; they are listless and eventually become blind. Within the first year of life a cherry-red spot appears in the macular region of the eye, and at about 2 years of age the head circumference reaches a size about 50% greater than normal. These children continue a progressively downhill course with feeding difficulties and repeated respiratory tract infections. They eventually die between the third and fourth year of life. There is no visceral organomegaly or involvement of the bony skeleton. The disease is inherited as an autosomal recessive trait.

Histological examination of the brain reveals swollen neuronal cells in various stages of degeneration, many of them containing concentrically layered electron-dense "membranous cytoplasmic bodies" (Fig. 2). The sections appear to show demyelination, although this may actually be due to the failure of adequate myelin formation. Chemical analysis of the brain reveals a large increase in the quantity of gangliosides caused primarily by a disproportionately high concentration of G_{M2}. An increase in the amount of the aminoglycolipid N-acetylgalactosaminylgalactosylglucosylceramide (asialo-Tay-Sachs ganglioside, Fig. 3a) also occurs, with levels of this lipid approximately one-fifth the concentration of G_{M2}. Late in the course of the disease there is a moderate accumulation of lactosylceramide (Fig. 3b) and a slight increase of glucoccrebroside (Fig. 3c). These accumulations occur almost exclusively in the central nervous system and, in contrast with other types of lipid storage diseases, peripheral organomegaly with excessive lipid accumulation does not occur.

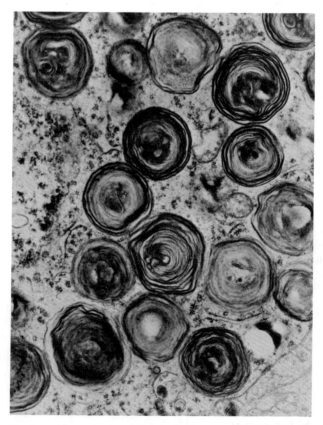

FIG. 2.—Electron photomicrograph of brain from a patient with Tay-Sachs disease. Note the concentrically laminated "membranous cytoplasmic bodies" within the swollen nerve cells.

(*a*) Aminoglycolipid: Ceramide — glucose — galactose-*N*-acetylgalactosa-
mine
(*b*) Lactosylceramide: Ceramide — glucose — galactose
(*c*) Glucocerebroside: Ceramide — glucose
(*d*) Globoside: Ceramide — glucose — galactose — galactose-*N*-acetylgalac-
tosamine
(*e*) Galactocerebroside: Ceramide — galactose

FIG. 3.—Structure of non-sialic acid-containing sphingoglycolipids.

The metabolic abnormality in Tay-Sachs disease has long perplexed investigators. However, within the past year, conclusive evidence of an enzymatic deficiency in patients with Tay-Sachs disease has been obtained. The
story is quite complicated, and the disordered reactions responsible for the
accumulation of Tay-Sachs ganglioside are still under active investigation.
Nevertheless, the following well-substantiated information is available at
this writing. In considering the site of a metabolic lesion in Tay-Sachs disease, it was suspected by analogy with all of the other lipid storage diseases that the disturbance would be due to a deficiency of a catabolic enzyme (Brady, 1966). As can be seen in Fig. 4, there are two terminal
components of G_{M2}: viz., *N*-acetylgalactosamine and *N*-acetylneuraminic
acid, and therefore two potential sites for a defective catabolic reaction
exist. The question of which pathway predominated in the enzymatic degradation of this substance—either the initial hydrolysis of the terminal
molecule of *N*-acetylgalactosamine or of *N*-acetylneuraminic acid—had to
be explored.
    In 1968, Sandhoff et al. showed through the use of the artificial sub-
strate *p*-nitrophenyl-β-D-*N*-acetylgalactosaminide that unfractionated homogenates of brain tissue from patients with Tay-Sachs disease contained
higher than normal total hexosaminidase activity. For this reason, we prepared G_{M2} labeled in the *N*-acetylneuraminic acid portion of the molecule
in order to investigate whether the catabolism of Tay-Sachs ganglioside occurred by the initial hydrolysis of the sialic acid residue, and to learn if
this reaction were impaired in tissues from patients with Tay-Sachs disease. Preparation of this substance involved a combination of biosynthesis
in vivo and selective enzymatic degradation of radioactive mixed brain
gangliosides to the desired G_{M2}-^{3}H (Kolodny et al., 1970a). Through the
use of this material, we were able to show that an enzyme is present in a
number of tissues which catalyzes the cleavage of the *N*-acetylneuraminic
acid moiety of Tay-Sachs ganglioside. The products of the reaction in
crude homogenates of intestinal tissue are free sialic acid and the corresponding asialoceramidetrihexoside (Kolodny et al., 1971). When this
information became available, we examined the activity of this enzyme in
muscle biopsies from control human sources and from patients with Tay-

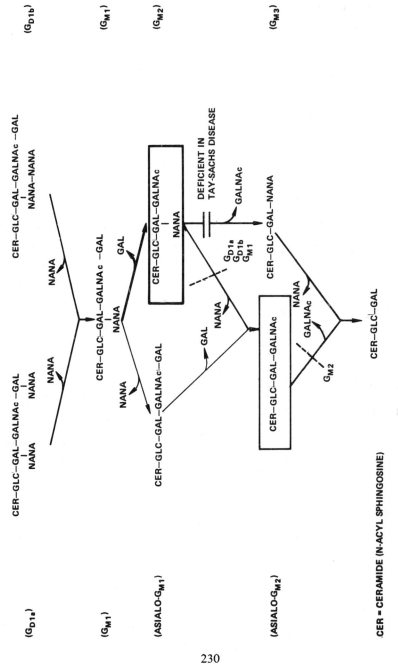

FIG. 4.—Pathways for the catabolism of gangliosides.

230

Sachs disease. There was no evidence of any diminution of activity of this enzyme in the tissue preparations from patients with Tay-Sachs disease (Kolodny et al., 1969a, 1969b). We therefore concluded that this was not the site of a metabolic lesion in Tay-Sachs disease and proceeded to prepare G_{M2} labeled in the N-acetylgalactosaminyl portion of the molecule.

While these studies were in progress, Okada and O'Brien (1969) showed through the use of the artificial substrate 4-methylumbelliferyl-β-D-N-acetylglucosaminide that most tissues had two enzymes (isozymes) which catalyzed the hydrolysis of this compound and that these enzymes could be separated from each other by starch gel electrophoresis. Furthermore, their investigations showed that the enzyme which migrated farther toward the anode was absent in tissues of patients with Tay-Sachs disease. Adopting the nomenclature of Robinson and Stirling (1968) who first described the electrophoretic separation of these two enzymes, they recognized the missing enzyme as hexosaminidase A. This observation has been amply confirmed. Shortly thereafter, we succeeded in preparing G_{M2} labeled in the N-acetylgalactosaminyl moiety and undertook studies of the catabolism of this substance again in homogenates of fresh muscle biopsy specimens. Normal human muscle preparations catalyzed the hydrolysis of G_{M2} labeled in the amino sugar portion, whereas no activity of this catabolic pathway could be demonstrated in biopsy specimens from patients with Tay-Sachs disease (Kolodny et al., 1969b).

These observations raise a number of important questions concerning ganglioside metabolism. The first and most obvious point to be clarified is why, in Tay-Sachs disease, the full ganglioside molecule with the sialic acid moiety intact accumulates and becomes the major compound in the brains of patients whereas the hydrolysis of the sialic acid portion of the molecule proceeds at a normal rate in in vitro preparations of tissues from patients. One would expect that G_{M2} would be hydrolyzed to the corresponding asialo compound, which would then accumulate due to the absence of a hexosaminidase required for the further catabolism of this substance. As indicated, this aminoglycolipid does accumulate in brain tissue of patients with Tay-Sachs disease but only to the extent of about one-fifth of that of the ganglioside. In addition, the uncomfortable observation has been made that both of the hexosaminidases, identified as A and B according to their migration on starch gel electrophoresis, catalyze the hydrolysis of this aminoglycolipid. Furthermore, there is usually a tremendous increase in hexosaminidase B activity in tissues of patients with Tay-Sachs disease. This compensatory increase is not unusual in lipid storage diseases, so that if hexosaminidase B can, in fact, catalyze the hydrolysis of the aminoglycolipid, why should it accumulate at all?

At the present time much current work is directed toward the solution of these unresolved aspects of Tay-Sachs disease. An indication of the direction of this work may be seen in the following observations. It has been known for some time that ganglioside turnover in mammalian brain is very active in the neonatal period of life. Thereafter ganglioside catabolism decreases to a low level. We indicate in Fig. 4 the pathway for the formation of G_{M2} from the two principal disialotetrahexosylganglioside precursors, G_{D1a} and G_{D1b}. The catabolism of each of these compounds is initiated by the hydrolysis of the one molecule of N-acetylneuraminic acid, resulting in each case in the formation of G_{M1}. This ganglioside is primarily hydrolyzed through the action of a ganglioside β-galactosidase forming free galactose and G_{M2}. Alternatively, a very limited amount of the sialic acid moiety of G_{M1} may be hydrolyzed to the corresponding tetrahexosylceramide. Then G_{M2} undergoes catabolism at least to some extent via the hydrolysis of the sialic acid portion of the molecule. The essential point which remains to be established at the present time is whether highly purified hexosaminidase A preparations will catalyze the hydrolysis of the galactosaminyl portion of intact G_{M2}. It is quite clear that this hexosaminidase is deficient in tissues of patients with Tay-Sachs disease, and it is therefore presumed that the catabolism of G_{M2} can occur only via the sialidase reaction in patients with this disease. However, this reaction is normally a rate-limiting step in ganglioside catabolism and is inhibited by other gangliosides such as G_{D1a}, G_{D1b}, and G_{M1} (Kolodny, 1970). Thus, the absence of the hexosaminidase pathway and the relative inhibition of the G_{M2}-sialidase pathway presumably accounts for the accumulation of this material in brain tissue of patients with Tay-Sachs disease.

Several additional observations may serve to explain why the asialo derivative of G_{M2} also accumulates. Some G_{M2} is catabolized by the sialidase reaction in spite of the natural limitation of this pathway and the additional constriction caused by the presence in vivo of the other ganglioside homologs. A small amount of asialo-G_{M2} may also arise through the action of β-galactosidase on the corresponding asialo-G_{M1}. The asialo-G_{M2} which accumulates is presumed to be catabolized through the action of hexosaminidases A and B. The activity of these hexosaminidases are in turn inhibited by the presence of G_{M2} (indicated by the dashed line in Fig. 4). Thus, we have a series of compounding effects. G_{M2} accumulates because of the relatively slow rate of hydrolysis by the sialidase pathway and inhibition of this pathway by higher gangliosides. As a secondary effect, the accumulated G_{M2} seems to inhibit the action of hexosaminidase on the corresponding asialo derivative.

Within the past three years a number of cases have been reported of a variant form of Tay-Sachs disease in which the clinical signs and symptoms are generally identical to those of the classic infantile form [Sandhoff et al., 1968], namely, a progressive, severe mental retardation, blindness, and a cherry-red spot in the macular region of the eyes. However, in contrast to most patients with classic Tay-Sachs disease, the patients with this condition have not been of Jewish ancestry. In this condition, there is a complete absence of hexosaminidase B as well as hexosaminidase A activity in the tissues of the afflicted children when assayed with p-nitrophenyl-β-D-N-acetylglucosaminide, 4-methylumbeliferyl-β-D-N-acetylglucosaminide, or the corresponding N-acetylgalactosaminide derivatives. An aminoglycolipid known as globoside (Fig. 3d) accumulates in the peripheral tissues of patients with this disease, while in the nervous system the amounts of G_{M2} and its asialo derivative are markedly increased.

In order to elucidate more clearly the etiology of this disease, recent studies have been performed on the catabolism of globoside by partially purified hexosaminidase A and hexosaminidase B preparations. We found in these experiments that only hexosaminidase B catalyzed the hydrolysis of globoside (Kolodny et al., 1970b). Hexosaminidase A was inactive in this regard. Therefore, the accumulation of globoside in this form of Tay-Sachs disease is most probably due to the absence of hexosaminidase B.

As a result of the enzyme findings in this disease, much current interest has been focused on a possible interrelationship between the two hexosaminidases. If hexosaminidase A is treated with neuraminidase, its electrophoretic mobility is then very similar to that of hexosaminidase B (Robinson and Stirling, 1968). This finding tends to support the hypothesis that hexosaminidase B is converted to hexosaminidase A through the action of a neuraminyl transferase, and that the absence of such an enzyme might explain the pathogenesis of the classical form of Tay-Sachs disease. Failure to form hexosaminidase B would then presumably lead to a simultaneous absence of hexosaminidase A, causing a dual enzyme deficiency such as occurs in the rare variant of Tay-Sachs disease. However, no definitive studies have yet appeared in support of this hypothesis. Work in progress has focused on the treatment of hexosaminidase A with neuraminidase and then an examination of the catalytic activity of the desialated enzyme using globoside as the substrate. So far, little conclusive information has been obtained in these experiments, although the matter is being pursued at this time.

We turn now to a consideration of the disease called G_{M1} gangliosidosis (generalized gangliosidosis), in which the monosialotetrahexosylceramide G_{M1} (Fig. 1e) accumulates in the central nervous system and a keratan sulfate-like mucopolysaccharide accumulates in the peripheral tissues of patients. In contrast with the classic form of Tay-Sachs disease, considerable organomegaly, particularly hepatomegaly, and bone marrow involvement is also usually present, along with severe, progressive mental retardation. The disease is extremely rare and occurs in infants of non-Jewish as well as Jewish ancestry. The nature of the metabolic defect in this condition was anticipated some years ago (Brady, 1966) and, through the use of specifically labeled G_{M1} ganglioside, has been shown to be that of a missing ganglioside β-galactosidase (Okada and O'Brien, 1968). Patients with generalized gangliosidosis have a 93-94% decrease in β-galactosidase activity in their tissues when assayed with p-nitrophenyl-β-D-galactopyranoside as substrate. Since leukocyte preparations from patients with this disease also reflect the enzyme deficiency, they have been employed in a convenient diagnostic procedure for this disease. The leukocyte assay also permits the detection of heterozygous carriers of this condition (Wolfe, et al., 1970).

Recently an interesting facet of these investigations has come to light. Due to the almost total absence of β-galactosidase activity in the tissues of these patients, it might be expected that other substances which have a terminal molecule of galactose such as galactocerebroside (Fig. 3e) or ceramidelactoside (Fig. 3b) might accumulate along with the G_{M1} ganglioside. This has not been shown to occur, and, in experiments in which the catabolism of authentic labeled galactocerebroside and ceramidelactoside have been performed on extracts of tissues of patients with generalized gangliosidosis, a four- to fivefold increase in the specific activity of these specific glycolipid galactosidases was observed (Brady et al., 1970a). These experiments clearly indicate that extreme caution must be observed when attempting to diagnose enzymatic deficiencies through the use of artificial substrates. However, such materials are certainly becoming increasingly useful for monitoring pregnancies and the detection of heterozygotes and homozygotes for both Tay-Sachs disease, the variant form of Tay-Sachs disease associated with visceral globoside accumulation, and G_{M1} gangliosidosis. Artificial substrates are of little use for the identification of patients with Krabbe's disease, which has been shown to be due to a missing galactocerebroside galactosidase (Suzuki and Suzuki, 1970), or the recently described condition in which ceramide lactoside accumulates (Dawson, 1970) due to a missing lactosylceramide β-galactosidase.

Now that specific quantitative methods are available patients with less drastic attenuation of these various enzymes are being identified in clinics, e.g., the juvenile form of Tay-Sachs disease (G_{M2} gangliosidosis). In these cases, enzyme assays reveal a level of activity between 10 and 20% of that in normal individuals. The rate of progression of the signs and symptoms of the pathological process is less rapid than in the classic forms of these diseases. It appears that there is a fairly sharp demarcation between the low levels of enzyme activity associated with pathological signs and symptoms in the lipid storage diseases and the moderately decreased enzyme activity in tissues of heterozygous carriers of these diseases. This seems to be a complicated phenomenon since the activity of certain sphingolipid hydrolases is decreased to 50 or 60% of normal in leukocytes or skin fibroblast preparations obtained from heterozygotes, whereas in these individuals there is no accumulation of the respective lipid nor any pathological abnormalities in the central nervous system or peripheral tissues. A probable exception to this generalization is seen in female carriers of Fabry's disease, in which there is late onset of some ocular manifestations. The level of activity of the ceramidetrihexoside galactosidase involved in this disease is really quite low in the heterozygote females (about 27% of normal). This is an X-linked disease and the hemizygous afflicted males show virtually no enzyme activity in this regard (Brady et al., 1967). Therefore, there seems to be a cutoff between the level of activity which is compatible with a normal life and that which is accompanied by the accumulation of various lipids which may be somewhere around 40-50% of the control values. It is also possible that a compensatory increase in the activity of the involved enzyme may occur in peripheral tissues of heterozygotes, since it has been shown that certain of these enzymes are indeed inducible (Kampine et al., 1967). It might be expected that this induction would not occur in leukocytes since they generally do not participate in the catabolism of cellular membranous materials from which sphingolipids arise, e.g., globoside (Fig. 3d) and hematoside (Fig. 1c) from the stroma of red blood cells and various gangliosides from the turnover of neural cell elements.

The therapy of patients with abnormalities related to the accumulation of gangliosides seems to be particularly difficult at the present time. Although serum contains considerable hexosaminidase A and hexosaminidase B activity, it seems likely that replacement therapy with fresh human plasma may not provide a very beneficial effect since it is unlikely that exogenously administered enzymes can reach the brain. Perhaps at the present moment the most logical form would be through the attachment of the proper DNA code to a lambda phage capable of human infection. This is a difficult feat, and it is hard to estimate how many cells must be transduced in this fashion before improvement would occur.

It therefore seems that the major hope now available to families at risk for ganglioside storage diseases is the detection of heterozygous carriers for these diseases through appropriate leukocyte or serum enzyme determinations now available so that pregnancies can be monitored in families where both parents are known to be heterozygous for one of these conditions. This determination can easily be done through enzyme assays on cultured fetal cells obtained by amniocentesis in the fourth month of pregnancy. Usually 20 ml of fluid is withdrawn by a transabdominal approach and the cells are collected by centrifugation. If the tap has been performed correctly, cells will be obtained which are exclusively of fetal origin and a small percentage of the cells in the pellet will be viable. These cells are then grown in tissue culture, and in about four weeks time a sufficient quantity of cells can be harvested for enzyme assays. Thus, if the family so elects, there is still sufficient time for termination of an affected pregnancy by standard accepted procedures. It should be remembered that these diseases have an autosomal recessive pattern of inheritance and therefore statistically only one in four pregnancies produced by two heterozygous carriers of these traits will be homozygous for the deficiency and hence clinically affected. It is our feeling that a pregnancy which results in a heterozygous fetus should not be terminated; in fact, there may be some slight survival value conferred by the heterozygous state, since the frequency of Tay-Sachs disease may actually be increasing (Shaw and Smith, 1969).

Recent investigations have revealed another type of genetic mismanagement of ganglioside metabolism also involving G_{M2} but quite opposite in nature to the human disease states to which we have already referred. Cells which have been transformed by the tumorigenic DNA viruses SV40 and polyoma virus show a drastic change in the pattern of gangliosides from that in normal cells (Mora et al., 1969). This alteration is characterized by a marked decrease in those gangliosides with an oligosaccharide chain larger than lactose. The major gangliosides in the normal mouse cell lines which were investigated were G_{D1a}, G_{M1}, and G_{M3}. In the virus-transformed cell lines, G_{M3} is the predominant ganglioside and all of the higher ganglioside homologs are missing (Fig. 5). In fact, the amount of G_{M3} in such transformed cells may actually increase.

It became important to determine whether the change in ganglioside composition in the transformed cells was due to increased catabolism of the higher ganglioside homologs or a failure to synthesize gangliosides larger than G_{M3}. Experiments with sialic-acid labeled gangliosides indicated that the catabolism of gangliosides such as G_{D1a} and G_{M1} proceeds at essentially a normal rate in the virus-transformed cell lines (Brady et al., 1970b). We therefore felt that excessively rapid catabolism could not account for the altered pattern. Ganglioside biosynthesis in the two types of cell lines was then investigated by adding radioactively labeled N-acetylated amino sugar precursors of gangliosides to the culture media. In the control cell lines the predominantly labeled gangliosides were G_{D1a} and G_{M1}, whereas the label was confined to G_{M3} in the virally transformed cells (Brady and Mora, 1970). These experiments indicated an impairment of the synthesis of gangliosides larger than G_{M3} in the transformed cell lines.

The biosynthesis of the next higher ganglioside homolog, G_{M2}, was therefore investigated in cellfree preparations of control and virus-transformed cell lines. The metabolic reaction involved at this step is the transfer of a molecule of N-acetylgalactosamine to G_{M3} (reaction 1).

Ceramide — glucose — galactose-N-acetylneuraminic acid (G_{M3})

$\quad$ + uridine diphosphate N-acetylgalactosamine $\xrightarrow{\text{transferase}}$ $\qquad$ (1)

Ceramide — glucose — galactose-N-acetylgalactosamine (G_{M2})

$\qquad\qquad$ |

$\qquad$ + N-Acetylneuraminic acid

$\qquad\qquad\qquad$ + uridine diphosphate

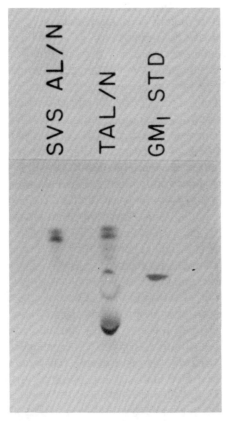

Fig. 5—Thin-layer chromatography of gangliosides in control (T AL/N) and simian virus 40-transformed (SVS AL/N) mouse cells. The major gangliosides in the control line are G_{D1a}, G_{M1}, and G_{M3} (cf. Fig 1), whereas only G_{M3} is present in the transformed cells. The double spots at each of the loci are due to the presence of N-acetylneuraminyl and N-glycolylneuraminyl (slower migrating) derivatives of the corresponding ganglioside. (Reproduced with permission from Mora et al., 1969).

The enzyme which catalyzes this reaction is quite active in normal and spontaneously transformed cell lines, but it was found to be virtually absent in SV40- and polyoma virus-transformed cell lines (Cumar et al., 1970). Confirmatory data were obtained from certain flat revertants of SV40-transformed cell lines whose phenotypic characteristics and growth properties resemble those of the control normal parent cell line. The ganglioside pattern in these revertant cells is normal, and there is full restitution of the hematoside: N-acetylgalactosaminyl transferase activity (Mora et al., 1971). Thus, we may deduce from these experiments that the presence of the oncogenic virus genome in the transformed cells brings about an impairment of this specific galactosaminyl transferase which in turn is responsible for the change in the ganglioside pattern. Since these glycolipids have been shown to be highly concentrated in the plasma membrane of cells, we may anticipate that changes in ganglioside composition would alter cell surface characteristics which may in turn cause a decrease in contact inhibition and alterations in the antigenic properties of the virus-transformed cells. It remains to be determined whether the attenuation of the N-acetylgalactosaminyl transferase activity is caused by a repression of the synthesis of this enzyme, the production of a modified, catalytically inactive enzyme, or even excessive catabolism of this particular enzyme in the transformed cell lines. This effect on ganglioside synthesis may be an obligatory concomitant of the propagation of the virus genome in the tumorigenic DNA virus-transformed cells. The change in the ganglioside pattern and the abnormal enzymology of the DNA virus-transformed cells stand now as one of the first demonstrations of an unambiguous biochemical difference between the virus-transformed cell lines and the parent cell lines. The importance and implications of these findings will be the subject of investigations for a long time to come.

It should be pointed out that this alteration of ganglioside pattern may not be a *sine qua non* of tumorigenicity. Certain cells transform spontaneously in tissue culture and become tumorigenic, and in such cells the ganglioside pattern appears to be relatively normal (Mora et al., 1969). However, there are indications of changes of the ganglioside pattern in tumorigenic cell lines produced by other agents. These alterations appear to be in the same general direction as those observed with the virus-transformed cells. For example, the ganglioside pattern of minimally deviated Morris hepatoma cells grown in tissue culture differs from that in well-differentiated hepatocytes. The higher ganglioside homologs in the former cells are decreased or absent, and there is an increased synthesis of G_{M2} in this chemically induced tumor cell line (Brady et al., 1969).

Some recent studies have also shown that the ganglioside composition of glial tumors is different from that of adjacent brain tissue (Kostic and Buchheit, 1970). This observation is very hard to interpret, since no one has yet been able to obtain a sufficient quantity of a homogeneous control glial cell preparation to determine the ganglioside pattern. A step in this direction has been made with human astrocytoma and human obligodendrocytoma cell lines grown in tissue culture. These lines have been cloned and show a homogeneous population of cells. Although both of these are derived from human malignant brain tumors, there is a significant difference in the ganglioside pattern between these two glial cell tumor lines (Snyder and Brady, 1970). Therefore, it is impossible to tell at the present time whether the observations regarding the ganglioside pattern of human glial tumors in situ actually represents a change from the normal ganglioside pattern of these cells.

CONCLUDING REMARKS

Within the past year and a half, exceptionally rapid progress has been made regarding abnormalities of ganglioside metabolism from two diametrically opposite directions. The first is a partial understanding of the pathogenesis of Tay-Sachs disease consequent to the preparation of G_{M2} (Tay-Sachs ganglioside) specifically labeled in the N-acetylneuraminic acid or the N-acetylgalactosamine portion of the molecule. Studies with these differentially labeled substrates have provided much information regarding the aberrant metabolism of gangliosides in Tay-Sachs disease. The enzymatic lesion in this condition appears to be a deficiency of a hexosaminidase which catalyzes the cleavage of the terminal molecule of N-acetylgalactosamine of G_{M2}. Some degree of uncertainty still exists as to why the entire molecule of ganglioside accumulates in the presence of a normal level of activity of the enzyme which catalyzes the hydrolysis of the sialic acid moiety from the molecule. Further studies are under way to try to clarify this ambiguity.

The demonstration that the activity of the hexosaminidase involved in Tay-Sachs disease can be conveniently assayed with artificial substrates such as 4-methylumbelliferyl-β-D-glucosaminide has provided for the facile diagnosis of homozygotes, the detection of heterozygous carriers, and the antenatal monitoring of fetuses at risk for Tay-Sachs disease. These are important contributions to medicine.

Second, a fuller understanding of the molecular biology of viral transformation of cells is beginning to merge from recent studies showing changes in the ganglioside pattern and a block of an obligatory step in ganglioside synthesis in SV40- and polyoma virus-transformed cell lines. These findings help to explain how alterations of cell membranes affect the oncogenic properties of transformed cells and provide meaningful new approaches for the investigation of tumorigenicity in man.

ACKOWLEDGMENT

Some of the work described in this review was supported in part by
Special Fellowship 2 F11 NB1849-02 NSRB from the National Institute
of Neurological Diseases and Stroke, Public Health Service, awarded to
E.H.K.

REFERENCES

Brady, R. O. 1966. The sphingolipidoses. New Eng. J. Med. 275:312-318.

———, C. Borek, and R. M. Bradley. 1969. Composition and synthesis of gangliosides in rat hepatocyte and hepatoma cell lines. J. Biol. Chem. 244:6552-6554.

———, A. E. Gal, R. M. Bradley, E. Martensson, A. L. Warshaw, and L. Laster.
1967. Enzymatic defect in Fabry's disease. Ceramidetrihexosidase deficiency.
New Eng. J. Med. 276:1163-1167.

———, and P. T. Mora. 1970. Alteration in ganglioside pattern and synthesis in SV
40 and polyoma virus transformed mouse cell lines. Biochim. Biophys. Acta.
218:308-319.

———, P. T. Mora, E. H. Kolodny, and C. Borek. 1970b. Ganglioside metabolism
in virally transformed and chemically induced hepatoma cell lines. Fed. Proc.
29:410 (abstract).

———, J. S. O'Brien, R. M. Bradley and A. E. Gal. 1970a. Sphingolipid hydrolases
in brain tissue of patients with generalized gangliosidoses. Biochim. Biophys.
Acta 210:193-195.

Cumar, F. A., R. O. Brady, E. H. Kolodny, V. W. McFarland, and P. T. Mora.
1970. Enzymatic block in the synthesis of gangliosides in DNA virus-transformed tumorigenic mouse cell lines. Proc. Nat. Acad. Sci. U.S.A. 67:757-764.

Dawson, G. Personal communication, Chicago, Ill., April, 1970.

Greene, H. L., G. Hug, and W. K. Schubert. 1969. Metachromatic leukodystrophy.
Treatment with Arylsulfatase A. Arch. Neurol. 20:147-153.

Kampine, J. P., J. N. Kanfer, A. E. Gal, R. M. Bradley, and R. O. Brady. 1967.
Response of sphingolipid hydrolases in spleen and liver to increased erythrocy-
torrhexis. Biochim. Biophys. Acta 137:135-139.

Kolodny, E. H. 1970. Studies on the metabolic defect in Tay-Sachs disease. Neurology. In press.

———, R. O. Brady, J. M. Quirk, and J. N. Kanfer. 1969a. Studies on the metabolism of Tay-Sachs ganglioside. Fed. Proc. 28:596.

———, ———, ———, and ———. 1970a. Preparation of radioactive Tay-Sachs
ganglioside labeled in the sialic acid moiety. J. Lipid Res. 11:144-149.

———, ———, and B. W. Volk. 1969b. Demonstration of an alteration of ganglioside metabolism in Tay-Sachs disease. Biochem. Biophys. Res. Commun.
37:526-531.

———, A. E. Gal, and R. O. Brady. 1970b. Unpublished observations.

———, J. N. Kanfer, J. M. Quirk, and R. O. Brady. 1971. Properties of a particle-
bound enzyme from rat intestine that cleaves sialic acid from Tay-Sachs ganglioside. J. Biol. Chem. 246:1426-1431.

Kostic, D., and Buchheit, F. 1970. Gangliosides in human brain tumors. Life Sci.
9:589-596.

Mora, P. T., R. O. Brady, R. M. Bradley, and V. W. McFarland. 1969. Gangliosides in DNA virus-transformed and spontaneously transformed tumorigenic mouse cell lines. Proc. Nat. Acad. Sci. U.S.A. 63:1290-1296.

Mora, P. T., F. A. Cumar, and R. O. Brady. 1971. A common biochemical change in SV_{40} and polyoma virus induced transformation of mouse cell coupled to changes in growth properties in culture. Virology. In press.

O'Brien, J. S., S. Okada, A. Chen, and D. L. Fillerup. 1970. Tay-Sachs disease. Detection of heterozygotes and homozygotes by serum hexosaminidase assay. New Eng. J. Med. 283:15-20.

Okada, S., and J. S. O'Brien. 1968. Generalized gangliosidoses: beta-galactosidase deficiency. Science 160:1002-1004.

———, and ———. 1969. Tay-Sachs disease: generalized absence of a beta-D-N-acetylhexosaminidase component. Science 165:698-700.

Robinson, D., and J. L. Stirling. 1968. N-Acetyl-β-glucosaminidases in human spleen. Biochem. J. 107:321-327.

Sachs, B. 1887. On arrested cerebral development, with special reference to its cortical pathology. J. Nerv. Ment. Dis. 14:541-553.

Sandhoff, K., U. Andrea, and H. Jatzkewitz. 1968. Deficient hexosaminidase activity in an exceptional case of Tay-Sachs disease with additional storage of kidney globoside in visceral organs. Life Sci. 7:283-288.

Shaw, R. F., and A. P. Smith. 1969. Is Tay-Sachs disease increasing? Nature 224:1214-1215.

Snyder, R. A., and R. O. Brady. 1970. Unpublished observations.

Suzuki, K., and Y. Suzuki. 1970. Globoid cell leukodystrophy (Krabbe's disease): deficiency of galactocerebroside β-galactosidase. Proc. Nat. Acad. Sci. U.S.A. 66:302-309.

Tay, W. 1884. A third instance in the same family of symmetrical changes in the region of the yellow spot in each eye of an infant closely resembling those of embolism. Trans. Ophthal. Soc. U.K. 4:158-159.

Wolfe, L. S., J. Callahan, J. S. Fawcett, F. Andermann, and C. R. Scriver. 1910. G_{M1}-gangliosidoses without chondrodystrophy or visceromegaly. β-Galactosidase deficiency with gangliosidoses and the excessive excretion of a keratan sulfate. Neurology 20:23-44.

CHAPTER 7

The Genetics of Short Stature

Charles I. Scott, Jr.

From the Departments of Pediatrics and Medicine, Johns Hopkins University School of Medicine, and The John F. Kennedy Institute, Baltimore, Maryland.*

HEREDITARY DISORDERS OF THE SKELETON are relatively rare, and yet they are of disproportionate interest and importance in relation to the development and the genetics of man. A significant number of these disorders is associated with shortness of stature, and nowhere in medicine are heterogeneity and pleiotropism better illustrated (Fig. 1). Uncertainty of diagnosis and multiplicity of terms, as well as incomplete documentation of many published series of cases, have created considerable confusion. For many years these disturbances of skeletal growth were vaguely classified as "chondrodystrophies." Clinically, the affected individuals were categorized as dwarfs or midgets; the term dwarf being applied to those of disproportionate short stature, while the label midget was reserved for those of proportionate but reduced height. Through the application of a combination of morphologic, genetic, and biochemical approaches, a large number and variety of specific, well-delineated entities has gradually emerged. Though the mode of inheritance is known for many, the fundamental biochemical fault is unknown in most. Genetic counseling must be based on accurate diagnosis and on familarity with the natural behavior of the specific disorder, not only in terms of its pattern of genetic transmission but also in terms of the range of manifestation, severity, and associated findings.

Many of those working in this area of medicine have been concerned with the lack of standardization of diagnostic terminology (Kozlowski et al., 1969). The nosology of bone dysplasias has been beset by a plethora

* This work was in part supported by the Department of Health, Education and Welfare, Maternal and Child Health Grant "Project 917."

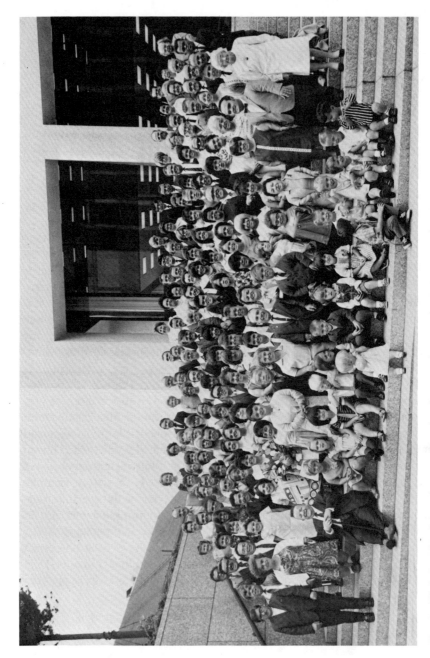

FIG. 1.—Little People of America annual national convention, Portland, Oregon, July, 1970.

of labels as well as systems of classification. According to O'Brien (1969), there are four levels of sophistication in the study of genetic disease, raised to five in the adapted list shown in Table 1. In the case of most bone diseases only the first two levels have been tackled. In an effort to promote uniform usage in the literature, a group met under the aegis of the European Society of Pediatric Radiology and proposed an international nomenclature for constitutional disorders of bone (Maroteaux, 1970) (Table 2). This system was not intended to be an exhaustive list-

TABLE 1.—*Levels of Understanding of Genetic Disorders**

Level 1 Clinical description of phenotype.
Level 2 Proof of Mendelian nature, including mode of inheritance.
Level 3 Identification of general nature of biochemical defect, by description of abnormality of urinary excretion or tissue accumulation or by other biochemical abnormality.
Level 4 Identification of defect in specific enzyme or other protein.
Level 5 Determination of the precise nature of the genetic change, e.g., structural gene mutation versus controller gene mutation

* Modified from O'Brien (1969).

TABLE 2.—*Constitutional (Intrinsic) Diseases of Bone**

Constitutional Diseases of Bone with Unknown Pathogenesis

Osteochondrodysplasia (Abnormalities of cartilage and/or bone growth and development)

I. Defects of growth of tubular bones and/or spine
  A. Manifested at birth
    1. Achondroplasia
    2. Achondrogenesis
    3. Thanatophoric dwarfism
    4. Chondrodysplasia punctata (formerly stippled epiphysis), several forms
    5. Metatropic dwarfism
    6. Diastrophic dwarfism
    7. Chondroectodermal dysplasia (Ellis-van Creveld)
    8. Asphyxiating thoracic dysplasia (Jeune)
    9. Spondyloepiphyseal dysplasia congenita
    10. Mesomelic dwarfism
      a. Nievergelt type
      b. Langer type
    11. Cleidocranial dysplasia (formerly cleidocranial dysostosis)
  B. Manifested in later life
    1. Hypochondroplasia
    2. Dyschondrosteosis
    3. Metaphyseal chondrodysplasia, Jansen type
    4. Metaphyseal chondrodysplasia, Schmid type
    5. Metaphyseal chondrodysplasia, McKusick type (formerly cartilage-hair hypoplasia)

6. Metaphyseal chondrodysplasia with malabsorption and neutropenia
7. Metaphyseal chondrodysplasia with thymolymphopenia
8. Spondylometaphyseal dysplasia (Kozlowski)
9. Multiple epiphyseal dysplasia (several forms)
10. Hereditary arthroophthalmopathy
11. Pseudoachondroplastic dysplasia (formerly pseudoachondroplastic type of spondyloepiphyseal dysplasia)
12. Spondyloepiphyseal dysplasia tarda
13. Acrodysplasia
    a. Rhinotrichophalangeal syndrome (Giedion)
    b. Epiphyseal (Thiemann)
    c. Epiphysometaphyseal (Brailsford)
II. Disorganized development of cartilage and fibrous components of the skeleton
    1. Dysplasia epiphysealis hemimelica
    2. Multiple cartilangenous exostoses
    3. Enchondromatosis (Ollier)
    4. Enchondromatosis with hemangioma (Maffucci)
    5. Fibrous dysplasia (Jaffe-Lichtenstein)
    6. Fibrous dysplasia with skin pigmentation and precocious puberty (McCune-Albright)
    7. Cherubism
    8. Multiple fibromatosis
III. Abnormalities of density or of cortical diaphyseal structure and/or of metaphyseal modeling
    1. Osteogenesis imperfecta congenita (Vrolik, Porak-Durante)
    2. Osteogenesis imperfecta tarda (Lobstein)
    3. Juvenile idiopathic osteoporosis
    4. Osteopetrosis with precocious manifestations
    5. Osteopetrosis with delayed manifestations
    6. Pyknodysostosis
    7. Osteopoikilosis
    8. Melorheostosis
    9. Diaphyseal dysplasia (Camurati-Engelmann)
    10. Craniodiaphyseal dysplasia
    11. Endosteal hyperostosis (Van Buchem and other forms)
    12. Tubular stenosis (Kenny-Caffey)
    13. Osteodysplasty (Melnick-Needles)
    14. Pachydermoperiostosis
    15. Osteoectasia with hyperphosphatasia
    16. Metaphyseal dysplasia (Pyle)
    17. Craniometaphyseal dysplasia (several forms)
    18. Frontometaphyseal dysplasia
    19. Oculodentoosseous dysplasia (formerly oculodentodigital syndrome)

Dysostoses (Malformation of individual bone, single or in combination)

I. Dysostoses with cranial and facial involvement
    1. Craniosynostosis, several forms
    2. Craniofacial dysostosis (Crouzon)
    3. Acrocephalosyndactyly (Apert)
    4. Acrocephalopolysyndactyly (Carpenter)
    5. Mandibulofacial dysostosis (Treacher-Collins, Franceschetti, and others)

      6. Mandibular hypoplasia (includes Pierre Robin syndrome)
      7. Oculomandibulofacial syndrome (Hallermann-Streiff-Francois)
      8. Nevoid basal cell carcinoma syndrome

II. Dysostoses with predominant axial involvement
      1. Vertebral segmentation defects (including Klippel-Feil)
      2. Cervicooculoacoustic syndrome (Wildervanck)
      3. Sprengel deformity
      4. Spondylocostal dysostosis (several forms)
      5. Oculovertebral syndrome (Weyers)
      6. Osteoonychodysostosis (formerly nail-patella syndrome)

III. Dysostoses with predominant involvement of extremities
      1. Amelia
      2. Hemimelia (several types)
      3. Acheiria
      4. Apodia
      5. Adactyly and oligodactyly
      6. Phocomelia
      7. Aglossia-adactylia syndrome
      8. Congenital bowing of long bones (several types)
      9. Familial radioulnar synostosis
    10. Brachydactyly (several types)
    11. Synphalangism
    12. Polydactyly (several types)
    13. Syndactyly (several types)
    14. Polysyndactyly (several types)
    15. Campodactyly
    16. Clinodactyly
    17. Biedl-Bardet syndrome
    18. Popliteal pterygium syndrome
    19. Pectoral aplasia-dysdactyly syndrome (Poland)
    20. Rubinstein-Taybi syndrome
    21. Pancytopenia-dysmelia syndrome (Fanconi)
    22. Thrombocytopenia-radial-aplasia syndrome
    23. Orofaciodigital (OFD) syndrome (Papillon-Leage)
    24. Cardiomelic syndrome (Holt-Oram and others)

Idiopathic osteolyses

   1. Acroosteolysis
     a. Phalangeal type
     b. Tarsocarpal form, with or without nephropathy
   2. Multicentric osteolysis

Primary disturbances of growth

   1. Primordial dwarfism (without associated malformation)
   2. Cornelia de Lange syndrome
   3. Bird-headed dwarfism (Virchow, Seckel)
   4. Leprechaunism
   5. Russel-Silver syndrome
   6. Progeria
   7. Cockayne syndrome
   8. Bloom syndrome

9. Geroderma osteodysplastica
.10. Spherophakia-brachymorphia syndrome (Weill-Marchesani)
11. Marfan syndrome

Constitutional Diseases of Bones with Known Pathogenesis

I. Chromosomal aberrations
II. Primary metabolic abnormalities
   A. Calcium phosphorus metabolism
      1. Hypophosphatemic familial rickets
      2. Pseudodeficiency rickets (Royer, Prader)
      3. Late rickets (McCance)
      4. Idiopathic hypercalciuria
      5. Hypophosphatasia (several forms)
      6. Idiopathic hypercalcemia
      7. Pseudohypoparathyroidism (normo- and hypocalcemic forms)
   B. Mucopolysaccharidosis
      1. Mucopolysaccharidosis I (Hurler)
      2. Mucopolysaccharidosis II (Hunter)
      3. Mucopolysaccharidosis III (Sanfilippo)
      4. Mucopolysaccharidosis IV (Morquio)
      5. Mucopolysaccharidosis V (Scheie)
      6. Mucopolysaccharidosis VI (Maroteaux-Lamy)
   C. Mucolipidosis and lipidosis
      1. Mucolipidosis I (Spranger-Wiedemann)
      2. Mucolipidosis II (Leroy)
      3. Mucolipidosis III (pseudo-Hurler polydystrophy)
      4. Fucosidosis
      5. Mannosidosis
      6. Generalized Gm_l gangliosidosis (several forms)
      7. Sulfatidosis with mucopolysacchariduria (Austin, Thieffry)
      8. Cerebrosidosis including Gaucher's disease
   D. Other metabolic extraosseous disorders
III. Bone abnormalities secondary to disturbances of extraskeletal systems
      1. Endocrine
      2. Hematologic
      3. Neurologic
      4. Renal
      5. Gastrointestinal
      6. Cardiopulmonary

---

* From Maroteaux (1970).

ing of bone diseases. Provisions were made for the addition of new conditions as they are described and for revisions as necessary. This review of the genetics of dwarfism will use the proposed international nomenclature. The conditions selected for discussion are the more common members of this category, as well as those which are firmly established. Many of these have been and are confused with achondroplasia, the most common primary bone dysplasia associated with short stature, and therefore the prototype.

ACHONDROPLASIA

The most common type of short limb dwarfism is achondroplasia. Estimates of its frequency differ widely. Mørch (1941) found one case in every 10,000 live births in Denmark. He believed that 80% of these died within the first year of life, giving a frequency of 20 per million in the general population. This estimate of incidence is high (Slatis, 1955; Silverman and Brunner, 1967). Review of some of Mørch's cases by Silverman and Brunner (1967) indicated inaccurate diagnosis; e.g., vitamin D-resistant rickets and pseudoachondroplastic dysplasia were labeled as acondroplasia. The incidence in the United States has been estimated to be 15 per million (Potter and Coverstone, 1948) and in Northern Ireland 28 per million (Stevenson, 1957). These studies were done prior to the identification of many of the chondrodystrophies which are specific entities distinct from achondroplasia. The high frequency of death in early life in Mørch's series strongly indicates the inclusion of cases of thanatophoric dwarfism, asphyxiating thoracic dysplasia, and other disorders which lead to early death. True achondroplasia is well tolerated and is not often a cause of early death.

The clinical manifestations of achondroplasia are evident at birth. The diagnosis can usually be made on clinical grounds and is confirmed by demonstration of characteristic radiologic findings (Langer et al., 1967). The typical achondroplasic has a large head with a prominent, bossed forehead, depressed or flat nasal bridge, and relative protrusion of the mandible. These changes are the result of restricted development of the chondrocranium. A small irregularly shaped foramen magnum and internal hydrocephalus contribute to the enlarged head (Dennis et al., 1961). Intelligence is generally within the normal range; however, mean intelligence is reduced and some achondroplasts are retarded as a result of arrested hydrocephalus.

The dwarfism is one of the short-limb variety and rhizomelic in type; the proximal arm and leg are shortened comparatively more than the distal segments. The trunk is essentially normal in size, and there is exaggerated lumbar lordosis with pelvic tilt leading to prominence of the buttocks. This tilt, accompanied by flat-roofed acetabula and bowed legs, leads to a ducklike gait. Limitation in extention of the elbows is the rule. Although the hands are short and stubby, they appear large in comparison to the more abbreviated limbs. Wide proximal phalanges lead to difficulty in opposing the fingers. A space between the third and fourth digits gives rise to the characteristic "trident" or three-pronged hand (Marie, 1900). The mean adult height for achondroplastic men is 51.81 inches, and for women 48.62 inches; the mean adult weights are 120.61 pounds for males, 100.62 pounds for females (Murdoch et al., 1970). Parental height in sporadic cases of achondroplasia does not significantly influence the dwarf's height.

The radiologic features of achondroplasia (Fig. 2) have been well defined (Rubin, 1964; Caffey, 1967) and include a shortened skull base, small foramen magnum, and large vault. The interpedicular distance from the thoracic vertebrae to the sacrum shows caudad narrowing, a reverse of the normal finding. Lumbar gibbus is common in infancy, but with weight bearing and ambulation the gibbus usually gives way to exaggerated lordosis. The narrowed spinal cord, which can be visualized on lateral as well as frontal roentgenographic views of the lumbar spine, predisposes to neurological problems caused by compression of the cord and nerve roots by osteophytes, prolapsed intervertebral discs, or deformity of the vertebral bodies (Vogl, 1962; Cohen et al., 1967). The long bones are short and thick with slight outward bowing, and the growth plates may be V-shaped. A short broad pelvis with horizontal acetabular margins and narrow, relatively deep greater sciatic notches are typical (Langer et al., 1967). The most striking changes in the hands are the short, broad, and conically shaped proximal and middle phalanges.

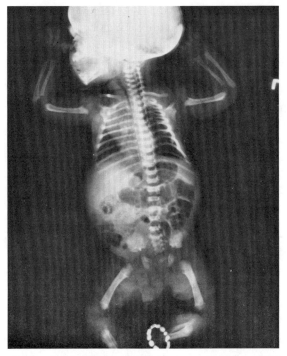

Fig. 2.—Newborn achondroplastic dwarf. Features include caudad narrowing of interpedicular distance, deep sciatic notches, and horizontal acetabular roofs.

Markedly disorganized endochondral ossification has generally been thought to be the histological explanation for the peculiar skeletal development in this type of short-limb dwarfism. In reviewing the published material, Rimoin et al. (1970) noted that the majority of these cases did not have classical achondroplasia but rather were misdiagnosed cases of thanatophoric dwarfism, metatropic dwarfism, or achondrogenesis. Rimoin and co-workers found morphologically regular, well-organized endochondral ossification in rib and iliac crest biopsies from patients with true achondroplasia. Similar results from iliac crest biopsies were shown by Ponseti (1970). He found that the fibular growth had cartilage cell clusters separated by wide fibrous septa which appeared to be slowly and irregularly resorbed at the vascular front. Bone formation was stunted in the fibular metaphysis but formed normally in the fibular head and in the periostium.

Classic achondroplasia is a simple autosomal dominant trait. A new mutation is thought to be the cause of over 80% of cases. In a study (Murdoch et al., 1970) of 148 achrondroplasics, of whom 117 were sporadic and 31 familial, a significant parental age effect on the occurrence of new mutations for the achondroplasia gene was shown. The paternal component of this parental age effect was the major factor. The increased maternal age and birth order only reflected this elevated paternal age. Reproductive fitness in achondroplasia is considerably reduced, in part because of social difficulties in finding a mate and in part because of obstetric problems created by the small pelvis. Reduced survivorship to reproductive age is not a major element in the reduced reproductive fitness.

Ethnic differences in achondroplasia may be associated with the later marriages of males of certain ethnic groups, resulting in greater paternal age, particularly if the sibship is large.

Hall et al. (1969) reported 2 infants, each with two achondroplastic parents, who probably were homozygous for the achondroplasia gene. Clinically and radiographically these children were more severely affected than heterozygous achondroplastic infants, and they died during the first 3 months of life. Murdoch et al. (1970) noted that, of 16 affected offspring of 23 marriages between achondroplastic dwarfs, 7 died in infancy and were presumably homozygous. The possibility of homozygous achondroplasia was suggested by Morgan et al. (1970), who reported a child of two achondroplastic dwarfs. This child was described as showing radiographic findings of classic achondroplasia (no illustrations were provided), marked mental retardation, and congenital heart disease with transposition of the great vessels. It is likely that homozygous achondroplasia has a characteristic radiographic picture distinct from that of heterozygous achondroplasia (Hall et al., 1969). If the radiographic changes were truly those of classic achondroplasia, it can be questioned that the case of Morgan et al. (1970) was homozygous.

The occurrence of two or more distantly related cases of achondroplasia in a single kindred was reported by Opitz (1969), and in two first cousins by Wadia (1969). This suggested to Opitz (1969) the hypothesis of inheritance of an "unstable premutation" in man in the sense of Auerbach (1956). Rimoin and McKusick (1969) described an achondroplastic dwarf whose left second through fifth fingers were normal in structure, in contrast to the typical chondrodystrophic involvement of the remainder of his skeleton. The possibility of somatic mosaicism was suggested. This could have been secondary to a back mutation, somatic crossing over, a small chromosal deletion, or a supressor mutation.

ACHONDROGENESIS

Few reports of achondrogenesis have been published since Parenti (1936) first described this rare form of short-limbed dwarfism, which is lethal. These infants survive at most only a few days. Fraccaro (1952) further identified the disorder, and Langer et al. (1969) described additional cases ascertained from the literature under a variety of diagnoses.

The head in achondrogenesis is strikingly large, the extremities disproportionately small, and the trunk abbreviated in length. The trunk appears nearly as wide as it is long (Gorlin and Sedano, 1970). Radiographic examination is diagnostic, revealing extreme underossification. This is especially obvious in the vertebral bodies of the lumbar spine, sacrum, and pubic and ischial bones. The degree of ossification of the long bones is variable, and they are markedly shortened (Fig. 3). When there is sufficient ossification, marked flaring at both ends of the humeri is seen. Achondrogenesis is inherited as an autosomal recessive trait. Saldino (1970) observed in a Gypsy family, in which the parents were second cousins, 2 offspring with well-documented achondrogenesis. Two other offspring may have been affected. Silverman (1970) also has information on a family with multiple affected sibs. Houston (1960) has observed 4 sibs with achondrogenesis out of a family of 9.

Confusion in usage of the term achondrogenesis has been pointed out by several workers. Under the same term, achondrogenesis, Grebe (1952, 1955) reported sisters of a consanguineous union who were identically affected with a type of short-limbed, nonlethal drarfism. Quelce-Salgado (1964, 1968) described 47 similar cases among a highly consanguineous group of Brazilian Indians. An isolated case of Greek extraction was reported by Scott (1969a).

The affected individuals are 39 to 42 inches tall and have a relatively normal-sized trunk. The extremities are short and deformed, this being most pronounced distally. The fingers are greatly shortened and often functionless. Half of the patients have polydactyly. The feet are deformed and short, in addition to valgus positioning. Intelligence is normal. The diminished height is due entirely to pronounced shortening of the long bones. Every bone element in the extremity is aplastic or hypoplastic (Quelce-Salgado, 1968).

Achondrogenesis of the Grebe or Brazilian type is inherited as an autosomal recessive trait. The use of this diagnostic term is not appropriately descriptive. It has no relation to the condition originally described by Parenti and Faccaro, and its continued use only serves to confuse the nomenclature further. Classification with the mesomelic dwarfs would be more logical.

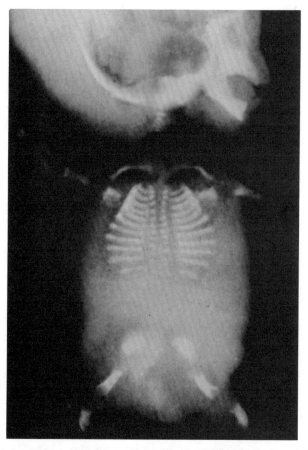

FIG. 3.—Achondrogenesis. Poor ossification and marked shortening of the extremities are typical findings.

Thanatophoric Dwarfism

The Greek word *thanatophoros* ("death bearing") was given to this specific chondrodystrophy by Maroteaux et al. (1967). Until their report thanatophoric dwarfs were unrecognized, buried in the literature with other congenital short-limbed dwarfs, under such diagnoses as achondrogenesis and achondroplasia. They described 4 cases and were able to find another 17 examples in the literature. Subsequently additional cases have been published by Giedion (1968), Langer et al. (1969), Huguenin et al. (1969), Beaudoing et al. (1969), Keats et al. (1970), and Kaufman et al. (1970). It seems clear that this chondrodystrophy represents a specific and quite distinct form of short stature.

Hydraminos is common, and in several cases paucity of fetal movements was mentioned by the mothers. Abnormal fetal proportions have been suspected on clinical examination and demonstrated in utero by radiographs (Cronberg, 1933; Wichtl, 1965; Keats et al., 1970). In utero fetal cranial decompression has been required in order to deliver the hydrocephalic head.

These infants may be stillborn or die within the first few hours of life. The longest survival reported in the literature is 25 days; however, an infant requiring continuous oxygen therapy is known to have survived 156 days (McKusick, 1970). Upon delivery, micromelia is striking while the trunk is essentially of normal length. Total body length has ranged between 36 and 47 cm. The thorax is small and narrow in all dimensions due to very short ribs. The skull is disproportionately large in comparison to the face, and is often associated with large fontanelles and prominence or bossing of the forehead. Nasal bridge depression and bulging eyes typify the facies. Numerous skin folds are present on the very short extremities which tend to extend outward from the trunk with the thighs abducted and externally rotated. Hypotonia is usually marked and the primitive reflexes absent. If born alive, severe respiratory distress is a constant feature. The infant has tachypnea, rib cage retractions, cyanosis, and periods of apnea. Death in respiratory acidosis and congestive heart failure rapidly ensue.

In addition to the abnormal skeletal findings, other malformations have been observed at autopsy. Patent ductus arteriosus, atrial septal defect, and herniation of the cerebellum through the falx tentorium were noted by Langer et al. (1969). Huguenin et al. (1969) reported absence of the corpus callosum and temporal abnormalities, including polymicrogyria and numerous subependymal neuronal heterotopias in the gray matter. Coarctation of the aorta and a patent foramen ovale, both associated with patent ductus arteriosis, were found at autopsy in 2 of the 3 cases reported by Keats et al. (1970).

The radiographic features in thanatophoric dwarfism are distinctive (Fig. 4). There are certain similarities with achondroplasia, particularly homozygous achondroplasia (Hall et al., 1969). In thanatophoric dwarfism the distinguishing features are extreme flatness of the vertebral bodies and excessive vertical dimensions of the intervertebral spaces. In frontal projection the bodies are very flat with the mid-point being the narrowest. The lumbar vertebrate have been an inverted U appearance. The interpediculate distances do not flare caudally, and there is relative lumbar canal stenosis. The nonossified spaces between the vertebral bodies are markedly increased in size throughout the spine. The pelvic configuration is generally short and broad with small sacrosciatic notches. The transverse diameter of the ilia is greater than the vertical, and the crests have a frayed appearance.

The ribs are short and have wide cupped anterior ends. The entire thorax is narrow in both transverse and anteroposterior measurements. The long bones of the extremities are short, broad, and bowed and have flared, irregular metaphyses. No epiphyseal ossification centers are present at the distal femur or proximal tibia, but they are present in the calcaneus

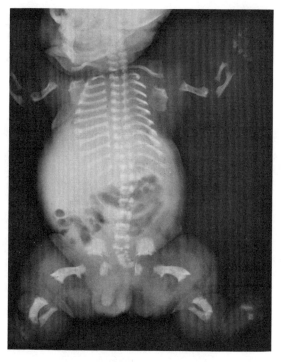

Fig. 4.—Thanatophoric dwarfism with extreme flatness of the vertebral bodies, short ribs, and abbreviated long bones.

and talus. The skull is disproportionately large with a small foramen magnum, depressed nasal bridge, and frontal bossing.

The cause of thanatophoric dwarfism is unknown. All reported cases have been sporadic, and parental age is not increased (Maroteaux et al., 1967). Nor is there evidence of parental consanguinity. Twin females discordant for thanatophoric dwarfism were published by Keats et al. (1970). Clearly it is not due to homozygosity of the achondroplasia gene. Since the parents are normal skeletally, one would have to postulate simultaneous mutations of two genes. The radiographic changes are quite different in the two conditions. Rimoin et al. (1969a) demonstrated disorganized endochondral ossification in thanatophoric dwarfism, while regular, well-organized endochondral bone formation characterized achondroplasia. Kaufman et al. (1970) pointed out the close clinical, skeletal, and pathological resemblance of thanatophoric dwarfism to the recessively inherited "achondroplasia mutant" of the rabbit and suggest that it more likely represents an animal homolog for thanatophoric dwarfism in man.

CHONDRODYSPLASIA PUNCTATA

Chondrodysplasia punctata has a bewildering array of names including the more commonly used terms: Conradi's disease, chondrodystrophia calcificans congenita, and stippled epiphyses (Melnick, 1965). In actual fact this form of chondrodystrophy does not appear to be a single entity but rather two or more, so that the nosology is as confused as the terminology. To complicate the matter further, stippling of the epiphyses has been demonstrated radiographically in a host of unrelated disorders: the cerebro-hepato-renal syndrome, generalized gangliosidosis, Smith-Lemli-Opitz syndrome, anencephaly, trisomy 21 syndrome, and cretinism.

There are over 110 cases of chondrodysplasia punctata in the medical literature (Melnick, 1965). Both autosomal dominant and recessive modes of inheritance have been described. The recessively determined form has received the most attention and is the best known. It is characterized by dwarfism of the short-limb type, the humeri and femora showing the more severe abbreviation (Allansmith and Senz, 1960). Joint contractures, limitations of movement, depression of the nasal bridge, bilateral cataracts, and skin and hair abnormalities are common (Comings et al., 1968). Death often occurs within the first year of life, the average age at death being 5 months (Allansmith and Senz, 1960). In survivors mental retardation is likely (Armaly, 1957). Radiographs in infants, in addition to stippled epiphyseal ossification centers (Figs. 5a, 5b, and 5c), show vertical clefting of the vertebral bodies on lateral projection, and rather marked metaphyseal involvement of the long tubular bones. The humeri and femora are short. Scoliosis is common.

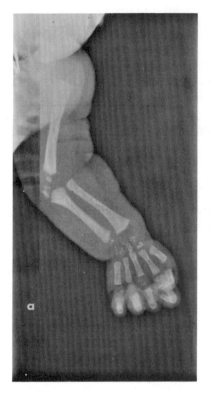

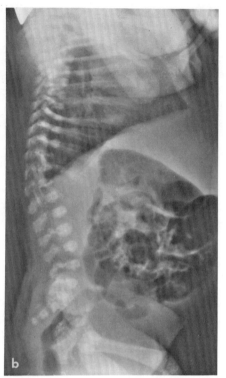

FIG.—5(*a, b, c*) Chondrodysplasia punctata, age 2 weeks. In addition to stippling of the epiphyses, note the rhizomelia.

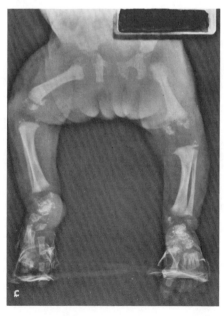

Though less clearly defined, an autosomal dominant type of chondro-dysplasia punctuta has been recognized (Spranger et al., 1971). Langer (1969) refers to the case (pp. 134-135) in Rubin's *Dynamic Classification of Bone Dysplasias* as being illustrative of this disorder. Those cases which Silverman (1961) described as epiphyseal dysplasia punctata probably also represent this form. The autosomal dominant form is not associated with rhizomelia nor severe metaphyseal changes but is frequently asymmetric in distribution and can be mild in clinical manifestation.

METATROPIC DWARFISM

Metatropic dwarfism for years was thought to be an atypical chondro-dysplasia, usually being reported as a variant of achondroplasia or Morquio's disease. Maroteaux et al. (1966) reported 6 cases and were able to gather another 12 from earlier reports.

At birth infants with this condition have a long, narrow thorax and trunk, and relatively short extremities as is found in achondroplasia. In the course of development, there is a reversal of body proportions. Rapidly progressing kyphoscoliosis results in short-spine dwarfism, while growth of the long bones is less disturbed. The condition in some ways comes to resemble Morquio's disease. Because of this reversal of body proportions, the Greek term *metatropos* ("changing pattern") was used to name the disorder.

The face is normal, though Fleury et al. (1966) noted one case with peculiar facies. The extremities are short and broad with enlarged joints and restricted movement. The hands and feet are rather plump, the fingers hyperextensible. Adult height is approximately 110-120 cm (44-48 inches). The diagnosis may be made in infancy by roentrographic examination. The spine displays severe underossification of the vertebral bodies which are reduced to narrow tongue-like structures. Occasionally there is a long double fold of tissue over the sacrum which is rather tail-like and reaches the upper anal fold. Kyphoscoliosis is apparent quite early and rapidly progresses. The ribs are short, and the pelvis has a peculiar battle-axe (or halberd) configuration due to marked flaring of the iliac crests.

Relative shortening of the long bones of the extremities confers a dumb-bell shape because of exaggerated metaphyseal widening and irregularity (Silverman, 1968). The epiphyses are also irregular and deformed. Representative radiographs are well illustrated by Rubin (1964) on pp. 380 and 381 as an "unresolved differential diagnostic problem."

The genetics of metatropic dwarfism is as yet incompletely understood. It appears most likely to be inherited as an autosomal recessive trait. The two brothers reported by Michail et al. (1956) probably had this condition. The disorder described by Kniest (1952) had some similarity to metatropic dwarfism but must be considered a separate entity which might be called metatropic dwarfism, type II, or the Kniest syndrome.

DIASTROPHIC DWARFISM

The recognition of a distinct entity previously mistaken for a variant form of achondroplasia with clubfeet or with arthrogryposis multiplex is credited to Lamy and Maroteaux (1960). In addition to short-limb dwarfism, they were impressed by certain anomalies including scoliosis, clubfeet, and abnormal hands and ears, and suggested the name from the Greek term for twisted or crooked. The first report of recognized diastrophic dwarfism in English literature was of two sibs of a consanguineous mating (Taybi, 1963). In a review of the world literature, Walker et al. (1971) were able to find 69 cases and reported an additional 51 cases.

In the newborn period this chondrodystrophy may be recognized by the unique constellation of malformations. With maturity additional features become apparent. The head and skull are normal, but there is a similarity of the facies due to a narrow root and broad midportion of the nose, long upper lip, and a rather square jaw. Midline frontal hemangiomas are common, and one-fourth have cleft palates. Deformity of the external ear typically develops within the first 2 or 3 weeks of life in 84% of the individuals (Walker et al. 1971). Initially there is acute inflammation and cystic swelling of the body of the pinna. The swelling subsides within 4 to 6 weeks, and the ear shows residual thickening, firmness, and cauliflower deformity. Later calcification and ossification can be demonstrated within this tissue. The external auditory canals may be small, but hearing is not often defective. Deformity of the ossicles, perhaps a feature of this disorder leading to decreased hearing, was reported by Maloney (1969). In addition to nasality to speech in those with cleft palates, many affected individuals have a characteristic timbre of the voice which is rasping or hoarse in nature. Stover et al. (1963) and Walker et al. (1971) noted the occurrence of a mesodermal defect of the anterior chamber of the eyes consisting of thick pectinate stands extending from the peripheral iris to the trabecular mesh. Similar observations have been reported in a variety of disorders, e.g., Marfan's syndrome and idiopathic scoliosis (Burian et al., 1960).

The mean adult height is 44 inches, with the range for males 34-50 inches, and for females 41-48 inches (Walker et al., 1971). The limbs are rhizomelic with the shortening most severe in the upper arms and lower legs. Stature is further reduced by the occurrence of kyphoscoliosis and major joint flexion contractures, especially at the hips and knees. There is a tendency to joint subluxation and dislocation (Rubin, 1964), particularly of the elbows, shoulders, hips, and patellas. The hips are normal at birth, but subsequent to weight bearing and ambulation hip dysplasia with subluxation or dislocation and coxa vara becomes evident. Gait is greatly disturbed. Also there is marked limitation of movement of all joints.

Scoliosis is manifest in early childhood, most frequently within the first year of life and is progressive in nature (Spranger and Gerken, 1967). Kyphosis of the cervical spine may lead to neurological complications (Kaplan et al., 1961; Stover et al., 1963; Langer, 1965).

Malformation of the hands is one of the hallmarks of diastrophic dwarfism; as well as being broad, short, and deviated ulnarward, the fingers of the hands are fixed due to proximal interphalangeal synphalangism. The hypermobile thumb is in a hitchhiker position due to deformity of the first metacarpal. The feet are severely deformed due to metatarsus varus and equinus which are progressive and exceedingly difficult to correct by the usual methods employed in clubfoot treatment. If partially or completely untreated, ambulation is additionally hindered by the extreme equinus foot position. Medial deviation of the broadened great toes is common. Intelligence is normal.

The roentgenographic findings are distinctive. The large tubular bones of the extremities are short and thick with broad, flared metaphyses. The epiphyses are delayed and irregular in development. Stippling of the epiphyses has been observed in a few cases (Silverman, 1968). The epiphyses of the proximal femurs are absent at birth, and when ossification does occur are flat and distorted. The proximal tibial epiphysis, which is medially located on the metaphysis, may be triangular in shape and is larger than the distal femoral epiphysis.

The pelvis appears short and broad with slight flaring of the iliac wings (Fig. 6a). In older individuals the femoral necks are short and wide. Coxa vara, subluxation, and dislocation are often present. Precocious ossification in the costal cartilages is another frequent finding.

The most characteristic changes in diastrophic dwarfism are in the bones of the hands and feet, particularly the hands. The first metacarpal is small, oval or triangular in shape, and set low on the carpus, often with subluxation of the metacarpophalangeal joint (Fig. 6b). More carpal and tarsal centers are ossified than is normal. Equinovarus deformity of the feet is present, sometimes with additional varus and broadening of the great toe (Fig. 6c).

Scoliosis is not present in early infancy, and the vertebrae are of normal height. With time, the scoliosis is manifest. The interpediculate distance may widen or narrow in caudad direction in the lumbar area or remain constant. Spinal canal stenosis is never of the degree seen in achondro-

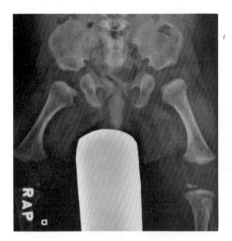 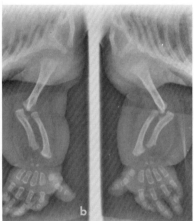

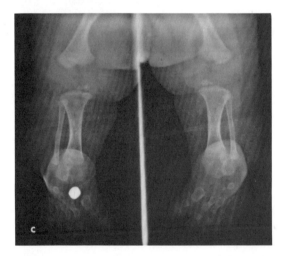

FIG. 6.—(a) Diastrophic dwarf. The pelvis is short and broad, the proximal femoral epiphyses nonossified, and the metaphyses are flared. (b) Hitchhiker thumb due to deformity of first metacarpal in diastrophic dwarfism. (c) Clubfoot deformity of diastrophic dwarfism.

plasia. Cervical spine kyphosis and subluxation can occur. The skull is normal, but calcification or ossification of the external ears may be demonstrated.

Poor columnization and calcification of cartilage cells in the femoral heads and in epiphyseal plates, with flattened and atrophic chondrocytes, have been observed (Kaplan et al. 1961). Diastrophic dwarfism is inherited as an autosomal recessive trait. Of 35 families studied by Walker et al. (1971), 12 kindreds had more than one affected child while the parents and 10 half-sibs were entirely normal. Each of two of the diastrophic women in that series was delivered of an unaffected child by Cesarean section. Consanguinity is rare in this disorder, and parental age is not advanced.

CHONDROECTODERMAL DYSPLASIA: THE ELLIS-VAN CREVELD SYNDROME

Until 1964 little more than 50 cases of the Ellis-van Creveld syndrome were recorded in the literature since its original description in 1940 (Ellis-van Creveld). McKusick et al. (1964) doubled this number and fully delineated the condition and its inheritance.

The clinical diagnosis can be made on inspection of the patient at birth. There is shortening of the extremities in a mesomelic fashion, e.g., the forearms and shanks are comparatively shorter than the proximal segments of the limbs. The hands are short and stubby; postaxial polydactyly is always present in the hands and, in approximately 10%, in the feet as well. The nails are hypoplastic, and the teeth show several anomalies, including natal teeth, precocious exfoliation, or missing or conical teeth. Multiple frenuli tend to obliterate the buccolabial sulcus and an upper, midline partial harelip is often present. Congenital heart disease, usually atrial septal defect, is present in over half of the cases.

Although the radiographic features are widespread (Fig. 7a and 7b), the most characteristic are in the extremities. The middle phalanges are short and broad, while the distal phalanges are hypoplastic. Cone-shaped epiphyses in the proximal and middle phalanges are seen in the older child. Polydactyly with fusion of the capitate and hamate and nearly pathognomic of the disorder. Also quite typical is slanting of the proximal tibial metaphysis, giving rise to knock-knee deformity.

Chondroectodermal dysplasia is inherited as an autosomal recessive trait. Consanguinity is frequent. In McKusick's studies of the inbred Old Order Amish, all parents of affected sibships, which now total 35, had one common ancestor, thus demonstrating the Founder Principle and the usefulness of studies of population isolates. Although very rare, chondroectodermal dysplasia has been described in persons of many different races or nationalities.

ASPHYXIATING THORACIC DYSPLASIA

Asphyxiating thoracic dysplasia is a rare, familial bone disorder in which early onset of respiratory distress may result in early death. It was

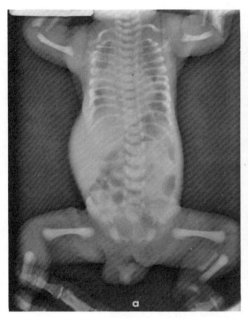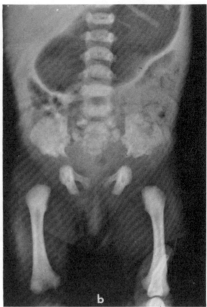

FIG. 7.—(*a*, *b*) Chondroectodermal dysplastic newborn who died at 6 days of age due to congenital heart disease. Note the normal interpedicular distances in the lumbar spine.

originally described by Jeune (1955) in 2 sibs who died during infancy. Subsequently other infants were reported with typical features by clinical and radiological examination but without respiratory problems and with survival into childhood (Neimann et al., 1963; Maroteaux and Savart, 1964; Pirnar and Neuhauser, 1966). It becomes gradually apparent that there was a rather wide spectrum of clinical and radiographic findings ranging from the relatively benign to the life-threatening.

Characteristic of the disorder is a small thorax, narrow in both the transverse and the anterioposterior diameter. The ribs are short and horizontally oriented. Not all infants with these findings show respiratory distress. Some die rapidly, while others seem to outgrow it. The fingers and toes are short, and the limbs are variable in this regard. Inconsistent abnormalities include hand and foot polydactyly, dental anomalies, clubfeet, jaundice, pectus carinatum, costal rosary, and situs inversus (Kohler and Babbitt, 1970). A number of these cases have developed progressive renal disease in childhood (Herdman and Langer, 1968). Initially this is demonstrated by proteinuria without urinary sediment abnormalities. Renal failure, hypertension, and death in uremia follows periods of illness of months to years. Histologically the changes in the kidney are nonspecific, showing interstitial fibrosis, round-cell infiltration, and tubular atrophy.

Apart from the dysplastic thorax (Fig. 8), the radiological findings include an unusual pelvic configuration with retarded ossification of the triradiate cartilage resulting in a double notch appearance. The metacarpals, metatarsals, and phalanges are short and splayed. The spine and skull are normal. Those infants with asphyxiating thoracic dysplasia and polydactyly may be indistinguishable on radiographic criteria alone from the Ellis-van Creveld syndrome (Langer, 1968). The correct diagnosis in these cases can be made by differences on physical examination.

Asphyxiating thoracic dysplasia has been described in multiple affected sibs with normal parents and is considered to be an autosomal recessive trait.

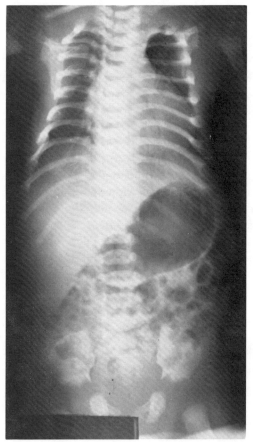

FIG. 8.—Newborn with asphyxiating thoracic dysplasia. Note the moderately small thorax and tendency towards horizontally positioned ribs.

Spondyloepiphyseal Dysplasia Congenita

Spranger and Wiedemann (1966) described a variety of short-trunk dwarfism with skeletal abnormalities manifest at birth. Because the major changes involve the spine and proximal epiphyses, they suggested the name spondyloepiphyseal dysplasia congenita. This same term had been used by Rubin (1964) to include both this condition and Morquio's disease (mucopolysaccharidosis, type IV). However, it is not an appropriate synonym for Morquio's disease since this disorder is not manifested in the newborn period and is a dystrophy rather than a dysplasia.

The earliest description of spondyloepiphyseal congenita was probably by Patel in 1901, but because of insufficient radiological documentation it is impossible to be certain. Spranger and Langer (1970) were able to gather 19 cases from the literature and contributed 29 new cases.

Growth disturbance in the form of disproportionate short-trunk dwarfism is apparent at birth or shortly thereafter. Clubfeet and cleft palate are frequent (Bach et al., 1967; Fraser et al., 1969). Moderately flat or dish-like facies are due to underdevelopment of the facial bones and relative accentuation of the lower face. The eyes may be wideset. The head is normal in size and seems to rest directly on the shoulders due to a very short neck. A broad or barrel-shaped chest may be associated with a pectus carinatum deformity as well as deep Harrison grooves.

The normal thoracic kyphosis and lumbar lordosis are exaggerated. Scoliosis may develop during adolescence but is usually mild and primarily involves the thoracic spine. Genu valgum is common, though genu varum also occurs. The extremities are comparatively long in relation to the trunk. Rhizomelic shortening of the limbs is present. The hands and feet are normal in shape and length. Muscular hypotonia can be present and, coupled with the abnormal body proportions, is a factor in delayed motor development. Intelligence is normal, and the gait is waddling. Adult height is quite variable, ranging from 37 to 52 inches, depending on the severity of platyspondyly (Spranger and Langer, 1970).

Ocular and visual defects occur in association with a number of osseous dysplasias such as Marfan's syndrome, osteogenesis imperfecta, chondrodysplasia punctata, and the mucopolysaccharidoses. Over half of the patients with spondyloepiphyseal dysplasia congenita have high myopia and/or retinal detachments. Not all of those with retinal detachment have had myopia. Areas of peripheral retinal degeneration have been observed to precede detachments. The corneas are clear. Fraser et al. (1969) observed one child who was blind due to associated buphthalmos. It is mandatory that individuals with this chondrodystrophy have regular ophthalmologic examination for early detection and treatment of retinal detachment.

Laboratory investigations have shown normal chromosomal analyses, urinary amino acid chromatograms, and mucopolysaccharides. Spranger and Wiedmann (1966b) found metachromatic inclusions in peripheral lymphocytes in several of their cases. Metachromosia is, of course, a non-specific finding. On roentenographic examination the striking lesions are in the spine, pelvis, and femoral heads and necks (Spranger and Langer, 1970). There is retarded ossification of the pubic bones, knee epiphyses, calcanei, and tali. Early, the vertebral bodies are flat and ovoid or pear-shaped and the thorax is broad and bell-shaped. The odontoid is hypo-plastic, and the pelvic ilia do not flare. Rhizomelic brachymelia and minor abnormalities of the hands and feet are present. The femoral head and neck ossification centers develop very slowly and may not appear until well into childhood. This often is confused with hip dislocation. Severe coxa vara can be demonstrated by hip arthrography. When ossified, the femoral head usually appears widely separated from the metaphysis. Ulti-mately there is extensive shortening of the spine with mild to moderate thoracic kyphoscoliosis and marked lumbar lordosis. The vertebral bod-ies are irregular and flat with narrow disc spaces. Of the tubular long bones, the humeri and femora are more severely shortened and wide than others. Epiphyseal centers may be flat, deformed, and have multiple foci of ossification. Changes in the hands are minor, the most frequent being multiple accessory epiphyses.

Spondyloepiphyseal dysplasia congenita appears to be inherited as an autosomal dominant trait. While most cases are sporadic, parent to child transmission has been reported in several instances (Spranger and Wiede-mann, 1966; Spranger and Langer, 1970). Increased paternal age, as evi-dence favoring new mutation in sporadic cases, was pointed out by Fraser et al., (1969).

HYPOCHONDROPLASIA

Though probably not rare, there have been remarkably few reports of hypochondroplasia. As with so many other chondrodystrophies, it too was long considered a mild or a typical form of achondroplasia. Probably the first description was by Ravenna (1913). The name was proposed by Leri and Linoissier (1924). The clinical and radiological characteristics were further delineated by Lamy and Maroteaux (1961) Kozlowski (1965), and Beals (1969). The exact limits are still not known, and it is suspected that the range of dwarfism might at the extreme of mildness approach the lower limits of normal physical size within minimal other stigmata.

Hypochondroplasia is difficult to diagnose in infancy. Birth weight and length may be within the lower limits of normal, and shortness of stature usually is not recognized until age 2 or 3. Clinically these patients have a relatively long trunk and disproportionately short limbs. The upper to lower segment ratio is greater than unity. The head appears normal; specifically the hallmarks of true achondroplasia are not present. There is no cranial enlargement, frontal bossing, depression of the nasal bridge, or mandibular protrusion. The spine usually shows mild to moderate lumbar lordosis and pelvic tilt. While short and stocky, the extremities may show mild genu varum which tends to disappear with age. The hands and feet are somewhat broad, but there is no trident hand deformity. In contrast to achondroplasia there are no major neurological complications. Aching in the knees, elbows, ankles, and low back occasionally is complained of older individuals. The adult height range is 52 to 58 inches. Mental retardation has been reported as fairly frequent (Kozlowski, 1965).

The typical radiographic findings are primarily in the spine, pelvis, and long bones. The skull is essentially normal, though there may be mild alterations. The long bones are mildly abbreviated, and there is slight flaring of the metaphyses, most noticeably at the knees. In younger patients, the distal femoral metaphysis may show a shallow V-shaped indentation, but this is not as pronounced as the chevron-shaped indentation seen in achondroplasia. The pelvis may appear basically normal or demonstrate mild changes such as reduced width of the greater sciatic notches and square, shortened ilia. In the spine, the interpedicular distance decreases from the first to the fifth lumbar vertebrae, but these alterations are not as profound as in achondroplasia. The vertebral bodies are not diminished in height, and there is concavity of the posterior border of the lumbar vertebrae.

Hypochondroplasia is inherited in an autosomal dominant manner. Beals (1969) reported one kindred in which transmission occurred through four generations. Most cases appear to be sporadic, presumably due to new mutations. Of 11 cases of hypochondroplasia described by Kozlowski (1965) there were two instances of hypochondroplastic adults mating with achondroplastic dwarfs. The resultant children were either achondroplastic or hypochondroplastic, but no intermediate forms were observed. Hypochondroplasia appears to be a separate and distinct genetic entity.

METAPHYSEAL CHONDRODYSPLASIAS

This group of disorders in the past has been referred to as metaphyseal dysotoses. The term dysostosis is misleading (Rubin, 1964) as these are alterations of bone form or modeling due to disturbances of intrinsic bone growth, e.g., dysplasias. Several distinct varieties are now recognized.

Metaphyseal Chondrodysplasia, Jansen Type

Since Jansen (1934) originally reported this very rare dysplasia, very few cases have been reported (De Haas et al., 1969; Lenz, 1969; Holt, 1969). All metaphyses including those of the hands and feet are severely involved. They are considerably enlarged and widened; their structure is irregular and sponge-like. Stature is dwarfed and the joints appear enlarged. Because of contracture deformities, stance is crouched and the arms are long and dangling. The legs are shortened to a greater degree than the arms. Jansen's original case was restudied by DeHaas (1969) and noted to be 125 cm tall at age 44 years. Remarkable spontaneous improvement towards more normal bony architecture had occurred, although there was considerably residual gross deformity. Partial deafness was observed, presumed to be due, at least in part, to sclerosis of the petrous temporal bone. Unexplained in these patients are the high serum calcium levels (13-15 mg%) without clinical symptomatology. Jansen's disease has been reported in mother and daughter (Lenz, 1969).

Metaphyseal Chondrodysplasia, Schmid Type

A second major type of metaphyseal chondrodysplasia is that described by Schmid (1949). Several large pedigrees have been reported (Stickler et al., 1962; Rosenbloom and Smith, 1965). Clinically these patients have shortness of stature of mild to moderate degree, enlarged wrists, bowing of the legs, a waddling gait, inability to fully extend the fingers, and flaring of the lower rib cages. Radiographically the characteristic changes involve the metaphyses and are less severe than those of Jansen's type. The abnormalities vary from mild scalloping to gross irregularity with widening and fragmentation of the metaphyses. Most frequently these findings are present at the ankle, knee, wrist, shoulder, and hip. The hands and feet show no irregularities or only minor ones.

Metaphyseal chondrodysplasia of the Schmid type has been reported in a large Mormon kindred in Utah as achondroplasia (Stephens, 1943). There has been a great deal of confusion of this dysplasia with vitamin D-resistant rickets. However, in the Schmid type of metaphyseal chondrodysplasia, there are no characteristic biochemical changes, no beneficial response to administration of vitamin D in any dosage, and there are a number of histological differences (Dent and Normand, 1964). These workers observed radiographic "healing" of the metaphyseal lesions with bed rest and recurrence on weight bearing. On radiologic examination there is no generalized osteomalacia or loss of definition at the metaphysis. Vitamin D-resistant rickets (familial hypophosphatemic rickets) is inherited as an X-linked dominant trait. Schmid's type of metaphyseal chondrodysplasia has an autosomal dominant mode of inheritance with variable expression, females tending to have less marked manifestations. Advanced paternal age may be a factor in sporadic cases (Rosenbloom and Smith, 1965).

Metaphyseal Chondrodysplasia, McKusick Type

McKusick et al. (1965a) defined the clinical and genetic characteristics of previously undescribed syndrome which they named cartilage-hair hypoplasia. Radiologically the conspicuous changes are those of metaphyseal chondrodysplasia.

The dwarfism of this syndrome is of the short-limb variety. Adult heights vary from 42 to 58 inches. The head and face are normal, and the hands and feet are short and pudgy. Loose-jointedness of the fingers and toes can be extraordinary. The nails are short but of nearly normal width. There is inability to extend the elbows fully, mild flaring of the lower ribs, prominence of the sternum, and ankle deformity due to the excessive length of the fibula distally relative to the short tibia. In the older individual mild bow leg deformity or unilateral knock-knee may occur. The hair is fine, sparse, light in color, and relatively fragile. In early childhood intestinal malabsorption and Hirschprung's disease have been reported, as well as a tendency to unusually severe varicella apparently due to a defect in the function of small lymphocytes. Lux et al. (1970) found that these individuals are able to synthesize antibodies to a variety of other viral and bacterial antigens. Persistent lymphopenia, normal serum immunoglobulins, diminished delayed skin hypersensitivity, and diminished responsiveness of lymphocytes in vitro are additional features. The mechanism of this relationship is unclear.

Biopsy of the metaphyseal area shows ossification per se to be normal, but the cartilage is hypoplastic. There are decreased numbers of chondrocytes and disorganized columnization. Microscopically the hairs are abnormally small in caliber and often lack a pigmented core. Serum calcium, phosphorus, and alkaline phosphatase are normal. Radiographically the metaphyses of the tubular bones are scalloped and regularly sclerotic, often with cystic areas. The entire width of the metaphyseal area is involved. Ankle deformity is usually present due to the excessive length of the fibula distally. The ribs are flared and cupped, and the vertebral bodies, though slightly decreased in height, are normal, as is the skull.

McKusick's type of metaphyseal chondrodysplasia is inherited as an autosomal recessive trait. It is particularly common among the Old Order Amish, a religious isolate. where the frequency is thought to be about 2 per thousand births.

The relationship of this dysplasia to that described by Burgert et al. (1965) is unclear. Their patients had aregenerative anemia, celiac syndrome and extremely elevated alkaline phosphatase levels in addition to metaphyseal dysplasia.

Metaphyseal Chondrodysplasia with Malabsorption and Neutropenia

Since Schwachman et al. (1964) described the syndrome of pancreatic insufficiency and bone marrow dysfunction, a number of similar cases have been published. Shmerling et al. (1969) and Taybi et al. (1969) extended the syndrome, which in complete form is manifest by (a) dwarfism with a height below the third percentile, (b) exocrine pancreatic insufficiency not due to cystic fibrosis of the pancreas, (c) constant or cyclical neutropenia, and (d) severe bilateral destructive metaphyseal dysplasia of the hips leading to coxa vara. These bony alterations are associated with only minor changes in other metaphyses. Apparently, adequate treatment of the exocrine insufficiency does not improve the neutropenia or the bone lesions. Diabetes mellitus has occurred in 2 of these patients. Evidence favors autosomal recessive inheritance. In 5 out of the 29 published families, more than one child was affected. There has been no instance of parental consanguinity, and both sexes are equally affected.

Metaphyseal Chondrosplasia with Thymolymphopenia

In this disorder, first described by Nahmias et al. (1967), there is inability to stimulate a lymphocyte response with certain antigens, a lack of cellular immunity, recurrent infections, thymic aplasia, and normal immunoglobulin levels. Some of these patients have the bony changes of metaphyseal dysostosis (Fulginiti et al., 1967). The radiologic findings are quite different from those in the McKusick-type metaphyseal chondrodysplasia. The mode of inheritance is autosomal recessive.

Kozlowski and Zychowicz (1962) reported a short-statured girl with bow legs and radiological findings which they believed were intermediate between the Jansen and Schmid types of metaphyseal chondrodysplasia. The changes in the elbow and shoulder were quite similar to the Schmid type, while those in the knee and ankle were suggestive of Jansen's type. The epiphyses were unaffected, and there were changes of a mild nature in the short tubular bones of the hands and feet. The long bones were long and slender, and the femoral head and necks normal. It appears that this intermediate form of metaphyseal chondrodysplasia is a separate entity. Its mode of inheritance is unknown.

Rimoin and McAlister (1971) described a family of 3 boys, all with short-limb dwarfism, conductive hearing loss, mental retardation, and radiographic demonstration of generalized dysplasia of the metaphyses of the tubular bones including the hands and feet. The parents, of Italian extraction, were first cousins. This interesting constellation may represent yet another metaphyseal chondrodysplasia which probably is transmitted as an autosomal recessive trait.

SPONDYLOMETAPHYSEAL DYSPLASIA

Spondylometaphyseal dysplasia is a poorly delineated condition which, until recently, was included with Morquio's disease but which is clearly different. It does not have associated visceral abnormalities, corneal clouding, deafness, or abnormal mucopolysaccharide elimination. The majority of case reports have appeared in the European literature (Kozlowski et al., 1967) Remy et al., 1970; Piffaretti et al., 1970; Michel et al., 1970). Kozlowski and co-workers described 3 unrelated children with short-trunk dwarfism. Radiographically the lesions predominated in the vertebral column and long bone metaphyses. They proposed the name spondylometaphyseal dysplasia to describe the entity.

The affected individual usually comes to medical attention between 1 and 4 years of age because of growth retardation or gait disturbance. Dwarfism is of the short-trunk type. The head and face are normal, and the neck may be somewhat short. There is mild sternal protrusion and moderate kyphosis or kyphoscoliosis. The hands are sometimes short and bulky. Joint movement tends to be limited, especially at the hip, knee, and elbow. Gait is waddling. The corneas are clear; there are no visceral abnormalities, and urine and blood chemistries are negative.

Platyspondyly is generalized, and interpedicular distances are normal. The vertebral bodies are biconvex in shape. Anterior hypoplasia of the first one or two lumbar vertebrae does not occur, a finding common in Morquio's disease. Kyphosis or kyphoscoliosis may also be present. The metaphyses are enlarged, irregular, and delayed in ossification. These lesions are most striking in the shortened femoral necks and adjacent trochanters but occur in variable degree in other metaphyses. The epiphyses are essentially normal in development. Deformity of the pelvis is characterized by roughly square ilia of decreased height, small greater sciatic notches, and horizontal acetabular roofs. Carpal and tarsal bones are retarded in development, and the short tubular bones are abbreviated with metaphyseal irregularities.

Inheritance has not been definitely established but has been considered to be an autosomal recessive trait (Kozlowski et al., 1967). However, in a recent paper Michel et al. (1970) reported 2 cases in which there was autosomal dominant transmission.

Schmidt et al. (1963) described a boy with metaphyseal dysostosis in whom gross vertebral changes were a cardinal feature. Sutcliffe (1965) also reported similar cases. These appear to be a separate entity. Compared to the Kozlowski type, there are less prominent platyspondyly, more severe peripheral metaphyseal lesions, and an entirely different pelvic configuration. The genetic transmission of this Schmidt type is not known at present.

MULTIPLE EPIPHYSEAL DYSPLASIA

Since Fairbank (1946, 1947) reviewed 26 cases of this disorder and established it as a clinical entity, there have been numerous reports and surveys. From this vast array of information it is obvious that considerable heterogeneity exists within this category of bone dysplasias. Reviewing the literature, it is impossible to segregate many of the cases into specific subgroups because of incomplete documentation of all parts of the skeleton, lack of serial studies, and failure to recognize normal variations. Despite these difficulties, it is possible to recognize a common pattern of epiphyseal disturbances.

Affected individuals are typically asymptomatic and unrecognized until 5 to 10 years of age, at which time the child is noted to be short for his age and have a waddling gait or difficulty with climbing stars and running. Joint pains and limitation of movement are common, especially in the lower limbs (Weinberg et al., 1960). In younger patients a mistaken diagnosis of bilateral Legg-Perthes disease is frequently made, while older patients often present as precocious osteoarthritis of the hips (Jacobs, 1968). The hands are sometimes short and stubby. Limitation of motion in the knees, hips, shoulders, and wrists can occur. Dwarfing is generally not severe, adult heights usually being in the range of 54 to 60 inches, and some affected persons are well over 5 feet tall. The trunk is normal, and the extremities are shortened to a variable degree. Many adults have minimal or absent symptoms, and aside from shortness of stature might escape detection (Fairbank, 1951; Weinberg et al., 1960). Intelligence is normal.

The radiological findings consist of bilateral, symmetrical irregularity and underdevelopment of the epiphyseal ossification centers. The centers may be mottled and contain occasional subsidiary centers, but there is no true stippling. The time of appearance and fusion may be retarded. The dysplasia is most severe in the hips, knees, and ankles with lesser involvement in the upper extremities. Mild shortening of the long tubular bones develops, and the metaphyses occasionally show minimal irregularity and fraying. Leeds (1960) drew attention to a deficiency in the lateral part of the distal tibial ossification center in children which causes a sloping, wedge-shaped distal tibial articular surface. This can be an important diagnostic sign when evaluating adults. Frequently a bipartite patella is present. The hands may be normal or show short stubby digits and metacarpals with irregularity of the epiphyses. Vertebral involvement is uncommon. If present, it consists primarily of Schmorl's nodes and anterior wedging of localized segments, principally in the lower thoracic or upper lumbar area (Lamy and Maroteaux, 1961). True platyspondyly does not occur in multiple epiphyseal dysplasia.

Silverman (1961) postulated a relationship between chondrodysplasia punctata (Conradi's disease) and multiple epiphyseal dysplasia. Cases which appear to represent multiple epiphyseal dyslasia in the adult sometimes present in infancy with Conradi's disease.

The familial incidence of multiple epiphyseal dysplasia was initially noted by Fairbank. Jackson et al. (1954) suggested autosomal dominant inheritance for the typical cases. Maroteaux et al. (1968) recognized autosomal recessive types. Juberg and Holt (1968) reported a family in which 4 of 15 sibs from normal parents were affected with multiple epiphyseal dysplasia. These authors reviewed the literature and found evidence supporting autosomal recessive inheritance in one form of this disorder. It is interesting that the recessively determined cases do not seem to differ from the dominantly inherited types either on clinical or radiological grounds. The generalization that recessive disorders tend to be more severe than their dominantly transmitted counterparts does not appear to be true in the multiple epiphyseal dysplasias.

PSEUDOACHONDROPLASTIC DYSPLASIA

Maroteaux and Lamy (1959) observed 3 dwarfed individuals who clinically looked very much like achondroplastic dwarfs. They termed this chondrodystrophy pseudoachondroplastic spondyloepiphyseal dysplasia. Further cases were added to the literature by Ford et al. (1961) and several others.

Dwarfism in pseudoachondroplastic dysplasia is seldom recognized until the second year of life or later, at which time the body proportions may resemble those of classical achondroplasia. The limbs show rhizomelic shortening, and the trunk is essentially of normal length. Lumbar lordosis and a waddling gait are conspicuous. Valgus deformity of the lower limbs is common although bow legs do occur. In contradistinction to achondroplasia the head and face are normal. There is no saddle-nose deformity, cranial enlargement, frontal bossing, trident hand deformity, or prominence of the mandible. Intelligence is normal.

The hands and feet are short and stubby with considerable laxity of ligaments of the wrists and fingers allowing for unusual positioning. Flexion contractures of the hips and knees are additional features. These patients do not have an increased incidence of rootlet or spinal cord compression but are often seriously handicapped by premature osteoarthritis.

X-ray examination allows for differentiation from achondroplasia. The skull and facial bones are normal, and the long bones have gross irregularities of the epiphysometaphyseal areas with fragmentation of the epiphyses and hypertrophic mushroom-type metaphyses. The vertebral bodies frequently show anterior tongue-like projections on lateral view. Platyspondyly is variable in degree, and the interpediculate distances do not narrow in the lumbar spine. The ilia tend to be large and straight-sided, the pubis and ishial bones are short and broad, and the greater sciatic notches are reduced in size. The metacarpals and phalanges are short and thick.

Hall and Dorst (1969) pointed out that there is considerable heterogeneity within this variety of dwarfism. They believe that at least four distinct forms of pseudoachondroplastic dysplasia can be recognized on clinical grounds. Inheritance is autosomal dominant in two types and autosomal recessive in two others. Roentgenologic differences further distinguish the entities.

Spondyloepiphyseal Dysplasia Tarda

Though several reports of spondyloepiphyseal dysplasia tarda can be found in the early literature under a number of diagnoses, it was first recognized as a specific disorder by Maroteaux et al. (1957).

Statural growth failure does not become evident until between 5 and 10 years of age; the shortness is primarily truncal. By adolesence it is particularly apparent and may be associated with complaints of pain and limited hip motion due to premature osteoarthritis. Low back pain and weakness are also common. Disabling arthritis and ankylosis occur in the fourth and fifth decades. The neck may be relatively short, and the chest is usually broad or barrel-shaped. Adult height varies from 4 feet, 4 inches, to 5 feet, 2 inches (Langer, 1964 a).

Radiological evaluation has been well described in the adult (Langer, 1964a) and child (Poker et al., 1965). The vertebral bodies have a distinctive configuration, most noticeable in the adult lumbar spine. Mild to moderate platyspondyly is generalized and there is a humping up, centrally and posteriorly, of bone in the ring apophysis areas. Thus the disc space appears narrowed. The thoracic cage is broad in all dimensions, while the pelvis is small and deep. Premature osteoarthrosis of the hips develops, and there are dysplastic changes in the epiphyses of the long bones. These are usually mild in degree, but can result in degenerative changes of the shoulders, knees, and ankles. The radiographic findings, coupled with the absence of metabolic and extraskeletal abnormalities, distinguish this condition from Morquio's disease, a common misdiagnosis.

Several large kindreds have been reported, establishing the X-linked recessive mode of inheritance. Jacobsen (1939) described 4 members of a family in which there were 20 affected males in four generations. He referred to the condition as Morquio's disease, but in fact they had spondyloepiphyseal dysplasia tarda. This kindred was restudied by Bannerman (1969) for evidence of Xg^a blood group linkage, and none was found.

Hypophosphatemic Familial Rickets

In childhood, familial hypophosphatemia is manifest as rickets resistant to unusually large doses of vitamin D. Infants with this disorder grow normally and have serum phosphorus concentrations in the normal range during the first months of life. At about 6 months of age, linear growth decreases and the serum phosphorus levels show a progressive fall to the very low range characteristic of familial hypophosphatemic rickets (Harrison et al., 1966). The disease clinically is manifested by disproportionate dwarfism of the short-limb type. The legs are more involved than the arm and in addition show anterior and lateral bowing deformities. The serum phosphorus level is low, serum calcium is usually normal, and in the active phase alkaline phosphatase is elevated but decreases during treatment. Archard and Witkop (1966) have drawn attention to the unusual dental abnormalities which consist of multiple gingival fistulas and periapical abscesses. The teeth show enlarged pulp chambers and elongated pulp horns extending to the dentinoenamel junction. Histologically there is globular dentin with clefts and tubular defects at the pulp horns communicating with the enamel surface. Through these defects microorganisms invade the pulp and give rise to abscess formation in the absence of carious destruction of the tooth. Skeletal features consist of radiolucency, cupping, and flaring of the metaphyses. These alterations are greatest at rapidly growing sites, especially the wrists and knees. They may be confused with the Schmid type of metaphyseal chondrodysplasia except for the abnormal metabolic parameters. With epiphyseal closure, the lesions of active rickets disappear but the deformities and dwarfism remain. Clinically the patients may bear a superficial resemblance to achondroplastic dwarfs, but this is easily dismissed on radiological examination.

A number of adults with familial hypophosphatemic rickets have been reported (Johnston et al., 1966; Steinhauser et al., 1970) with severe progressive bony proliferation including ankylosis of the spine. Between 2 and 20 years after adult height is reached, these individuals experience slowly increasing restriction of joint mobility, especially in the axial skeleton. The gait is waddling and stiff. Cord compression and other neurological complications may occur. Radiographic findings at this time include osteomalacia with a coarse trabecular pattern, dwarfism, genu varum, coxa vara, spurs or excrescences in areas of ligament and tendon insertion, and spondylosis. Osteophytes of the vertebral bodies with sclerosis and fusion of the apophyseal facets give rise to a bamboo-like spine. Pseudofractures, particularly of the proximal femurs, and radioulnar and tibiofibular synostoses are other features.

Familial hypophosphatemic rickets is inherited as an X-linked dominant trait (Winters et al., 1958). Clinically and radiologically males are on the average more severely affected than females, presumably due to the effects of Lyonization in the heterozygous female. Hypophosphatemic rickets, which clinically, radiographically, and chemically closely simulates X-linked hypophosphatemic familial rickets, has been reported as an autosomal dominant trait with male to male transmission by Bianchine et al. (1971). The basic biochemical defect is as yet incompletely understood. It has been postulated that there is a defect in the conversion of vitamin D to its biologically active form, 25-hydroxycholecalciferol. Recent work by Earp et al. (1970) indicates that such a defect does not appear to be solely responsible for the metabolic disturbances seen in this disease. Ordinarily treatment consists of vitamin D in massive doses adjusted for the individual in order to promote maximal healing with minimal risk of hypercalcemia and renal damage. When combined with oral phosphate supplements the dosage of vitamin D can be reduced. Since the biochemical defect is lifelong, and since disabling manifestations develop in some affected adults, lifelong treatment is indicated. This is particularly true in affected males (Steinhauser et al., 1970).

Mucopolysaccharidoses

The nosology of the mucopolysaccharidoses became more complicated as a result of finding metachromasia and increased mucopolysaccharides in fibroblasts cultured from patients with diseases not previously related to the mucopolysaccharidoses (reviewed by McKusick, 1969). Hitherto by combining clinical, morphologic, genetic, and biochemical approaches at least six types of genetic mucopolysaccharidoses had been recognized (McKusick, 1966).

Mucopolysaccharidosis Type I, Hurler's Syndrome

Children with Hurler's syndrome are often large at birth. Growth during the first year of life may be accelerated but subsequently deteriorates, resulting in severe dwarfism and bony deformities. Subtle changes in the facies, corneal clouding, thoracolumbar gibbus formation, and claw deformity are evident by one year of age. Developmental landmarks are retarded, and mental deterioration is severe. The facies become coarse and grotesque, and cardiac involvement, hepatosplenomegaly, hernias, continuous rhinorrhea, defective hearing, macroglossia, and hirsutism are other features. Death due to respiratory or cardiac complications usually occurs between 5 and 10 years of age. Severe skeletal changes are seen on radiological examination and include an enlarged, slipper or J-shaped sella, spatulate ribs, breaking of the lumbar vertebral bodies, and kyphosis with gibbus formation in the thoracolumbar area and abnormally short and broad long bones. There is poor modeling of the metacarpals, which have pointed proximal ends. The phalanges are also broad and reduced in length contributing to the claw hand deformity. Large quantities of acid mucopolysaccharides are excreted in the urine. Fractionation shows primarily dermatan sulfate and heparan sulfate. Peripheral white blood cells contain metachromatic granules. Similar granulations are present in reticular and plasma cells of the bone marrow. Cultured fibroblasts are filled with metachromatic granules (Danes and Bearn, 1965) and contain 10 times as much mucopolysaccharides as do normal cells, with the major increase in dermatan sulfate. Ganglioside accumulation in brain tissue and fibroblast cultures has been demonstrated (Dorfman and Matalon, 1969). A marked deficiency of a specific thermolabile β-galactosidase isoenzyme was shown by Ho and O'Brien (1969). The concept that there is a defect in degradation is supported by kinetic studies utilizing radioactive sulfate (Frantantoni et al., 1968a). The defect in Hurler's syndrome, as well as in Hunter's syndrome, can be corrected in vitro by a factor released into the fibroblast culture medium (Frantantoni et al., 1968b). Coupled with labeled sulfate this technique has been used for prenatal diagnosis of Hurler's syndrome (Frantantoni et al., 1969).

Mucopolysaccharidosis type I is inherited as an autosomal recessive trait. Using fibroblast cultures Danes and Bearn (1967a) traced heterozygous carriers through two unaffected generations.

Mucopolysaccharidosis Type II, Hunter's Syndrome

In all respects mucopolysaccharidosis type II is less severe than type I. Clinical features may not be appreciated until 2 or 3 years of age. and evolution of the clinical disease is more gradual. Mental development and linear growth slowly decline, with mental abilities plateauing by 6 years (Leroy and Crocker, 1966). Coarse facies, stiffness and contractures of the joints, claw hands, hepatosplenomegaly, hernias, cardiac complications, hirsutism, and progressive deafness develop. Clouding of the cornea is not clinically evident, though in older patients a slight haze may be observed by slit lamp examination. Lumbar gibbus does not occur. Occasionally a nodular pebble-like rash can be seen over the scapular area and upper arms. Radiological features are very similar to those in Hurler's syndrome, but are less pronounced. The urine contains increased amounts of dermatan sulfate and heparan sulfate, relatively more heparan than dermatan (Spranger, 1969). Metachromatic inclusions are present in peripheral white blood cells. Cultured fibroblasts contain similar metachromatic granules along the elevated levels of intracellular mucopolysaccharides (Matalon and Dorfman, 1966). As in the Hurler and Sanfilippo syndromes, lysosomal β-galactosidase activity is deficient, in particular the slow-moving components. Hurler and Hunter fibroblast cultures show mutual cross-correction of the metabolic defect (Frantantoni et al., 1968).

Mucopolysaccharidosis type II is inherited as an X-linked recessive trait. Clones derived from affected males contain uniform populations of metachromatic staining cells with increased cellular uronic acid. Clones derived from fathers of affected males do not show these properties. Clones from the heterozygous mothers and sisters show two cell populations: one with metachromasia and elevated uronic acid content, and a second population of normal cells (Danes and Bearn, 1967b). These studies nicely demonstrate X-linked inheritance, as well as providing evidence in favor of the Lyon hypothesis.

Mucopolysaccharidoses Type III, Sanfilippo's Syndrome

Sanfilippo et al. (1963) drew attention to children with mental retardation, mild physical abnormalities suggestive of Hurler's syndrome, and increased concentrations of heparan sulfate in the urine. Subsequently many cases were discovered, frequently in institutions for the retarded. Growth and development are usually normal until age 2 or 3 or even later, when mental retardation first becomes evident. By adolescence intellectual function has profoundly deteriorated. Shortness of stature is mild to moderate, and there is limitation of joint mobility, though not so severe as in mucopolysaccharidosis type I. The facial features are only slightly coarse, and the corneas are usually clear. Hepatosplenomegaly is slight to moderate. Behavioral management is difficult because of minimal physical impairment and severe mental retardation. Survival is into the third decade in some cases (McKusick, 1966). Radiologically the skeleton shows minimal deviations from normal (Langer, 1964b). Typically the skull is large and dolicocephalic, the calvaria thick, the sella omega-shaped, and the mastoids underpneumatized. The ribs may be oar-shaped, and the pelvis has flared ilia, narrowed acetabula, and usually coxa valga. In childhood the lower dorsal and upper lumbar vertebral bodies have a biconvex shape. The metacarpals are undermolded, and have thin cortices and prominent trabecular patterns. In the laboratory metachromatic granules can be found in peripheral lymphocytes as well as in cultured fibroblasts, which also contain large amounts of intracellular mucopolysaccharides (Dorfman and Matalon, 1969). Excess quantities of heparan sulfate are in the urine. A marked deficiency of the slow-moving components of lysosomal β-galactosidase has been shown by Ho and O'Brien (1969).

Mucopolysaccharidosis type III is inherited as an autosomal recessive trait. Heterozygote fibroblast cultures contain metachromatic inclusions (Danes and Bearn, 1967a).

Mucopolysaccharidosis Type IV, Morquio's Syndrome

Since the original description by Morquio (1929) and Brailsford (1929), a wide variety of dwarf conditions have been reported under the diagnosis of Morquio's disease. It became a catchall for most dwarfs with universal platyspondyly. On the basis of recent studies, diagnostic criteria were established.

Physical abnormalities are not apparent at birth, and mental and motor development is normal for the first year or two. The diagnosis can be made before one year of age by radiological examination in the absence of clinical signs and symptoms (Robins et al., 1963). Affected children usually present at age 1 or 2 because of awkward gait, failure to grow well, knock-knees, sternal bulging, flaring of the rib cage, flat feet, prominent joints, or dorsal kyphosis. With advancing age, all of these deformities increase and growth failure is marked. It tends to cease by 10 or 12 years, resulting in short-trunk dwarfism. Adults rarely exceed 4 feet in height. Corneal clouding is seen between 5 and 10 years of age. Slit lamp examination may be necessary to demonstrate this in younger children; frequently it is clinically apparent in adults but is never as striking as the corneal clouding of Mucopolysaccharidosis type I. Both deciduous and permanent teeth are abnormal (Garn and Hurme, 1952; Maroteaux and Lamy, 1963; Langer and Carey, 1966). The teeth are gray in color, have thin, easily fractured enamel, and are carious. The joints tend to be lax, most notably at the wrists. Severe genu valgum may interfere with ambulation. Hearing may be defective, and intelligence is generally normal. Aortic regurgitation and spinal cord compression are complications which lead to death before 20 years of age, although survival into the fourth decade has occurred.

The osseous abnormalities of mucopolysaccharidosis IV have been delineated by Langer and Carey (1966). Universal platyspondyly is characteristic, and of a specific pattern which varies with age. Early the dorsal vertebrae are oval in shape. Growth in height is very slow between 2 and 5 years of age, and is associated with an anterior projection or tongue. These changes progress in severity and lead to flattened rectangular bodies with wide disc spaces in the adult. The lumbar vertebral bodies are beaked or hook-shaped. The odontoid process is hypoplastic or absent with fitting of the posterior arches of the first cervical vertebra into the foramen magnum. Flared ilia with a long narrow configuration are typical of the pelvic changes. Early in development the capital femoral epiphyses are normal or only slightly flattened. However, progressive flattening and fragmentation occurs and coxa valga becomes more prominent. Coxa vara does not occur in Morquio's syndrome. The femoral heads in the adolescent and adult frequently disappear, resulting in erosion and widening of the necks. The carpal centers are small and retarded in appearance. Growth plates of the distal radius and ulna slope towards each other, and the metaphyses are wide and irregular. The long bones are short and poorly turbulated, especially in the upper extremities. Spatulate ribs, dorsal kyphosis, and sternal protrusion are other findings. The urine usually contains increased amounts of keratan sulfate. Perhaps this phenomenon is related to age. Campailla and Martinella (1969) found that mucopolysacchariduria in three sibs with Morquio's syndrome decreased with age and disappeared after puberty. Peripheral blood smears may show metachromasia of the white blood cells. Enzymatic defects have not been determined. The mode of inheritance is autosomal recessive.

Mucopolysaccharidosis Type V, Scheie Syndrome

This disorder of mucopolysaccharide metabolism was originally described by Scheie et al. (1962), and relatively few cases have been recognized (Emerit et al., 1966; McKusick, 1966). There is little or no impairment of intellect though psychosis may develop in adulthood. Stature may be normal or only mildly affected. Facial features are heavy with a broad mouth and full lips evident by 5 to 8 years. The corneas are clouded with the greatest density peripherally. Other features include: hirsutism, mild joint stiffness, pes cavus, retinal pigmentation, aortic regurgitation, and carpal tunnel syndrome. Radiologic examination shows remarkably little in the way of gross changes. The ribs tend to be spatulate, and there are cystic changes at the wrists, Large amounts of dermatan sulfate are excreted in the urine, and there is metachromasia of peripheral lymphocytes. No enzyme defects have been determined. Evidence points to autosomal recessive inheritance.

Mucopolysaccharidosis Type VI, Maroteaux-Lamy Syndrome

Maroteaux et al. (1963) delineated a new entity among the mucopolysaccharidoses, the major clinical features of which were normal intelligence and severe skeletal malformations. Additional patients have been reported by McKusick et al. (1965b), Sarrauy et al. (1965), and Rampini and Maroteaux (1966).

In infancy umbilical or inguinal hernias and recurrent respiratory infections are common. Psychomotor development is normal. On learning to walk the gait is wobbling and awkward. Statural growth ceases by 7 or 8 years resulting in rather marked dwarfism. Joint motion is restricted, particularly at the knees, hips, and elbows and posture is crouched. Gargoyle-like facies gradually develop by 5 or 6 years of age; these changes vary from moderate to grotesque within a sibship (McKusick, 1965; Scott, 1969b). Claw hand deformities, sternal prominence, a flared and grooved rib cage, short trunk, hepatosplenomegaly, and corneal clouding are regular features. Aortic and mitral valvular involvement is frequent. The skin is hirsute and has a firm or tight quality. Hearing may be deficient. Hydrocephalus has also been reported (Goldberg and Scott, 1970). The similarity to Hurler's syndrome is remarkable except for one important item. These children are normal intellectually, at least until late in the course of the disorder.

Skeletal examination reveals striking abnormalities. The skull is large and often dolicocephalic with great enlargement of the sella. The odontoid process is hypoplastic, and the lumbar vertebrae tend to have anterior beaks. In the pelvis the iliac wings are flared and the body poorly developed, producing obliquity of the acetabula. The femoral heads are irregular in ossification, and the elongated necks are overconstricted and in valgus position. The distal radius and ulna epiphysis and metaphyses are deformed and slant towards each other. The short tubular bones of the hands and feet are wide and reduced in length. Small, irregular carpal bones and proximal pointing of the metacarpals are typical findings. As in the other mucopolysaccharidoses the ribs are spatulate. Urinary mucopolysaccharide excretion is increased, with the major component dermatan sulfate. Peripheral blood cells, bone marrow cells, and cultured fibroblasts demonstrate metachromasia. Lysosomal enzyme studies have not been published. The Maroteaux-Lamy syndrome is inherited as an autosomal recessive trait. The existence of heterogeneity within this category has been proposed by Spranger (1969) based primarily on the degree of dysplasia in the hands.

Mucolipidoses and Lipidoses

With the development of sophisticated laboratory techniques within the past few years, a group of storage diseases has emerged which has signs, symptoms, and biochemical characteristics of both the mucopolysaccharidoses and the sphingolipidoses. Often these cases were reported as atypical or variant forms of Hurler's syndrome. With the exception of the Austin type of juvenile sulfatidosis, urinary mucopolysaccharide excretion is generally normal; at times mucopolysaccharide screening tests may be weakly positive, however. Although insufficient cases are reported, evidence favors autosomal recessive inheritance in each type.

Spranger and Wiedemann (1970) have proposed that this group of inherited metabolic diseases be classified as a separate group of thesaurismoses: the mucolipidoses, types I, II, and III. In addition, the generalized gangliosidoses, Austin-type juvenile sulfatidosis, fucosidosis, and mannosidosis are included because of the similarity of clinical, radiographic, and biochemical findings.

Mucolipidosis, Type I (Formerly Lipomucopolysaccharidosis)

Formerly these cases were considered under the name of lipomucopolysaccharidosis (Spranger et al., 1968). These children are normal until about 6 months of age when psychomotor retardation occurs; the mental retardation is not as severe as in Hurler's syndrome. Gargoyle-like clinical features appear in the second or third year of life. Cherry-red macular spots may be present. Increasing neurologic deterioration with hypotonia and ataxia is apparent in the preschool age. Urinary mucopolysaccharide excretion is normal, there are vacuolated lymphocytes in the peripheral blood smears, and fibroblast cultures show unusual cytoplasmic inclusions. The bone marrow contains coarsely vacuolated and granulated storage cells. Abnormal amounts of mucopolysaccharides and glycolipids can be demonstrated by histochemistry and electronmicroscopy. Lysosomal enzyme deficits have not been shown. Radiologic examination reveals changes similar to those in the Sanfilippo type of mucopolysaccharidosis. The disorder appears to be inherited as an autosomal recessive trait. Pincus et al. (1967) and Spranger et al. (1968) found vacuolated lymphocytes in peripheral blood and bone marrow cells in unaffected parents suggesting heterozygote manifestation.

Mucolipidosis, Type II (Formerly I-Cell Disease)

This disorder was described by Leroy et al. (1969) under the title I-cell disease. Clinical involvement may be noted at birth or shortly thereafter. Early features are congenital hip dislocation, hyperplasia of the gingival ridges, hernias, and a tightness of the skin making it impossible to pick up a fold of skin. These children are considered to be "good"; they do little fussing and have a generally placid nature. Developmental landmarks are slow, and mental retardation is severe. Hurler-like facial features and dwarfing become pronounced. Additional features include clear cornea, restricted joint mobility, and hepatosplenomegaly. Urinary mucopolysaccharide levels are normal. Peripheral blood smears demonstrate vacuolization of the lymphocytes; similar cells are also present in the bone marrow. Cultured fibroblasts contain coarse inclusions similar to those in Hurler's syndrome but with unusual staining properties (Matalon et al., 1968). Storage of abnormal amounts of both mucopolysaccharides and glycolipids is suggested, but the exact nature of the storage substances is unknown. Lysosomal enzyme defects have not been delineated. Radiographically there are striking changes which are quite like those of mucopolysaccharidosis type I (Hurler's syndrome). An autosomal recessive mode of inheritance is likely, based on multiple affected sibships, parental consanguinity, and discovery of coarse fibroblast inclusions in heterozygotes (Spranger and Wiedmann, 1970).

Mucolipidoses, Type III (Formerly Pseudo-Hurler Polydystrophy)

Under the designation of "pseudo-polydystrophie," Maroteaux and Lamy (1966) described 4 children with many features of Hurler's syndrome but with normal mucopolysaccharide levels in the urine and a slower clinical course.

Relatively few cases have reached the literature (McKusick et al., 1965; Steinbach et al., 1968; Scott and Grossman, 1969; Scott, 1971).

Clinical signs and symptoms are detected between 2 and 4 years of age. Medical consultation is sought because of short stature, gait disturbance, joint contractures, or restriction of joint motion. Mild gargoyle-like facial features are present, and mental retardation is mild to moderate. The corneas are clinically clear but show fine opacities by slit lamp examination. Cardiac involvement, most characteristically aortic regurgitation, occurs.

No vacuolization or metachromatic inclusions are present in peripheral blood smears although the bone marrow has vacuolated plasma cells suggesting glycolipid storage. Metachromatic inclusions have been demonstrated with alcian blue stains in cultured fibroblasts. The urinary excretion of mucopolysaccharides is normal. Radiological examination reveals irregularity and immaturity of the vertebral bodies, oar-shaped ribs, hypoplasia of the odontoid process, and pelvic deformity with low iliac wings and hypoplasia of the body. Coxa valga and flattened irregular proximal femoral epiphyses are typical. The hands have pointed proximal metacarpals and claw deformities. Inheritance is autosomal recessive.

Fucosidosis

Three patients have been reported with mental and motor retardation noted between 1 and 3 years, followed by progressive neurological deterioration and death by 4 to 6 years of age (Durand et al., 1969; Loeb et al., 1969). Mild gargoyle features become apparent, but the corneas remain transparent. Peripheral blood lymphocytes have vacuolated cytoplasm but no metachromatic granules. No abnormalities are seen in bone marrow cells, and urinary mucopolysaccharides are normal. Activity of α-fucosidase, a lysosomal enzyme, is absent in all tissues (Van Hoof and Hers, 1968a, 1968b), and fucose containing glycolipids accumulate in the liver and brain. Increased amounts of hexuronic acid are also found indicating storage of mucopolysaccharides. The pattern of inheritance is unknown, however an autosomal recessive mode is probable.

Mannosidosis

Öckerman (1967) reported the only case of mannosidosis. His patient was a boy with retarded growth and development, recurrent respiratory infections, facial features of Hurler's syndrome, mild hepatomegaly, hypotonia, and lumbar gibbus. The corneas were not clouded. Skeletal changes were mildly suggestive of a mucopolysaccharidosis. PAS-positive inclusions and vacuoles were demonstrated in lymphocytes. Urinary mucopolysaccharides were normal. Histological examination of the brain showed neuronal distention by PAS-positive material, the nature of which is undetermined. Total mannose levels in the liver were greatly increased. Lysosomal α-mannosidase levels were very low in liver, spleen, and brain. There is no information concerning inheritance.

Generalized GM_1 Gangliosidosis

The generalized GM_1 gangliosidoses are inherited neurovisceral storage diseases in which both gangliosides and mucopolysaccharides accumulate. Two types are recognized. Type I, the classic form, has been published under 12 or more designations including familial neurovisceral lipidosis (Landing et al., 1964) and Tay-Sachs disease with visceral involvement (Norman et al., 1959). O'Brien (1969) and Spranger and Wiedemann (1970) have reviewed over 24 reported cases. From birth these infants fail to thrive. They present with weakness, dependent edema, poor feeding, and weight gain. Physical examination reveals coarse facial features characterized by frontal bossing, depressed nasal bridge, a long full upper lip, gingival hypertrophy, and macroglossia, all of which give the impression of Hurler's syndrome. Half of the children have macular cherry-red spots and occasionally corneal opacities are found. Hepatosplenomegaly is present in all cases by 6 to 8 months of age. Short, stubby hands, dorsolumbar kyphoscoliosis, and multiple flexion contractures of the joints occur. Mental-motor retardation is apparent from birth, and neurological deterioration rapidly develops after the first year of life. Seizures, blindness, and swallowing difficulties precede death, which generally happens by age 2. Severe skeletal lesions are present, and hypoplastic, beaked vertebral bodies are typically found in the area of the lumbar gibbus. During the first few months of life symmetrical periosteal new bone formation cloaks the long bones. With increasing age the externally thickened cortical walls are thinned by expansion of the medulary cavity. The ribs are paddle-shaped, and the proximal metacarpals are bullet-shaped. Bone trabeculation is coarse, and maturation is retarded.

Urinary mucopolysaccharide excretion is normal. Peripheral lymphocytes and bone marrow histiocytes are vacuolated. Similar vacuoles are seen in Kupffer cells and renal glomerular epithelial cells. Neuronal lipidosis occurs throughout the brain and spinal cord. There is a generalized accumulation of GM_1 gangliosides and visceral and mesenchymal storage of an acid mucopolysaccharide similar to keratan sulfate. The activity of lysosomal acid β-galactosidase isoenzymes A, B, and C is absent in all tissues including fibroblasts, urine (Thomas, 1969), and peripheral white cells (Singer and Schafer, 1970).

Generalized GM_1 gangliosidosis type I is inherited as an autosomal recessive trait. Reduced β-galactosidase activity has been reported in heterozygotes (O'Brien, 1969).

Type II generalized gangliosidosis, due to abnormal cerebral accumulation of GM_1 ganglioside and visceral storage of an undersulfated keratan sulfate, has been described in 9 patients (Spranger and Wiedemann, 1970). The clinical manifestations are primarily those of severe neurological deterioration beginning at less than one year of age and rapidly progressing to convulsions and death between 3 and 10 years of age. Hurler-like facies, corneal opacities macular lesions, and hepatosplenomegaly do not occur. Although mild skeletal features suggestive of early type II mucopolysaccharidosis are present, there is normal urinary excretion of uronic acid containing mucopolysaccharides. Only the brain contains unusual amounts of GM_1 ganglioside while the liver and spleen accumulate large amounts of an undersulfated keratan sulfate-like mucopolysaccharide. Though the activity of β-galactosidase activity is markedly deficient in the brain, liver, fibroblasts, and white blood cells, it is only the isoenzymes B and C which show reduced activity in the liver. Inheritance is thought to be as an autosomal recessive trait.

Sulfatidosis with Mucopolysacchariduria

Three patients have been described (Austin, 1965; Thieffry et al., 1967) with juvenile metachromatic leukodystrophy, physical findings of mucopolysachariduria, and radiological changes of a gargoyle nature. These children are retarded in development. Slowly, progressive neurological deterioration begins around the second year of life, and death occurs in the early teens. The facies suggest a mild Hurler's syndrome, but the corneas are not clouded and there is no hepatosplenomegaly. Growth failure develops, and the individuals are short in stature. Increased amounts of sulfated mucopolysaccharides are found in the urine. Peripheral nerve biopsies may show metachromatic myelin degeneration. In contradistinction to the classic type of metachromatic leukodystrophy where there is absence of only arylsulfatase A, in the Austin type of metachromatic leukodystrophy all three arylsulfatases, A, B, and C, are absent. Autosomal recessive inheritance is likely but not established.

HYPOPITUARY DWARFISM

In 1902 Gilford proposed the term ateliosis ("not perfected") for those dwarfs with normal body proportions. He further distinguished sexual and asexual forms of ateliosis, depending on whether sexual development was or was not normal. After a number of years, the role of the pituitary in growth was established but progress in understanding human growth hormone was impeded by technical problems in its assay. The development of specific radioimmunoassays for human growth hormone led to new interest in the various forms of hypopituitary dwarfism, popularly known as midgets. Those individuals with sexual ateliosis were found to have isolated deficiency of growth hormone (Rimoin et al., 1966), and the asexual ateliotics were due to multiple hormone deficiencies, i.e., panhypopituitarism.

In isolated human growth hormone deficiency birth weight and length are usually normal. Growth retardation is not apparent until 6 months to 1 year of age. Although puberty is spontaneous, the onset of sexual maturation is delayed until 15 to 25 years of age in both sexes. Growth spurts of 7.5 to 20.5 cm often accompany puberty (Rimoin et al., 1968b). Adult weights range from 26.0 to 57.9 kg and their heights from 110 to 140 cm. Upper/lower segment ratios are over 1.0; thus body proportions are childlike with a relatively long trunk and short legs. Females menstruate and breast-feed their offspring (Rimoin et al., 1968a). The skin is soft, finely wrinkled, and appears thicker than normal, possibly due to increased subcutaneous fat. Their voices are high pitched with an unusual, distinctive tone.

Currently the genetic defects resulting in a monotropic deficiency of human growth hormone are not fully defined, but at least four types can be classified on a metabolic and hormonal basis (Merimee et al., 1969). In type I there is less than 5.0 ng/ml of human growth hormone in the plasma after provocative stimuli. Hypoglycemia after insulin is prolonged. Insulinopenia is found after arginine or glucose administration, and these individuals are responsive to exogenous human growth hormone. Autosomal recessive inheritance has been established in several families (Rimoin et al., 1966). Genetic evidence of the existence of two separate types of insulinopenic growth hormone deficiency is provided by a mating in which a phenotypically indistinguishable growth hormone-deficient mother and father produced 2 normal offspring (Rimoin et al., 1968c).

Human growth hormone levels are less than 5.0 ng/ml after arginine infusion or insulin-induced hypoglycemia in type II growth hormone deficiency, but these individuals are not hypersensitive to administered insulin. Insulin levels are normal or greater than normal in response to glucose or arginine, and there is resistance to exogenous human growth hormone. Though more rare than the autosomal recessive type, type II appears to be inherited as an autosomal dominant trait. An affected mother and daughter (with affected persons in other generations) have been studied, as well as sporadic cases (McKusick, 1968).

Type III growth hormone deficiency was described by Laron et al. (1966) in Yemenite Jews in Israel. An isolated case reported by Merimee et al. (1969) may be the same disorder. These individuals have relatively high basal levels of plasma growth hormone which are not suppressed by oral glucose and are further augmented by hypoglycemia and by arginine infusion. These patients have decreased response to exogenous human growth hormone. These observations suggest either than the endogenous growth hormone was immunologically active but biologically inactive, or that the metabolic action of growth hormone was blocked at the peripheral tissue level. Studies of Daughaday et al. (1969) indicate that the defect in the Laron-type midget involves the synthesis of sulfation factor in response to growth hormone. The pattern of inheritance is clearly autosomal recessive in the Yemenite cases of Laron.

A fourth type of asexual ateliosis is represented by the Babinga pygmies of Africa. Pygmies attain normal plasma concentrations of growth hormone after both arginine infusion and insulin-induced hypoglycemia like type I human growth hormone-deficient individuals, and show hypoglycemic unresponsiveness after arginine and glucose ingestion. Administration of exogenous human growth hormone leads to none of the usual metabolic responses. Sulfation factor activity is normal, however. Rimoin et al. (1969b) postulated that pygmies have end-organ subresponsiveness to the metabolic effects of human growth hormone.

Panhypopituitarism is most frequently idiopathic and not genetic. However, evidence of a rare autosomal recessive form has been presented by McKusick and Rimoin (1967). Six people in three families of an inbred religious sect, the Hutterites, had panhypopituitarism with deficiencies of gonadotropins, thyrotropin, ACTH, and human growth hormone. They had childlike body proportions, short stature, sexual infantilism, signs and symptoms of hypothyroidism, and adrenal insufficiency. In addition skeletal maturation was retarded, with open epiphyses, even in one patient age 36. Two of these patients, age 4 and 24, responded satisfactorily to exogenous human growth hormone. Hanhart (1925) described a type of dwarfism occurring in an inbred group on the island of Krk in the Adriatic. Zergollern (1971) restudied these people and concluded that they have panhypopituitarism apparently inherited as an autosomal recessive trait. Schimke et al. (1971) have evidence of X-linked recessive inheritance of panhypopituitarism. Their family consists of 2 affected half brothers with the same mother. Phelan et al. (1971) reported 4 affected males in three sibships related through carrier females.

Scott and Mengel (1971) reported 2 unrelated males each with idiopathic hypopituitarism and osteogenesis imperfecta. Family histories revealed no other affected individuals and no parental consanguinity. It is likely that damage to the hypothalamo-pituitary axis during birth or at some other early stage, secondary to the primary connective tissue disorder, is responsible for the hypopituitarism. Undoubtedly the classes of hereditary hypopituitarism listed above do not exhaust all the heterogeneity in this category. There are many steps in the pathways of growth hormone synthesis, release, and action which can be interrupted by gene mutation.

CONCLUSION

The material discussed in this review illustrates a number of genetic principles. The most obvious of these is heterogeneity. Achondroplasia, as the prototype of short-limb dwarfs, for a long time included a number of "atypical forms" and "variants." With careful scrutiny and attention to phenotypic variation, diastrophic dwarfism, the metaphyseal chondrodysplasias, thanatophoric dwarfism, and a host of other entities were delineated Exaggeration of skeletal deformities which are incompatible with survival beyond the neonatal period or early infancy are possible consequences of homozygosity in autosomal dominantly inherited traits, such as achondroplasia. The relation of negative selection and mutation equilibrium are demonstrated by dwarfism. Despite low reproductive fitness, achondroplasia remains the most common type of hereditary intrinsic bone disease resulting in drawfism. The majority of the cases are sporadic presumably due to new mutation. The effect of paternal age was discussed in both achondroplasia and spondyloepiphyseal dysplasia congenita. The principle of fitness and its relationship to clinical variability were also illustrated. When the mode of transmission is autosomal dominant and fitness is reduced, there is very little variability of the phenotype; conversely, there is greater variability when fitness is little affected.

The multiple effects of a single gene, or pleiotropism, are portrayed in many extraskeletal tissues. They are not only of general interest but can be important for diagnosis, prognosis, and treatment. Eye abnormalities occur in the mucopolysaccharidoses and spondyloepiphyseal dysplasia congenita; skin and nail lesions are features of chondrodysplasia punctata and McKusick's type of metaphyseal chondrodysplasia; dental lesions and congenital heart disease are frequent in chondroectodermal dysplasia; and kidney disease is associated with asphyxiating thoracic dysplasia.

As would be predicted, females affected with certain rare X-linked dominant traits, such as hypophosphatemic familial rickets, outnumber affected males. On the average the disorder is more severe in males, related to the hemizygous state of males and to the heterozygous state of affected females. Furthermore, because of Lyonization of the X-chromosome, heterozygous females show greater variability of phenotype than affected males. Studies in the Hunter type of mucopolysaccharidosis (MPS II) have not only established the X-linked mode of inheritance but have afforded laboratory support for the Lyon principle. The Founder effect was demonstrated by pedigree analysis of an inbred community in which all parents of multiple sibships affected with chondroectodermal dysplasia could be shown to have a common progenitor. The usefulness of study of inbred groups to the nosology of recessive disorders is illustrated by the McKusick type of metaphyseal chondrodysplasia. The axiom that autosomal recessive traits tend to be due to enzyme deficiencies has been exemplified by generalized gangliosidosis, fucosidosis, hypophosphatasia, and, tentatively, by certain mycopolysaccharidoses.

REFERENCES

Allansmith, M., and E. Senz. 1960. Chondrodystrophia congenita punctata (Conradi's disease). Review of literature and report of case with unusual features. Amer. J. Dis. Child. 100:109-116.

Archard, H. O., and C. J. Witkop. 1966. Hereditary hypophosphatemia presenting primary dental malformations. Oral Surg. 22:184-193.

Armaly, M. F. 1957. Ocular involvement in chondrodystrophic calcificans congenita punctata. Arch. Ophthal. 57:491-502.

Auerbach, C. 1956, A possible case of delayed mutation in man. Ann. Hum. Genet. 20:266-269.

Austin, J. H. 1965. Mental retardation. Metachromatic leucodystrophy. In Carter, C. C. (Ed.), Medical Aspects of Mental Retardation. Springfield, Ill., Thomas.

Bach, C., P. Maroteaux, P. Schaefer, A. Bitan, and C. Crumiere. 1967. Dysplasic spondylo-epiphysaire congénitale avec anomalies multiples. Arch. Franc. Pediat. 24:23-33.

Bannerman, R. M. 1969. X-linked spondyloepiphyseal dysplasia tarda (SDT). The Clinical Delineation of Birth Defects, Part 5, Birth Defects: Original Article Series. New York, National Foundation–March of Dimes.

Beals, R. K. 1969. Hypochondroplasia. A report of five kindreds. J. Bone Joint Surg. (Amer.) 51:728-739.

Beaudoing, A., M. Bost, and J. Pont. 1969. Nanisme thantophore. Une observation anatomo-clinique. Pédiatrie 24:459-461.

Bianchine, J. W., A. A. Stambler, and H. E. Harrison. 1971. Familial hypophosphatemic rickets showing autosomal dominant inheritance. Clinical Delineation of Birth Defects, Part 9, Birth Defects: Original Article Series. Baltimore, Williams & Wilkins.

Brailsford, J. F. 1929. Chondro-osteo-dystrophy, roentgenographic and clinical features of child with dislocation of vertebrae. Amer. J. Surg. 7:404-410.

Burgert, E. O., Jr., J. C. Dower, and W. N. Tauxe. 1965. A new syndrome—argenerative anemia, malabsorption (celiac), dyschondroplasia, and hyperphosphatemia. J. Pediat. 67:711-712.

Burian, H. M., G. K. von Noorden, and I. V. Ponseti. 1960. Chamber angle anomalies in systemic connective tissue disorders. Arch. Ophthal. 64:671-680.

Caffey, J. 1967. Pediatric X-Ray Diagnosis, ed. 5. Chicago, Year Book.

Campailla, E., and B. Martinelli. 1969. Morquio's disease: modification of mucopolysacchariduria with advancing age: report of three cases The Clinical Delineation of Birth Defects, Part 5, Birth Defects: Original Article Series. New York, The National Foundation–March of Dimes.

Cohen, M. S., A. D. Rosenthal, and D. D. Matson. 1967. Neurological abnormalities in achondroplastic children. J. Pediat. 71:367-376.

Comings, D. E., C. Papazian, and H. R. Schoene. 1968. Conradi's disease (chondrodystrophia calcificans congenita, congenital stippled epiphyses). J. Pediat. 72:63-69.

Cronberg, N. E. 1933. A case of chondrodystrophia foetalis, diagnosed by x-ray examination before delivery. Acta Obstet. Gynec. Scand. 13:275-282.

Danes, B. S., and A. G. Bearn. 1965. Hurler's syndrome: demonstration of an inherited disorder of connective tissues in cell culture. Science 149:987-989.

—, and —. 1967a. Cellular metachromasia: a genetic marker for studying the mucopolysaccharidoses. Lancet 1:241-243.

—, and —. 1967b. Hurler's syndrome: a genetic study of clones in cell culture with particular reference to the Lyon hypothesis. J. Exp. Med. 126:509-522.

Daughaday, W. H., Z. Laron, A. Pertzelan, and J. N. Heins. 1969. Defective sulfation factor generation: a possible etiological link in dwarfism. Trans. Ass. Amer. Physicians 82:129-140.

De Haas, W. H. D., W. DeBoer, and F. Griffioen. 1969. Metaphysial dysostosis. A late follow-up of the first reported case. J. Bone Joint Surg. (Amer.) 51:290-299.

Dennis, J. P., H. S. Rosenberg, and E. C. Alvord. 1961. Megalencephaly, internal hydrocephalus and other neurological aspects of achondroplasia. Brain 84:427-445.

Dent, C. E., and I. C. S. Normand. 1964. Metaphyseal dysostosis, type Schmid. Arch. Dis. Child. 39:444-454.

Dorfman, A., and R. Matalon. 1969. The Hurler and Hunter syndromes. Amer. J. Med. 47:691-707.

Durand, P., C. Barrone, and G. Della Cella. 1966. A new mucopolysaccharidelipid storage disease? Lancet 2:1313-1314.

———, ———, and ———. 1969. Fucosidosis. J. Pediat. 75:665-674.

Earp. H. S., R. L. Ney, H. J. Gitelman, R. Richman, and H. F. DeLuca. 1970. Effects of 25-hydroxycholecalciferol in patients with familial hypophosphatemia and vitamin-D-resistant rickets. New Eng. J. Med. 283:627-630.

Ellis, R. W. B., and S. van Creveld. 1940. A syndrome characterized by ectodermal dysplasia, polydactyly, chondro-dysplasia and congenital morbus coris: report of three cases. Arch. Dis. Child. 15:65-84.

Emerit, I., P. Maroteaux, and P. Vernant. 1966. Deux observations de mucopolysaccharidose avec atteinte cardio-vasculaire. Arch. Franc. Pediat. 23:1075-1087.

Fairbank, H. A. T. 1946. Dysplasia epiphysealis multiplex. Proc. Roy Soc. Med. 39:315-317.

Fairbank, T. 1947. Dysplasia epiphysialis multiplex. Brit. J. Surg. 34:225-232.

———. 1951. An Atlas of General Affectations of the Skeleton. Edenburg, Livingstone.

Fallis, N., F. L. Barnes, and N. DiFerrante. 1968. A case of polydystrophic dwarfism with urinary excretion of dermatan sulfate and heparan sulfate. J. Clin. Endocr. 28:26-33.

Fleury, J., C. H. deMenibus, and E. C. Hazard. 1966. Un cas singulier de dystrophic osteochondrale congenitale (Nanisme metatropique de Maroteauz). Ann Pediat. 13:453-456.

Ford, N., F. N. Silverman, and K. Kozlowski. 1961. Spondylo-epiphyseal dysplasia (pseudoachondroplastic type). Amer. J. Roentgen. 86:462-472.

Fraccaro, M. 1952. Contributo allo studio delle malattie del mesenchima osteopoietico: l'acondrogenesi. Folia Hered. Path. 1:190-208.

Fratantoni, J. C., C. W. Hall, and E. F. Neufeld. 1968a. The defect in Hurler's and Hunter's syndrome: faulty degredation of mucopolysaccharide. Proc. Nat. Acad. Sci. U.S.A. 60:699-706.

———, ———, and ———. 1968b. Hurler and Hunter syndromes: mutual correction of the defect in cultured fibroblasts. Science 162:570-572.

———, E. F. Neufeld, B. W. Uhlendorf, and C. B. Jacobson. 1969. Intrauterine diagnosis of the Hurler and Hunter syndromes. New Eng. J. Med. 280:686-688.

Frazer, G. R., and A. I. Friedmann. 1967. The Causes of Blindness in Childhood. Baltimore, Hopkins.

———, ———, P. Maroteaux, A. M. Glen-Bott, and U. Mitwoch. 1969. Dysplasia spondyloepiphysaria congenita and related generalized skeletal dysplasias among children with severe visual handicaps. Arch. Dis. Child. 44:490-498.

Fulginiti, V. A., W. E. Hathaway, D. S. Perlman, and C. H. Kempe. 1967. Agammaglobulinemia and achondroplasia. Brit. Med. J. 2:242.

Garn, S. M., and V. O. Hurme. 1952. Dental defects in three siblings afflicted with Morquio's disease. Brit. Dent. J. 93:210-216.

Giedion, A. 1968. Thanatrophoric dwarfism. Helv. Paediat. Acta 23:175-183.

Goldberg, M. F. and C. I. Scott. 1970. Hydrocephalus and papilledema in the Maroteaux-Lamy syndrome (mucopolysaccharidosis type VI). Amer. J. Ophthal. 69:970-975.

Gorlin, R. J., and H. Sedano. 1970. Achondrogenesis. Mod. Med. 38:144-145.

Grebe, H. 1952. Achondrogenesis ein einfaches rezessives Erbmerkmal. Folia Hered. Path. 2:23-28.

———. 1955. Chondrodysplasie. Rome, Institute Gregor Mendel.

Hall, J. G., and J. P. Dorst. 1969. Four types of pseudoachondroplastic spondyloepiphyseal dysplasia (SED). The Clinical Delineation of Birth Defects, Part 5, Birth Defects: Original Article Series. New York, National Foundation–March of Dimes.

———, ———, H. Taybi, C. I. Scott, L. O. Langer, and V. A. McKusick. 1969. Clinical Delineation of Birth Defects, Part 5, Brith Defects: Original Article Series. New York, National Foundation–March of Dimes.

Hanhart, E. 1925. Über heredodegenerativein Zwergwuchs mit Dystrophia Adiposogenitalis. An Hand von Untersuchungen bei drei Sippen von proportionierten Zwergen. Arch. Klaus Stift. Vererbungsforsch. 1:181-257.

Harrison, H. E., H. C. Harrison, F. Lifshitz, and A. D. Johnson. 1966. Growth disturbance in hereditary hypophosphatemia. Amer. J. Dis. Child. 112:290-297.

Herdman, R. C., and L. O. Langer. 1968. The thoracic asphyxiant dystrophy and renal disease. Amer. J. Dis. Child. 116:192-201.

Ho, M. W., and J. S. O'Brien. 1969. Hurler's syndrome: deficiency of a specific beta galactosidase isoenzyme. Science 165:611-613.

Holt, J. F. 1969. Discussion: Jansen's metaphyseal dysostosis. Clinical Delineation of Birth Defects, Part 4, Birth Defects: Original Article Series. New York, National Foundation–March of Dimes.

Houston, C. S. 1970. Personal communication, Saskatoon, Saskatchewan.

Huguenin, M., C. Godard, P. E. Ferrier, and F. Bamatter. 1969. Two different mutations within the same sibship: thanatophoric dwarfism and Ullrich-Feichtiger syndrome. Helv. Paediat. Acta 24:239-245.

Jackson, W. P. U., J. Hanelin, and F. Albright. 1954. Metaphyseal dysplasia, epiphyseal dysplasia, diaphyseal dysplasia, and related conditions. II: Multiple epiphyseal dysplasia; its relation to other disorders of epiphyseal development. Arch. Intern. Med. 94:886-901.

Jacobs, P. A. 1968. Dysplasia epiphysialis multiplex. Clin. Orthop. 58:117-128.

Jacobsen, A. W. 1939. Hereditary osteochondrodystrophia deformans: family with 20 members affected in 5 generations. J.A.M.A. 113:121-124.

Jánsen, M. 1934. Über atypische chondrodystrophic (Achondroplasie) und über eine noch nicht beschriebene angeborene Wachstumstörung des Knochensystems: metaphysäre Dysostosis. Z. Orthop. Chir. 61:253-286.

Jeune, M., C. Beraud, and R. Carron. 1955. Dystrophic thoracique asphyxiante de caractère familial. Arch. Franc. Pédiat. 12:886-891.

Johnston, C. C., G. J. Kurlander, D. M. Smith, J. M. Goodman, and R. L. Campbell. 1966. Familial vitamin D resistant rickets in untreated adult. Arch. Intern. Med. 117:141-147.

Josephson, B. M., and M. D. Oriatti. 1961. Chondrodystrophia calcificans congenita. Report of a case and review of the literature. Pediatrics 28:425-435.

Juberg, R. C., and J. F. Holt. 1968. Inheritance of multiple epiphyseal dysplasia, tarda. Amer. J. Hum. Genet. 20:549-563.

Kaplan, M., J. Sauvegrain, F. Hayem, P. Drapeau, F. Maugey, and J. Boulle. 1961. Etude d'un nouveau cas de nanisme diastrophique. Arch. Franc. Pediat. 18:981-1001.

Kaufman, R. L., D. L. Rimoin, W. H. McAlister, and J. M. Kissane. 1970. Thanatophoric dwarfism. Amer. J. Dis. Child. 120:53-57.

Keats, T. E., H. O. Riddervold, and L. L. Michaelis. 1970. Thanatophoric dwarfism. Amer. J. Roentgen. 108:473-480.

Kniest, W. 1952. Zur Abgrenzung der Dysostosis Enchondralis von der Chondrodystrophie. Z. Kinderheilk. 70:633-640.

Kohler, E. and D. P. Babbitt. 1970. Dystrophic thoraces and infantile asphyxia. Radiology 94:55-62.

Kozlowski, K. 1965. Hypochondroplasia. Pol. Rev. Radiol. Nucl. Med. 29:450-459.

————, P. Maroteaux, and J. Spranger. 1967. La dysostose spondylo-metaphysaire. Presse Med. 75:2769-2774.

————, ————, F. Silverman, H. Kaufmann, and J. Spranger. 1969. Classification des dysplasies osseuses. Table ronde. Ann. Radiol. 12:965-1007.

————, and C. Zychowicz. 1962. Metaphyseal dysostosis of mixed type in a female child. Amer. Roentgen. 88:443-449.

Lamy, M. E. 1969. Hereditary disorders of bones—an overview. Clinical Delineation of Birth Defects, Part 5, Birth Defects: Original Article Series. New York, National Foundation–March of Dimes.

Lamy, M., and P. Maroteaux. 1960. La Nanisme diastrophique. Presse Med. 68:1977-1980.

————, and ————. 1961. Les chondrodystrophies génotypiques. Paris, L'expansion Scientifique Francaise.

Landing, B. H., F. N. Silverman, M. M. Craig, M. D. Jacoby, M. E. Lahey, and D. L. Chadwick. 1964. Familial neurovisceral lipidosis. An analysis of eight cases of a syndrome previously reported as "Hurler-Variant," "Pseudo-Hurler Disease" and "Tay-Sachs Disease" with visceral involvement. Amer. J. Dis. Child. 108:503-522.

Langer, L. O. Jr., 1964a. Spondyloepiphyseal dysplasia tarda. Hereditary chondrodysplasia with characteristic vertebral configuration in the adult. Radiology 82:833-839.

————. 1964b. The radiographic manifestations of the HS-mucopolysaccharidosis of Sanfilippo. Ann. Radiol. 7:315-325.

————. 1965. Diastrophic dwarfism in early infancy. Amer. J. Roentgen. 93:399-404.

————. 1968. Thoracic-pelvic-phalangeal dystrophy: asphyxiating thoracic dystrophy of the newborn, infantile thoracic dystrophy. Radiology 91:447-456.

————. 1969. Short stature. Check list of conditions associated with retarded longitudinal growth. Clin. Pediat. 8:142-153.

————, P. A. Baumann, and R. J. Gorlin. 1967. Achondroplasia. Amer. J. Roentgen. 100:12-26.

————, and L. S. Carey. 1966. The roentgenographic features of the KS-mucopolysaccharidosis of Morquio (Morquio-Brailsford's disease). Amer. J. Roentgen. 97:1-20.

————, J. W. Spranger, I. Grienacher, and R. C. Herdman. 1969. Thanatophoric dwarfism. Radiology 92:285-303.

Laron, Z., A. Pertzelan, and S. Mannheimer. 1966. Genetic pituitary dwarfism with high serum concentration of growth hormone. A new inborn error of metabolism? Israel J. Med. Sci. 2:152-155.

Leeds, N. E. 1960. Epiphysial dysplasia multiplex. Amer. J. Roentgen. 84:506-510.

Lenz, W. D. 1969. Discussion: Murk Jansen type of metaphyseal dysostosis. Clinical Delineation of Birth Defects, Part 4, Birth Defects: Original Article Series. New York, National Foundation–March of Dimes.

Léri, A., and (Mille) Linoissier. 1924. Hypochondroplasia héréditaire. Bull. Soc. Med. Hop. Paris 48:1780.

Leroy, J. G., and A. C. Crocker. 1966. Clinical definition of the Hurler-Hunter phenotypes. A review of 50 patients. Amer. J. Dis. Child. 112:518-530.

——, R. I. DeMars, and J. M. Opitz. 1969. I-cell disease. The Clinical Delineation of Birth Defects, Part 5, Birth Defects: Original Article Series. New York, National Foundation–March of Dimes.

Loeb, H. M. Tondeur, G. Jonniaux, S. Mockel-Pohl, and E. Vamez-Hurwitz. 1969. Biochemical and ultrastructural studies in a case of mucopolysaccharidosis "F" (fucosidosis). Helv. Paediat. Acta 24:519-537.

Lux, S. E., R. B. Johnston, C. S. August, B. Say, V. B. Penschaszadeh, F. S. Rosen, and V. A. McKusick. 1970. Chronic neutropenia and abnormal cellular immunity in cartilage-hair hypoplasia. New Eng. J. Med. 282:231-236.

Maloney, F. P. 1969. Diastrophic dwarfism in infant, teenager and adult (case E-2). The Clinical Delineation of Brith Defects, Part 4, Birth Defects: Original Article Series. New York, National Foundation–March of Dimes.

Marie, P. 1900. L'achondroplasie dans l'adolescence et l'age adulte. Presse Med. 2:17-23.

Maroteaux, P. 1970. Nomenclature internationale des maladies osseuses constitutionnelles. Ann. Radiol. 13:455-464.

——, and M. Lamy. 1959. Les formes pseudo-achondroplasiques de dysplasies spondylo-epiphysaires. Presse Med. 67:383-386.

——, and ——. 1963. La maladie de Morquio: étude clinique, radiologique et biologique. Presse Med. 71:2091-2094.

——, and ——. 1966. La pseudopolydystrophie de Hurler. Presse Med. 74:2889-2892.

——, and ——. 1968. Le diagnostic des nanismes chondrodystrophiques chez les nouvequ-nés. Arch. Franc. Pediat. 25:241-261.

——, ——, and J. Bernard. 1957. La dysplasie spondylo-epiphsaire tardive; description clinique et radiologique. Presse Med. 65:1205-1208.

——, ——, and J. M. Robert. 1967. Le nanisme thanatophore. Presse Med. 75:2519-2524.

——, B. Levêque, J. Marie, and M. Lamy. 1963. Une nouvelle dysostose avec élimination urinaire de chondroitine-sulfate B. Presse Med. 71:1849-1852.

——, and P. Savart. 1964. La dystrophie thoracique asphyxiante: etude radiologique et rapports avec le syndrome d'Ellis et van Creveld. Ann. Radiol. 7:332-338.

——, J. Spranger, and H. R. Wiedemann. 1966. Der metatropische zwergwuchs. Arch. Kinderheilk 173:211-226.

——, R. Wiedeman, J. Spranger, K. Kozlowski, and L. Lenzi. 1968. Essai de classification des dysplasies spondylo-epiphysaires. Monographies de genetique medicale. Lyon, France.

Matalon, R. J. A. Cifonelli, H. Zellweger, and A. Dorfman. 1968. Lipid abnormalities in a variant of the Hurler Syndrome. Proc. Nat. Acad. Sic. U.S.A. 59:1097-1102.

————, and A. Dorfman. 1966. Hurler's syndrome: biosynthesis of acid mucopolysaccharides in tissue culture. Proc. Nat. Acad. Sci. U.S.A. 56:1310-1316.

McKusick, V. A. 1966. Heritable Disorders of Connective Tissue, ed. 3. St. Louis, Mosby.

————. 1968. Genetic disorders involving growth hormone in man. In Progress in Endocrinology: Proceedings of the Third International Congress of Endocrinology, Mexico, D. F.

————. 1969. The nosology of the mucopolysaccharidoses. Amer. J. Med. 47:730-747.

————. 1970. Personal communication, Baltimore, Maryland.

————, J. A. Egeland, R. Eldridge, and D. E. Krusen. 1964. Dwarfism in the Amish. I. The Ellis-Van Creveld syndrome. Bull. Hopkins Hosp. 115:306-336.

————, R. Eldridge, J. A. Hostetler, U. Ruangivit, and J. A. Egeland. 1965a. Dwarfism in the Amish. II. Cartilage-hair hypoplasia. Bull. Hopkins Hosp. 116:285-326.

————, D. Kaplan, D. Wise, W. B. Hanley, S. B. Suddarth, M. E. Sevick, and A. E. Maumanee. 1965b. The genetic mucopolysaccharidoses. Medicine 44:445-483.

————, and D. L. Rimoin. 1967. General Tom Thumb and other midgets. Sci. Amer. 217:102-110.

Melnick, J. C. 1965. Chondrodystrophia calcificans congenita (chondrodysplasia epiphysialis punctata, stippled epiphyses). Amer. J. Dis. Child. 110:218-225.

Merimee, T. J., J. D. Hall, D. L. Rimoin, and V. A. McKusick. 1969. A metabolic and hormonal basis for classifying ateliotic dwarfs. Lancet 1:963-965.

Michail, J., J. Matsovkas, S. Theodorou, and K. Houliaras. 1956. Maladie de Morquio (osteochondrodystrophie polyepiphysaire deformante) chez deux freres. Helv. Paediat. Acta 11:403-413.

Michel, J., B. Grenier, J. Castaing, J. L. Augier, and G. Desbuquois. 1970. Deux cas familiaux de dysplasie spondylo-metaphysaire. Ann. Radiol. 13:251-254.

Mørch, E. T. 1941. Chondrodystrophic Dwarfs in Denmark. Opera Ex Domo: Biologiae Hereditariae Humanae, Vol. 3. Copenhagen, Ejnar Munksgaard.

Morgan, B. C., J. M. Aase, and C. B. Graham. 1970. Homozygosity for achondroplasia? Report of a possible case, with congenital heart disease and severe mental deficit. Pediatrics 45:112-115.

Morquio, L. 1929. Sur une forme de dystrophie osseuse familiale. Bull. Soc. Pediat. 27:145-152.

Murdoch, J. L., B. A. Walker, J. G. Hall, H. Abbey, K. K. Smith, and V. A. McKusick. 1970. Achondroplasia—a genetic and statistical survey. Ann. Hum. Genet. 33:227-244.

Nahmias, A. J., D. Griffith, C. Salbury, and K. Yoshida. 1967. Thymic aplasia, with lympopenia, plasma cells and normal immunoglobulins. J.A.M.A. 201:729-734.

Neimann, N., M. Manciaux, G. Rayber, C. Pernot, and M. C. Bretagne-De-Kersuson. 1963. Dystrophie thoracique asphyxiante du nourisson. Pediatrie 18:387-397.

Norman, R. M., H. Urich, A. H. Tingey, and R. A. Goodbody. 1959. Tay-Sachs disease with visceral involvement and its relationship to Nieman-Pick's Disease. J. Path. Bact. 78:409-421.

O'Brien, J. S. 1969. Generalized gangliosidosis. J. Pediat. 75:167-186.

Ockerman, P. A. 1967. A generalized storage disorder resembling Hurler's syndrome. Lancet 2:239-241.

Opitz, J. M. 1969. Delayed mutation in achondroplasia? Clinical Delineation of Birth Defects, Part 5, Birth Defects: Original Article Series. New York, National Foundation–March of Dimes.

Parenti, G. C. 1936. La anosteogenesi (una varieta della osteogenesi imperfectta). Pathologica 28:447-461.

Parrot, J. M. 1878. Sur les malformations achondroplasiques et le dieu Ptah. Bull. Soc. Antropol., Paris 1:296-310.

Phelan, P. D., J. Connelly, F. I. R. Martin, and H. N. B. Wettenhall. 1971. X-linked recessive hypopituitarism. The Clinical Delineation of Birth Defects, Part 10, Birth Defects: Original Article Series. Baltimore, Williams & Wilkins.

Piffaretti, P. G., H. Delgado, and D. Nussle. 1970. La dysostose spondylo-métaphysaire de Kozlowski, Maroteaux et Spranger. Ann. Radiol. 13:405-417.

Pincus, J. H., J. P. Rossi, and R. B. Daroff. 1967. Delayed development of disturbed mucopolysaccharide metabolism in a Hurler variant. Arch. Neurol. Chicago 16:244-253.

Pirnar, T., and E. B. D. Neuhauser. 1966. Asphyxiating thoracic dystrophy of the newborn. Amer. J. Roentgen. 98:358-364.

Poker, N., N. Finby, and R. N. Archibald. 1965. Spondloepiphyseal dysplasia tarda. Four cases in childhood and adolescence, and some considerations regarding platyspondyly. Radiology 85:474-480.

Ponseti, I. 1970. Skeletal growth in achondroplasia. J. Bone Joint Surg. (Amer.) 52:701-716.

Potter, E. L., and V. A. Coverstone. 1948. Chondrodystrophy fetalis. Amer. J. Obstet. Gynec. 56:790-793.

Quelce-Salgado, A. 1964. A new type of dwarfism with various bone aplasias and hypoplasias of the extremities. Acta Genet. (Basel) 14:63-66.

———. 1968. A rare genetic syndrome. Lancet 1:1430.

Rampini, S., and P. Maroteaux. 1966. Ein ungewoehnlicher Phaenotyp des Hurler-Syndroms. Helv. Paediat. Acta 21:376-386.

Ravenna, F. 1913. Achondroplasie et chondrohypoplasie. Contribution clinique. Nouvelle inconographis de la Salpetriere, (N. Iconogr. Salpet.) Clin. Malad. Syst. Nerv. 26:157-184.

Remy, J., J. P. Nuyts, E. Bompart, and A. Rembert. 1970. La dysostose spondylometaphysaire. A propos de deux observations. Ann Radiol. 13:419-425.

Rimoin, D. L., G. B. Holzman, T. J. Merimee, D. Rabinowitz, A. C. Barnes, J. E. A. Tyson, and V. A. McKusick. 1968a. Lactation in the absence of human growth hormone. J. C.in. Endocr. 28:1183-1188.

———, G. N. F. Hughes, R. L. Kaufman, and W. H. McAlister. 1969a. The chondrodystrophies—clinical and histopathological correlations. J. Lab. Clin. Med. 74:1002.

———, ———, ———, R. E. Rosenthal, W. H. McAlister, and R. Silberberg. 1970. Endochondral ossification in achondroplastic dwarfism. New Eng. J. Med. 283:728-735.

———, and W. H. McAlister. 1971. Metaphyseal dysostosis, conductive hearing loss and mental retardation. Clinical Delineation of Birth Defects, Part 9, Birth Defects: Original Article Series. New York, National Foundation–March of Dimes.

————, and V. A. McKusick. 1969. Somatic mosaicism in an achondroplastic dwarf. Clinical Delineation of Birth Defects, Part 5, Birth Defects: Original Article Series. New York, National Foundation–March of Dimes.

————, T. J. Merimee, and V. A. McKusick. 1966. Growth hormone deficiency in man. An isolated recessively inherited defect. Science 152:1635-1637.

————, ————, D. Rabinowitz, L. L. Cavalli-Sforza, and V. A. McKusick. 1968b. Genetic aspects of isolated growth hormone deficiency. In Growth Hormone, Proceedings of International Symposium, Sept. 11-13, Milan, Italy, pp. 418-432.

————, ————, ————, ————, and ————. 1969b. Peripheral subresponsiveness to human growth hormone in the African pygmies. New Eng. J. Med. 281:1383-1388.

————, ————, ————, and V. A. McKusick. 1968a. Genetic aspects of clinical endocrinology. Recent Progr. Hormone Res. 24:365-437.

Roaf, R., J. B. Longmore, and R. M. Forrester. 1967. A childhood syndrome of bone dysplasia, retinal detachment and deafness. Develop. Med. Child. Neurol. 9:464-473.

Robins, M. M., H. G. Stevens, and A. Linker. 1963. Morquio's disease: an abnormality of mucopolysaccharide metabolism. J. Pediat. 62:881-889.

Rosenbloom, A. L., and D. W. Smith. 1965. The natural history of metaphyseal dysostosis. J. Pediat. 66:857-868.

Rubin, P. 1964. Dynamic Classification of Bone Dysplasias. Chicago. Year Book.

Saldino, R. M. 1970. Personal communication, San Francisco, California.

Salle, B., C. Picot, J. L. Vauzelle, P. Diffrenne, P. Monnet, R. Francois, and J. M. Robert. 1966. Le nanisme diastrophique. À propos de trois observations chez le nouveau-né. Pediatrie 21:311-327.

Sanfilippo, S. J., R. Podosin, L. O. Langer, Jr., and R. A. Good. 1963. Mental retardation associated with acid mucoplysacchariduria (heparitin sulfate type). J. Pediat. 63:837-838.

Sarrouy, C., S. Farouz, M. T. Roche, S. Sabatini, J. C. Vaillaud, and A. Revol. 1965. A propos d'une nouvelle observation de maladie de Hurler. Presse Med. 73:3219-3222.

Scheie, H. G., G. W. Hambrick, Jr., and L. A. Barness. 1962. A newly recognized forme fruste of Hurler's disease (gargoylism). Amer. J. Ophthal. 53:753-769.

Schimke, R. N., J. J. Spaulding, and J. G. Hollowell. 1971. X-linked congenital panhypopituitarism. The Clinical Delineation of Birth Defects, Part 9, Birth Defects: Original Article Series. Baltimore, Williams & Wilkins.

Schmid, F. 1949. Beitrag zur Dysostosis Enchondralis Metaphysaria. Monats. Kinderheilk. 97:393-397.

Schmidt, B. J., W. Becak, M. L. Becak, I. Soibleman. A. Da Silva Queiroz, A. P. Lorga, F. Secaf, C. F. Antonio, and A. DeAndrade Carvalho. 1963. Metaphyseal dysostosis. J. Pediat. 63:106-112.

Schwachman, H., L. K. Diamond, F. A. Oski, and K. T. Khaw. 1964. The syndrome of pancreatic insufficiency and bone marrow dysfunction. J. Pediat. 65:645-663.

Scott, C. I., Jr., 1969a. Achondrogenesis type II (Grebe or Brazilian type). Clinical Delineation of Birth Defects, Part 5, Birth Defects: Original Article Series. New York, National Foundation–March of Dimes.

Scott, C. I. 1969b. Maroteaux-Lamy syndrome in four sibs. The Clinical Delineation of Birth Defects, Part 5, Birth Defects: Original Article Series. New York, National Foundation–March of Dimes.

Scott, C. I. 1971. Pseudo-Hurler polydystrophy. Clinical Delineation of Birth Defects, Part 8, Birth Defects: Original Article Series. Williams & Wilkins.

Scott, C. I., Jr., and M. S. Grossman. 1969. Pseudo-Hurler polydystrophy. The Clinical Delineation of Birth Defects, Part 5, Birth Defects: Original Article Series. New York, National Foundation–March of Dimes.

Scott, C. I., and M. C. Mengel. 1971. Osteogenesis imperfecta and panhypopituitarism in two unrelated males. The Clinical Delineation of Birth Defects, Part 9, Birth Defects: Original Article Series. Baltimore, Williams & Wilkins.

Shmerling, D. H., A. Prader, W. H. Hitzig, A. Giedion, B. Hadorn, and M. Kühni. 1969. The syndrome of exocrine pancreatic insufficiency, neutropenia, metaphyseal dysostosis and dwarfism. Helv. Paediat. Acta 24:547-575.

Silverman, F. 1968. A differential diagnosis of achondroplasia. Radiol. Clin. N. Amer. 6:223-237.

———. 1970. Personal communication, Cincinnati, Ohio.

———, and S. Brunner. 1967. Errors in the diagnosis of achondroplasia. Acta Radiol. (Diag.) (Stockholm) 6:305-321.

Silverman, F. N. 1961. Dysplasies épiphysaires: entité protéiforme. Ann. Radiol. 4:833-867.

Singer, H. A., and I. A. Schafer. 1970. White-cell β-galactosidose activity. New Eng. J. Med. 282:571.

Slatis, H. M. 1955. Comments on the rate of mutation to chondrodystrophy in man. Amer. J. Hum. Genet. 7:76-79.

Spranger, J. W. 1969. The genetic mucopolysaccharidoses. The Clinical Delineation of Birth Defects, Part 5, Birth Defects: Original Article Series. New York, National Foundation–March of Dimes.

———, and H. Gerken. 1967. Diastrophischer zwerwuchs. Z. Kinderheilk. 98:227-234.

———, and L. O. Langer, Jr. 1970. Spondyloepiphyseal dysplasia congenita. Radiology 94:313-322.

———, M. Tolksdorf, E. Graucob, and R. Caesar. 1968. Lipomucopolysaccharidose. Kinderheilk. 103:285-306.

———, and H. R. Wiedemann. 1966. Dysplasia spondyloepiphysaria congenita. Helv. Paediat. Acta 21:598-611.

———, and H. R. Wiedemann. 1970. The genetic mucolipisoses. Humangenetik 9:113-139.

———, J. M. Optiz, and W. Bidder. 1971. Heterogeneity of chondrodysplasia punctata. Humangenetik 11:190-212.

Steinbach, H. L., L. Preger, H. E. Williams, and P. Cohen. 1968. The Hurler syndrome without abnormal mucopolysacchariduria. Radiology 90:472-478.

Steinhauser, R. K., C. I. Scott, J. A. Mays, and V. A. McKusick. 1970. Ankylosing spondylosis in familial hypophosphatemia. In Proceedings of the 51st Annual Session of the American College of Physicians, April 12-17, 1970, Philadelphia, pp. 26-27.

Stephens, F. E. 1943. An achondroplasic mutation and the nature of its inheritance. J. Hered. 34:229-235.

Stevenson, A. C. 1957. Achondroplasia: an account of the condition in northern Ireland. Amer. J. Hum. Genet. 9:81-91.

Stickler, G. B., F. T. Maher, J. C. Hunt, E. C. Burke, and J. W. Rosevear. 1962. Familial bone disease resembling rickets (hereditary metaphyseal dysostosis). Pediatrics 29:996-1004.

Stover, C. N., J. T. Hayes, and J. F. Holt. 1963. Diastrophic dwarfism. Amer. J. Roentgen. 89:914-922.

Taybi, H. 1963. Diastrophic dwarfism. Radiology 80:1-10.

———, A. D. Mitchell, and G. Friedman. 1969. Metaphyseal dysostosis and the associated syndrome of pancreatic insufficiency and blood disorders. Radiology 93:563-571.

Thieffry, S., G. Lyon, and P. Maroteaux. 1967. Encephalopathie metabolique associant une mucopolysaccharidose et une sulfatidose. Arch. Franc. Pediat. 24:425-432.

Thomas, G. H. 1969. β-D-Galactosidase in human urine: deficiency in generalized gangliosidosis. J. Lab. Clin. Med. 74:725-731.

Van Hoff, F., and H. G. Hers. 1968a. Mucopolysaccharidoses by absence of α-fucosidase. Lancet 1:1198.

———, and H. G. Hers. 1968b. The abnormalities of lysosomal enzymes in mucopolysaccharidoses. Europ. J. Biochem. 7:34-44.

Vogl, A. 1962. The fate of achondroplastic dwarf (neurological complications of achondroplasia). Exp. Med. Surg. 20:108-117.

Wadia, R. 1969. Achondroplasia in two first cousins (mothers and sisters): all four parents normal and neither pair related. Clinical Delineation of Birth Defects, Part 5, Birth Defects: Original Article Series. New York, National Foundation–March of Dimes.

Walker, B. A., C. I. Scott, Jr., J. G. Hall, J. L. Murdoch, and V. A. McKusick. 1972. Diastrophic dwarfism. Medicine, Vol. 51.

Weinberg, H., M. Frankel, and M. Makin. 1960. Familial epiphyseal dysplasia of the lower limbs. J. Bone Joint Surg. 42:313-332.

Wichtl, O. 1965. Zur pränatalen Diagnose der Chondrodystrophie (Achondroplasie). Fortschr. Rontgenstr. 103:114-116.

Winters, R. W., T. F. Williams, and J. Graham. 1958. Genetic study of familial hypophosphatemia and vitamin D resistant rickets with a review of the literature. Medecine 37:97-127.

Zergollern, L. 1971. A follow-up on Hanhart's dwarfs of Krk. Clinical Delineation of Birth Defects, Part 9, Birth Defects: Original Article Series. Baltimore, Williams & Wilkins.

Author Index

301

Subject Index

Page numbers followed by t refer to tables.

Anti-D immunoglobulin
  anticipated requirements, 217-218
  clearance acceleration, 195-197
  clinical trials, 182-190
  dose-stimulus relation, 200-204, 202t,
    203t
  dose–transplacental hemorrhage rela-
    tion, 192-195
  effective dose, 199
  after first pregnancy, 177, 178
  half-life, 198
  intravenous vs. intramuscular adminis-
    tration, 195-197t
  in male volunteers, 193t
  potency, 203
  during pregnancy, 191-192
  RhoGAM, 186, 187t, 193t, 198, 202t
  risks, 204
Anti-D immunoglobulin production, 213-
  218
  immunization route, 215
  immunization safety, 215
  plasmapheresis, 215-217
  primary immunization, 213
  red cells for immunization, 214-215
  secondary immunization, 213-214
Anti-D plasma, 187, 195
  risks, 204
Anti-D serum, 171, 173
Antigenic drift, 42, 44, 48
Antigenic system, 105, 119
Antigens
  Australian, 171
  change in, 37, 38, 42
  in complementation, 23
  genetic control of response, 33
  in genetic recombination, 14, 15, 16
  influenza virus, 38, 41, 42, 43, 44
  in phenotype mixing, 24, 25
  T, 14, 15
  transplantation, 14, 31
  viral envelope, 23, 24, 28, 41, 42, 44,
    48
Antilymphocyte serum, 31, 205
Argininosuccinate synthetase, 135
Arylsulfatase, 130-131, 160, 286
Asphyxiating thoracic dysplasia, 262-264
Ataxia telangiectasia, 80-82
Atomic-bomb survivors, 65-67
Atropinesterase, 125
Australian antigen, 171
Australian wild rabbits, 38, 40

Bacterial protein synthesis, 140
Bacteriophage, 10, 25, 29, 46
Benign tumor, single-cell origin, 63

Benzene exposure, 68
BHK21 cells, 15
Bikini, 67
Bilirubin, 143-144
Biological distance, 109, 110
Blood groups, 33
Blood types, 156
Bloom's syndrome, 72-77
  biochemical defect, 76
  cancer in, 69, 74
  chromosomes in, 69, 74-76, 91
  –Fanconi's anemia comparison, 78-79
  leukemia in, 93
  marker chromosome, 74
  mitosis in, 75-76
  pseudodiploid clones in, 76
  Qr formation in, 75, 76
  sun sensitivity in, 74, 76
Bone disease, constitutional (intrinsic),
  245t-248t
Brain, in Tay-Sachs disease, 227-228
5-Bromodeoxyuridine, 12

Cancer
  in Bloom's syndrome, 69, 74
  as cataclysmic event, 90
  chromosomal instability and, 61-101
  chromosomal mutation in etiology, 61,
    65, 89, 91
  chromosomes and, 92-93
  clones in, 63, 65
  cytogenic classes, 92-93
  environmental factor, 65, 90
  fetal irradiation and, 67
  ganglioside metabolism and, 238, 239
  human "experiments," 65-69
  karyotype in, 61, 65, 90, 95
  in Louis-Bar syndrome, 70, 81, 91
  marker chromosome, 63, 89, 93, 95
  mitosis in, 94
  origin in single cell with chromosomal
    mutation, 62-65, 89
  pleomorphism in, 94
  progenitor cell, 65
  in radiologists, 68
  risk, 72
  stemline, 63, 64, 89
  variant cell-types, 63
  viruses in, 14, 22, 28, 31-32, 47, 68-69,
    93
  in xeroderma pigmentosum, 70, 84, 88,
    154
Carbamyl phosphate synthetase, 153
Carrier detection, 108
Catalase, 127, 137
Chondrodysplasia punctata, 256-258, 273